Forthcoming Monographs

THE RADIOLOGY OF VERTEBRAL TRAUMA

John A. Gehweiler, Jr., M.D., Raymond L. Osborne, Jr., M.D., and R. Frederick Becker, Ph.D.

ARTHROGRAPHY: PRINCIPLES AND TECHNIQUES

Tom W. Staple, M.D.

CLINICAL PEDIATRIC AND ADOLESCENT UROGRAPHY

Alfred L. Weber, M.D., and Richard C. Pfister, M.D.

PEDIATRIC ORTHOPAEDIC RADIOLOGY

M. B. Ozonoff, M.D.

XEROMAMMOGRAPHIC PATHOLOGY

Michael D. Lagios, M.D., H. Joachim Burhenne, M.D., and F. Margolin, M.D.

E. JAMES POTCHEN, M.D., *Consulting Editor*

Professor and Chairman
Department of Radiology
Michigan State University
East Lansing, Michigan

Published

Volume 1 in the Series
SAUNDERS
MONOGRAPHS
IN CLINICAL
RADIOLOGY

SECOND EDITION

GASTROINTESTINAL ANGIOGRAPHY

STEWART R. REUTER, M.D.

Professor and Vice Chairman,
Department of Radiology,
University of California,
Davis, California;
Professor of Radiology,
University of California,
San Francisco, California;
Chief, Diagnostic Radiology Service,
Veterans Administration Hospital,
Martinez, California;
Formerly, Professor of Radiology,
University of Michigan School of Medicine,
Ann Arbor, Michigan

HELEN C. REDMAN, M.D.

Associate Chief, Department of Radiology,
Mt. Zion Hospital, San Francisco, California;
Clinical Associate Professor of Radiology,
University of California School of Medicine,
San Francisco, California;
Clinical Associate Professor of Radiology,
Stanford University School of Medicine,
Palo Alto, California;
Formerly, Associate Professor of Radiology,
University of Michigan School of Medicine,
Ann Arbor, Michigan

1977

W. B. SAUNDERS COMPANY • *Philadelphia* • *London* • *Toronto*

W. B. Saunders Company: West Washington Square
Philadelphia, PA   19105

1 St. Anne's Road
Eastbourne, East Sussex BN21 3UN, England

1 Goldthorne Avenue
Toronto, Ontario M8Z 5T9, Canada

Library of Congress Cataloging in Publication Data

Reuter, Stewart R

Gastrointestinal angiography.

(Saunders monographs in clinical radiology; v. 1)

Includes bibliographies and index.

1. Digestive organs — Blood-vessels — Radiography.
   I. Redman, Helen C., joint author.   II. Title. [DNLM:
   1. Angiography.   2. Gastrointestinal system —
   Radiography. WI141 R447g]

RC804.A5R48 1977   616.3'07'572   76–50156

ISBN 0–7216–7566–2

Gastrointestinal Angiography   ISBN   0-7216-7566-2

Last digit is the print number: 9   8   7   6   5   4   3   2   1

FOREWORD

Five years ago, *Gastrointestinal Angiography,* by Stewart R. Reuter and Helen C. Redman, initiated the Saunders Monographs in Clinical Radiology series. To the delight of authors, editor and publisher, it was rapidly and widely accepted as an authoritative source of information about an area of clinical medicine that had become increasingly important. In addition, the book set a standard of excellence for subsequent volumes in the series.

Now, in the Second Edition, the authors have added to the basic discussion of the subject newer developments in application and technique of gastrointestinal angiography, including interventional angiographic procedures, and thus once again have prepared an up-to-date, definitive monograph for radiologists, gastroenterologists and abdominal surgeons.

Dr. Reuter is now Professor and Vice Chairman of Radiology at the University of California, Davis and Professor of Radiology at the University of California, San Francisco. Dr. Redman is Assistant Chief of the Department of Radiology at Mt. Zion Hospital in San Francisco. Both have contributed to the development of techniques of gastrointestinal angiography and are now widely recognized as the leaders in the field. It is a pleasure to welcome this Second Edition of the first Saunders Monograph in Clinical Radiology, in anticipation that it will be as well received as its predecessor. The authors have again provided us with a remarkable opportunity to keep abreast of a rapidly changing field.

E. JAMES POTCHEN, M.D.

PREFACE

The years between the publication of the first and second editions of this monograph have witnessed the rapid development of trends that were discernible, though inchoate, at the time of the initial writing. Perhaps the most important has been the improved accuracy of noninvasive diagnostic imaging modalities in the abdomen. These techniques have placed angiography in a proper, if diminished, role in the diagnosis of visceral disease. In the past, angiography was used too frequently as a diagnostic screening method in the pancreas, the liver and throughout the abdomen generally. As late as 1973, a widely respected chairman of a university surgery department stated that all patients with suspected carcinoma of the pancreas should have pancreatic angiography. Now this has changed. Most patients coming to pancreatic angiography have had a diagnosis established; pancreatic angiography is being done primarily to determine resectability of carcinomas and to establish a diagnosis in those few patients in whom the diagnosis remains equivocal. Another major change has been the rapid expansion of therapeutic angiography in all parts of the body. In the abdomen, this has been primarily in the control of massive gastrointestinal hemorrhage.

The second edition has been modified to reflect these changes. Although the disease orientation of chapters has been maintained, those diseases in which the use of angiography has increased or become better defined have been expanded. Those diseases in which angiography now plays a smaller role have been contracted. Throughout the book, the number of illustrations has been increased and improved.

Finally, there has been a general request for the inclusion of a section on superselective catheterization technique. Although these techniques were adequately developed at the time of the first edition, a description was excluded because it was felt that most physicians to whom the book would appeal would not perform or have interest in these examinations. We underestimated the sophistication of our audience and therefore have added a section on superselective angiographic technique. This section is to be read with the caveats that the selection of a particular angiographic technique is personal and that techniques are difficult to describe. Therefore, although we have described techniques developed and used by other angiographers, those receiving the greatest emphasis have been our own.

We were delighted with the response to the first edition and with the knowledge that it filled a gap in the angiographic literature. The second edition is directed toward the same audience as the first. We hope the field of visceral angiography has now stabilized to the point where this edition will not become obsolete so rapidly.

CONTENTS

Chapter 1

EQUIPMENT AND TECHNIQUE USED IN CATHETERIZATION OF THE VISCERAL ARTERIES

Selection of the proper catheterization equipment and development of a facile catheterization technique are essential in obtaining a successful angiogram, in decreasing the discomfort of the patient and in keeping angiographic complications to a minimum. This chapter is detailed because an overall discussion of catheterization equipment and technique is not easily available to the beginning angiographer. In this discussion the principles involved in selectively catheterizing the visceral vessels are stressed. Recommendations of the equipment of one or another manufacturer are specifically avoided. By stressing the principles that are important for producing excellent angiograms while minimizing the complications of the procedure, the equipment and technique acceptable to most visceral angiographers can be described. Varying experience, of course, leads to a variety of techniques, and other methods are also acceptable in many instances.

CATHETERIZATION EQUIPMENT

Catheterization of the visceral arteries is done exclusively by the percutaneous transarterial technique devised by Seldinger (1953). The necessary equipment consists of a needle, a guide wire and a catheter.

1

These must be compatible with each other so that there is a good fit between needle and guide wire, and between guide wire and catheter. The units of measurement for the catheterization equipment are confusing since they are given variously in inches, millimeters or the French scale. Needle sizes are generally stated as Stubs needle gauge, guide wires as thousandths of an inch and catheters as French, inches or millimeters. Both inner and outer diameters for catheters must be known. Table 1–1 gives the conversion equivalents for commonly used guide wire and catheter sizes.

While extensive changes have occurred in radiographic tubes and generators during the past 25 years, only relatively minor developments have occurred in equipment for catheterization. The most important change has been the use of smaller needles, guide wires and catheters. The early angiographers used approximately 15 gauge needles, 0.052 inch guide wires and 8 French outer diameter catheters. The needles now used are 18 gauge or smaller, the guide wires are about 0.038 inch and the catheters are 7 French outer diameter or less. The use of smaller equipment is one of the most important factors in the decreased incidence of complications with angiography today compared with 15 years ago.

Needles

The needle generally used for arterial puncture in the Seldinger method has two parts—an outer, blunt cannula and an inner, pointed trocar. For adults, the thin-walled 18 gauge needle is used; for children, the thin-walled 19 gauge. Conventional thick-walled needles should not be used in angiography. The use of a smaller thin-walled needle causes a smaller puncture hole in the artery and still permits passage of the same diameter guide wire. Several types of trocars are available. Some are two-piece, and others are single. Most trocars are beveled, but some have a central point. The bevel or point should be short. No difference exists in the amount of arterial damage caused by short-bevel or central-pointed needles.

Guide Wires

The guide wire has two basic functions. First, it provides support for passage of the catheter through the soft tissues at the puncture site, through the arterial wall and into the arterial lumen. Second, it passes from the puncture site into the abdominal aorta, providing a path for the catheter to follow through atherosclerotic and tortuous iliac arteries. Both of these functions are extremely important in preventing the complications of angiography, most of which occur at the puncture site or in an atherosclerotic, tortuous iliac artery. The standard guide wire is straight and has a soft, flexible end measuring about 1½ inches. Two wires are present inside the coil. One, with a very small diameter, extends from tip to tip and is welded at both ends. This is the safety wire, which should be part of all guide wires. Its development has prevented breakage of guide wires in the patient, a complication of angiography

TABLE 1–1. Conversion Table for Measurements of Guide Wires and Outer Diameters of Thin-walled Catheters Commonly Used in Visceral Angiography

GUIDE WIRES		
Inches	Millimeters	Pass Through Thin-walled Needle Gauge
.028	0.711	19
.038	0.956	18
.045	1.143	16
.052	1.321	15

CATHETERS		
French (mm diameter × 3)	Inches (diameter)	Millimeters (diameter)
3	.039	1.00
4	.053	1.34
4.1	.054	1.37
5	.065	1.67
5.3	.070	1.78
6	.079	2.00
6.3	.083	2.11
6.6	.087	2.20
7	.092	2.33
7.2	.094	2.40
8	.104	2.67
8.4	.110	2.80
9	.118	3.00

in the past (Dotter et al., 1966). The second, thicker wire fills the remainder of the coil and provides stiffness to the body of the guide wire, which supports the catheter during its introduction into the artery. Without this support, the catheter would buckle, the guide wire would kink and the artery might be torn. The stiffening wire should be tapered as it approaches the flexible end so that there is a smooth transition between the stiff body and the soft end of the wire. The largest diameter guide wire that passes freely through the puncture needle should be used, both to provide maximum support and to allow passage of the largest possible catheter end hole. For a thin-walled 18 gauge needle this is a 0.038 inch wire (see Table 1–1). Many shapes and diameters of guide wires are available. Most of these have been designed to advance through tortuous iliac arteries, and their design and use are discussed under catheterization technique.

Catheters

The catheter materials used for angiography are polyethylene, polyurethane and polytetrafluoroethylene (Teflon). These plastics are generally made radiopaque with barium, bismuth or lead salts. In the early days of angiography, many examiners used nonopaque catheters because the catheters were frequently positioned in the aorta without the benefit of fluoroscopy. With the currently available equipment, no catheter should be positioned in the aorta or one of its branches without image-intensified fluoroscopic monitoring. There is, therefore, no longer a place for nonopaque catheters in visceral angiography.

Of the three types of catheter material mentioned, polyethylene has some advantages over the other two for visceral angiography. It is easy to shape and, therefore, allows the angiographer a great deal of flexibility in designing a shape suitable for the catheterization problem at hand. This is particularly important in superselective angiography. Polyethylene not only has good torque control but also is flexible enough to avoid damage to the intima. Also, even thin-walled polyethylene catheters with inner diameters in the range of 1.4 mm withstand flow rates up to 20 cc per second without rupturing. Since the injection rates used in visceral angiography are in the range of 5 to 15 cc per second, this is entirely adequate. Finally, most of the polyethylene catheters on the market have excellent radiopacity.

Teflon can withstand high injection pressures and has been useful in aortography. It is stiff, however, and when used to catheterize branches of the aorta can easily tear intima or perforate arteries. Moreover, Teflon is difficult to shape and taper, requiring exact temperatures. The injection rates and pressures required for visceral angiography are low enough so that Teflon catheters are unnecessary.

Polyurethane also has limitations as a catheter material. It has a high coefficient of friction, and unless specially coated, polyurethane catheters generate a great deal of resistance as they pass through the skin and as guide wires are passed through them during catheter exchange. For this reason Teflon-coated guide wires should always be used with polyurethane catheters. One possible advantage of polyurethane compared with other catheter materials is its smooth surface, particularly when coated. Although the relationship between the surface of a catheter and its thrombogenicity has not yet been demonstrated, polyurethane has been shown to be less thrombogenic than polyethylene (Durst et al., 1974). However, catheter thrombosis may soon become a less frequent complication of angiography. The use of total body heparinization has decreased the incidence of catheter-related thrombosis (Wallace et al., 1972), and heparin-bonded polyethylene catheters will soon become available commercially.

Recently, polyethylene and polyurethane catheters with excellent torque control have been introduced. Torque control has been achieved by placing a metallic mesh between the layers of extruded plastic. This mesh extends throughout the body of the catheter, ending several centimeters before the tip, so that the tip of the catheter can be formed into the desired shape. The degree of torque control offered by these catheters is unnecessary for most visceral procedures but may be helpful in certain superselective catheterization procedures, in patients with tortuous iliac arteries or ectatic aortas and in the catheterization of visceral arteries using the axillary approach.

Shaping Catheters

The tips of polyethylene catheters may be tapered over an alcohol lamp or hot air blower using the trocar of a thin-walled 18 gauge needle in the lumen (Fig. 1–1). Although a guide wire of the same size to be used for the catheterization can also be utilized, the resulting fit between catheter tip and guide wire is frequently too tight, causing the tip to bind as it is passed over the wire. With the trocar in place, the catheter material is rotated 360 degrees over an alcohol flame until the polyethylene begins to soften and expand slightly. The catheter is then removed from the flame, and the tip is pulled slowly and steadily. Drawing the tip while still over the flame generally results in the catheter material melting as it

becomes thinner. If the rotation over the flame is not made through a complete 360 degrees, the catheter material softens unevenly, and the resulting tip will deviate to one side. When the desired taper is achieved, the trocar is removed; the catheter material is dipped in cold water to harden the plastic and sliced with a razor blade at the narrowest point. The end of the catheter is then slipped over a wire which has the desired curve, and the combination is dipped into boiling water (Fig. 1–2). When the catheter material is soft, it is removed from the water and placed in cold water to fix the shape. The forming wire is removed, and the distal part of the catheter is ready for use. The final step is flanging the proximal end of the catheter by holding it perpendicular to the alcohol flame and moving it in and out of the flame.

Blowers which direct a hot air jet of variable temperature for softening and shaping the catheter are available commercially. Also, a funnel can be inverted over a tea kettle of boiling water and the catheter sof-

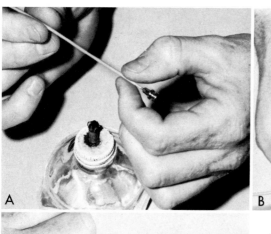
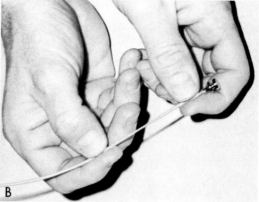
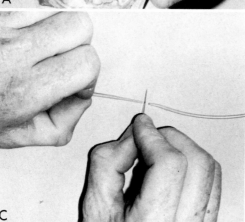

Figure 1–1. Forming catheter tips.

A. With a trocar of a thin-walled 18 gauge needle or a 0.038 guide wire in the lumen, the catheter is rotated through 360 degrees over an alcohol lamp until the catheter material begins to soften and swell.

B. The catheter is then removed from the flame and steadily and slowly drawn until the desired taper is achieved. The tip is dipped in cold water to fix the taper and the trocar or guide wire is removed.

C. The catheter is then sliced with a sharp razor blade at the desired point.

Figure 1–2. Forming bends in catheters.

A soft metal wire of approximately 0.035 inch in diameter is placed in the lumen of the catheter and the combination is bent into the desired shape. They are then dipped into boiling water for 2 to 3 seconds. It is important to keep the tapered tip out of the water, since it will soften and dilate if heated. The catheter and forming wire are finally dipped in cold water to fix the shape and the forming wire is removed.

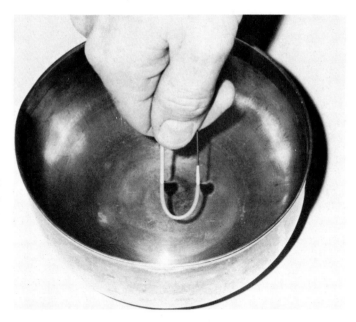

tened over the resulting steam jet. The latter technique works particularly well with the thin-walled polyethylene catheters made by Becton-Dickenson.

The catheter shapes suitable for gastrointestinal angiography are shown in Figure 1–3. The same shape can be used for celiac, superior mesenteric and renal artery catheterizations. Distal to the renal arteries, the aorta tapers and is much narrower at the origin of the inferior mesenteric artery. The curve for the inferior mesenteric artery catheter, therefore, must have a shorter radius and a shorter distal limb.

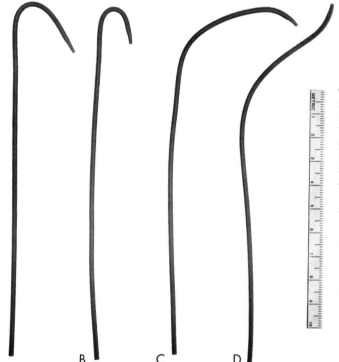

Figure 1–3. Shapes of distal catheter bends for visceral angiography.

A. Shape for celiac, superior mesenteric and renal angiography in an average patient. The distal limb must be lengthened for a patient with a dilated aorta and shortened for a child or small woman.

B. Shape for inferior mesenteric angiography in an average patient.

C. Shape for superselective angiography of the hepatic, splenic or gastroduodenal arteries.

D. Shape for left gastric artery or a dorsal pancreatic artery arising from the superior mesenteric artery.

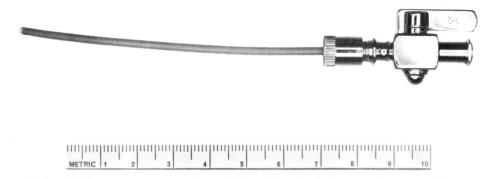

Figure 1–4. Combination of stopcock and flanged polyethylene catheter used in visceral angiography.

Stopcocks

The final piece of equipment necessary for performing the catheterization is the stopcock. This is best combined with the catheter as shown in Figure 1–4. Alternatively, a two-way stopcock can be attached to a female adapter. The latter combination is less desirable because a clot can form in the empty space between the adapter and the catheter.

GENERAL CATHETERIZATION TECHNIQUE

Over the years many different methods have been used for introducing contrast medium into visceral arteries. Until the development of the percutaneous transarterial Seldinger method, most of these procedures relied on introducing large doses of contrast medium into the aorta. The contrast medium would then flow into the aortic branches. These methods included translumbar aortography (dos Santos et al., 1931), large volume intravenous arteriography (Bernstein et al., 1960) and retrograde brachial artery injections (Sweet and Grismer, 1967). None of these methods have a place in modern visceral angiography because the concentration of contrast medium delivered to the visceral arteries from an aortic injection is inadequate to demonstrate the subtle vascular abnormalities of gastrointestinal diseases (Fig. 1–5). The only acceptable method is the selective injection of contrast medium into the celiac, superior mesenteric or inferior mesenteric artery.

Preangiographic Preparation of the Patient

The afternoon before the angiographic examination, the procedure should be explained to the patient, and he must be informed about both the potential diagnostic benefits to be derived and the potential complications which can occur. A mild sedative and an analgesic are given approximately a half hour prior to the examination. The combinations of drugs used are legion, but they should not be used to excess. They should also be used cautiously in children, old people and people with hepatic disease and jaundice. It is important that the patient be alert during the examination so that he can cooperate in holding his breath during the filming, and is able to complain of unusual pain that would indicate a complication. General anesthesia is not needed in visceral angiography. A few patients are hypersensitive to pain, and when this situation arises or if an older patient is extremely uncomfortable lying on his back for the duration of the examination, it is better to give small doses of a minor tranquilizer such as Valium during the examination rather than oversedate the patient prior to the examination.

Excessive withholding of fluids from the patient prior to the examination is dangerous. If left on their own, many nurses give the patient nothing by mouth after midnight, and the patient is dehydrated by the time he reaches the angiographic suite the following morning. It is preferable to specifically order a clear fluid breakfast. By doing so the increased dangers of high doses of contrast medium in dehydrated

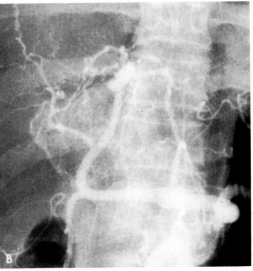

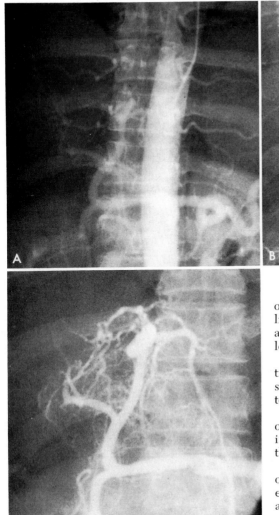

Figure 1–5. Demonstration of the value of selective angiography. Aortography, celiac angiography and hepatic angiography in a 56 year old man with hepatoma in the left lobe of the liver.

A. Aortogram. The concentration of contrast medium in the left hepatic artery resulting from an aortic injection is inadequate to allow a diagnosis of tumor.

B. Celiac angiogram. The concentration of contrast medium in the left hepatic artery is good and tumor vessels are demonstrated throughout the hepatoma.

C. Hepatic angiogram. The concentration of contrast medium in the hepatic artery is excellent. A definite diagnosis can be made and the extent of the lesion can be evaluated.

patients, particularly those with diminished renal function, are avoided.

Sites for Catheter Introduction

The technique in general use for catheterization of the visceral arteries was described by Seldinger in 1953. The method is shown in Figure 1–6 and can be used to introduce a catheter into any peripheral artery or vein. The arteries which have been used for gastrointestinal angiography have been the femoral, axillary and brachial. Of these, the femoral approach is by far the most preferable. It is the largest of the three arteries, and the catheter, when in place, compromises local blood flow the least. The patient can lie comfortably on his back during the examination, and a draw-sheet can be placed over the lower part of the angiographic table to maintain sterility. This artery is easily compressed and observed following the examination.

Occasionally, because of severe iliac atherosclerosis or the presence of aortofemoral grafts, the femoral artery cannot be used. The artery of choice then becomes the left axillary artery (Bron, 1966). This has several disadvantages when compared with the femoral approach but is still preferable to the brachial approach. The patient must lie with his arm behind his head during the

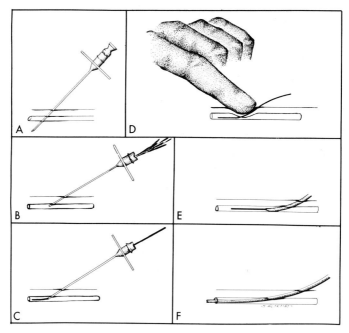

Figure 1–6. Seldinger technique for percutaneous angiography.

A. The needle is decisively thrust through both walls of the artery at an angle of approximately 45 degrees.

B. The trocar is removed and the cannula slowly withdrawn and depressed until blood spurts from the needle.

C. The guide wire is introduced through the cannula and passed into the aorta.

D. The cannula of the needle is removed from the guide wire and the puncture site compressed.

E. The catheter is advanced over the guide wire until the guide wire appears through the stopcock of the cathete:. The guide wire and catheter are then advanced together into the artery. The guide wire is then held stationary while the catheter is fed over the guide wire into the aorta.

F. Finally, the guide wire is removed and the catheter is ready for positioning in the desired aortic branch.

examination. This position is tiresome and often results in decreased circulation to the hand and a sensation of the hand "going to sleep," which is difficult to differentiate from decreased circulation caused by spasm around the catheter. The axillary artery is smaller than the femoral artery, and the catheter may partially interfere with the blood flow. The puncture must be made through the brachial plexus. This is frequently painful and, rarely, results in nerve damage. The axillary artery is much more mobile than the femoral artery and is harder to puncture. Finally, compression of the axillary artery following the examination may be difficult, and if a hematoma does occur, it is more difficult to control.

The brachial artery is the favored approach of the cardiac angiographer, who uses a cut-down technique. It is not suit-able for selective visceral catheterization, however, because of the great distance and the large number of bends between the arterial puncture site and the artery to be catheterized. The more bends a catheter makes, the more difficult the tip is to control. Also, the brachial artery is small, and spasm frequently occurs around the catheter. Spasm may prevent advancing the catheter into the subclavian artery and may also cause thrombosis at the puncture site.

Arterial Puncture

The first step in catheterization is the palpation and marking of the pulse distal to the puncture site so that it can be monitored during the examination. This is the

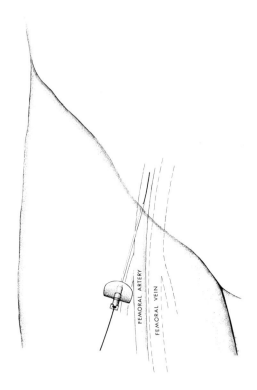

Figure 1-7. Femoral puncture site. The puncture should be made into the femoral artery at the inguinal crease or within 1 cm below the crease. The needle should be angled approximately 45 degrees in order to assure that the puncture is made into the common femoral artery.

dorsalis pedis, posterior tibial or radial artery, depending upon the approach. Monitoring may be done by intermittent palpation or with an inexpensive Doppler unit, which provides a continuous signal indicating the presence and quality of the pulse. The puncture site is then selected by palpating in the groin or axilla for the pulse. In the groin the best site for puncture is the inguinal crease (Fig. 1-7). A more caudal puncture may enter the superficial femoral artery, resulting in an increased incidence of thrombosis at the puncture site, especially in older patients. In an obese patient it is especially important to make the puncture into the inguinal crease since this is the shortest distance between the skin and the artery. Problems associated with passing a catheter to the artery through a great deal of fat are thereby lessened. The ax-

illary artery should be punctured distally (laterally in the axilla), since it is difficult to compress the artery following a puncture made medially, toward the chest wall (Fig. 1-8).

When the puncture site is selected, the area is shaved, washed with Betadine and isolated with sterile towels and drapes. The area around the puncture site is then anesthetized with 10 to 15 cc of local anesthetic. A skin wheal is first made with a 25 gauge needle over the puncture site. The remaining anesthetic is placed on either side of the artery with a 22 or 23 gauge needle; 5 to 7 cc is deposited deep, behind the artery. The most important part is the deep deposition of local anesthetic; infiltration above the artery alone is not adequate to prevent pain. Finally, a 3 mm incision is made in the skin with a scalpel blade. This should extend through the subcutaneous tissues.

Some debate has occurred about the relative value of a through-and-through puncture of the artery versus puncture of the anterior arterial wall only. A through-and-through puncture does not increase the complication rate and generally can be done with one attempt; an anterior wall puncture may require more attempts and in inexperienced hands can lead to subintimal guide wire passage. In general, an anterior wall puncture in an elderly, thin patient with an ectatic femoral artery is fairly easy, and we generally do this in such a patient.

The puncture technique is as follows: the index and middle fingers of the left hand are placed below and above the puncture site respectively, and the pulse is palpated. The needle is then advanced steadily along the course of the artery at approximately a 45 degree angle to the artery. When the needle comes up against the artery, the pulsation will be transmitted through the needle. If the thumb of the right hand is against the needle hub, the pulsation can be felt, permitting central positioning of the needle. When central placement of the needle is obtained, the examiner makes a short, decisive thrust of the needle through both arterial walls. The trocar is removed, and the hub is depressed slightly. The needle is slowly withdrawn until blood spurts through the needle. If the needle is positioned well in the lumen of the artery, the blood spurt is strong and

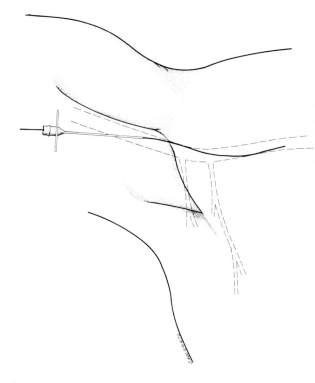

Figure 1–8. Axillary puncture site. The puncture of the axillary artery should be made as far laterally in the axillary crease as the artery is well palpated. The axillary artery is more mobile than the femoral artery and extending the arm over the head helps stretch and straighten the artery. With the arm over the head, the axillary artery generally lies just under the pectoral fold.

continues, though diminished, through diastole. If the needle is too near a wall or the tip is partially occluded by an atherosclerotic plaque, the spurt of blood is short and ceases during diastole. Another indication of a puncture too near the lateral wall of the artery is a single spurt of blood through the needle as it is withdrawn. If either of these situations occurs, the needle should be completely withdrawn and the artery compressed for 5 minutes. The process should then be repeated at a slightly different angle of insertion. One should not reinsert the trocar and make an immediate repuncture of the artery, as is frequently done for veins, since a hematoma may develop during the procedure. Occasionally, venous blood will return as the needle is withdrawn. The examiner should not assume that he is medial to the artery and quickly pull out the needle. He should continue slow withdrawal, since the vein occasionally lies behind the artery.

Guide Wire Insertion

The soft end of the guide wire is inserted through the needle into the artery. No at-tempt should be made to pass a guide wire through a poorly positioned needle, since this may result in the raising of a subintimal flap or laceration of the artery. The passage should be perfectly smooth into the abdominal aorta. If any resistance is encountered during the passage of the guide wire, fluoroscopy should be used immediately to determine what is hindering the passage. Occasionally, a slight withdrawal of the wire and reinsertion will result in a free passage into the aorta. The guide wire should never be forced forward against resistance. If the standard guide wire cannot be passed through a tortuous iliac artery or past atherosclerotic plaques, then a specially shaped wire should be substituted. Prior to exchanging the guide wire, the needle should be advanced over the wire so that it has a position in the lumen of the femoral artery well beyond the puncture site. On occasion, when advancing the guide wire is difficult or painful, fluoroscopic observation reveals that it is passing laterally into the deep circumflex iliac artery instead of medially. This generally causes the patient pain at the point of resistance. When this occurs, the guide wire should be drawn back into the needle and

Coping with Tortuous Iliac and Subclavian Arteries

Several methods have been devised to negotiate atherosclerotic and tortuous iliac arteries. The original method described by Baum and Abrams (1964) used a catheter with a tight J-shaped tip. A J-shaped guide wire was later substituted for the catheter (Judkins et al., 1967), eliminating a catheter exchange. The tightly curved end of the tip of the J-shaped guide wire bounces off atherosclerotic plaques and follows tortuous vessels very well, while the standard, straight tip tends to catch on the irregular surfaces of the iliac vessels (Fig. 1–10). Another wire which has been used for negotiating tortuous or atherosclerotic iliac or subclavian arteries has a 10 to 20 cm soft end (Rossi and Verdu, 1966). When the tip of this guide wire catches in an irregular area, it buckles into a "J," which then freely passes the atherosclerotic area.

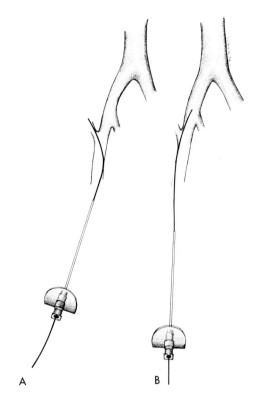

Figure 1–9. Redirecting a guide wire entering the deep circumflex iliac artery.

A. Occasionally the guide wire passes cranially and laterally, entering the deep circumflex iliac artery.

B. By directing the needle and guide wire slightly laterally, the guide wire bounces off the common femoral artery before reaching the deep circumflex iliac artery and is directed medially, passing freely up the iliac artery to the aorta.

Catheter Insertion

When the guide wire reaches the upper abdominal aorta, the needle is removed. The distal three fingers of the left hand should compress the artery at the puncture site as soon as the needle is withdrawn. The thumb and forefinger firmly grasp the guide wire so that it is not pulled out as the needle is taken off or the catheter put on. The guide wire is then wiped free of blood with a dry sponge. Guide wires should always be wiped free of blood after needles and catheters are removed from the artery during puncture or catheter exchange to help prevent clotting on the wire during reinsertion of the catheter. Many examiners prefer the use of a wet sponge for this purpose, but we use dry sponges for two reasons. First, wet sponges on the field soak through to the nonsterile underlying sheets and decrease the sterility of the field. Second, it is easier to manipulate the catheter when all the equipment is dry. The catheter is advanced over the guide wire until the tip is at the skin. The guide wire must have appeared through the stopcock. To introduce the catheter through the soft tissues into the artery it should be grasped

the tip of the needle directed laterally (Fig. 1–9). Although it seems contradictory, this maneuver generally causes the guide wire to bounce off the lateral wall of the femoral artery and to point medially toward the common iliac artery.

With the axillary approach, the guide wire occasionally passes down the subscapular or lateral thoracic artery instead of continuing into the subclavian artery. When this occurs, the arm can be brought into more of a right angle position relative to the body, putting the axillary and subclavian arteries more in a straight line and resulting in smooth passage of the guide wire centrally.

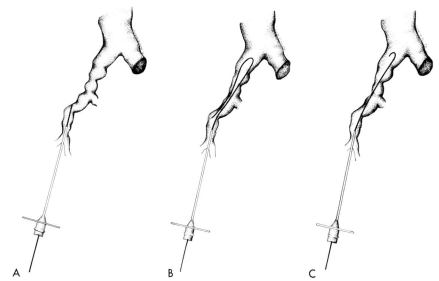

Figure 1–10.   Negotiating atherosclerotic iliac arteries with the guide wire.

A. The conventional straight guide wire frequently catches on atherosclerotic plaques and passage of the wire becomes impossible. Instead of continuing with this guide wire, which may result in subintimal dissection by the wire, a long "floppy-tipped" or J-shaped guide wire should be substituted.

B. Long "floppy-tipped" guide wire. This wire has a 10 to 20 cm flexible tip and when the tip catches on an atherosclerotic plaque, the long soft portion of the guide wire buckles. As the wire is advanced, a loop forms and progresses up the tortuous artery. When the stiff portion of the wire enters the artery, it follows the loop and generally passes easily into the aorta.

C. J-shaped guide wire. As the guide wire tip exits from the needle, a tight bend is formed and this bounces off atherosclerotic plaques. The wire generally passes freely through even severely atherosclerotic iliac vessels.

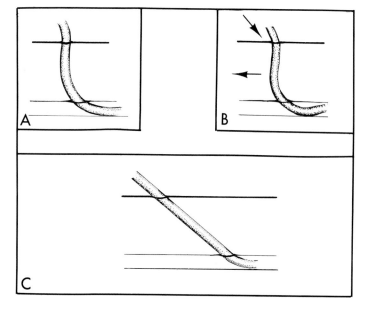

Figure 1–11.   Buckling of catheter in the soft tissues of the groin in obese patients.

A. There is a tendency for beginning angiographers to make too vertical a puncture of the femoral artery in obese patients.

B. When an attempt is made to advance the catheter, it may buckle in the soft tissue; therefore, the tip of the catheter becomes very difficult to control.

C. This buckling can be corrected by maintaining the correct 45 degree angle for the puncture so that forward force is transmitted in a straighter line. This helps to avoid such buckling.

close to the skin and should be advanced with small, firm thrusts using slight rotation during each thrust. If the catheter does not pass freely into the lumen of the artery, either because of obesity or atherosclerosis, a dilating catheter should then be used. This is a short Teflon catheter of approximately the same outer diameter as the catheter being used. It is stiff and makes a track through the soft tissues into the artery. When it is removed, the initial catheter generally passes freely along the path made by the dilator catheter. As the catheter is advanced into the aorta, the guide wire should be held stationary.

In extremely obese patients, the catheter tends to buckle in the soft tissues, particularly when the distal tip of the catheter and the distal curve have already passed through the skin. This can usually be avoided by making the puncture in the depths of the inguinal crease. It is especially important to angle the needle puncture to 45 degrees in obese patients. A more vertical puncture will lead to a vertical position of the catheter in the soft tissues and to great difficulty manipulating the catheter once it is in place (Fig. 1–11). It is imperative that the catheter move forward when advanced instead of buckling in the soft tissues.

Systemic Heparinization

The technique of subclinical systemic heparinization (Wallace et al., 1972) has gained increasing clinical acceptance. As soon as the catheter has been introduced into the abdominal aorta, approximately 3000 units of heparin are given through the catheter. The use of heparin in this manner prevents accumulation of thrombus on the catheter and eliminates almost all the thrombotic complications of catheterization. In addition, the time required for compression necessary to control bleeding at the puncture site following the catheterization is not significantly increased. A bleeding problem encountered following catheterization can be controlled by the injection of 10 mg of protamine sulfate for every 1000 units of heparin used during the procedure. This systemic heparinization technique has merit, since most of the complications at the puncture site are related to thrombosis during the procedure, particularly in old people and young women. Alternatively, heparin-bonded catheters are being developed and should soon be available commercially.

Catheterization of the Abdominal Aorta from the Axillary Approach

If the axillary approach must be used, the abdominal aorta can best be entered from the left axilla. In young patients, the left subclavian artery forms a straight line with the descending thoracic aorta, and a guide wire introduced from the left axilla can generally be directed into the abdominal aorta. With the guide wire held stationary, a catheter having an appropriately shaped tip can be advanced into the abdominal aorta and then into the desired visceral branch. In order to have good control of the catheter tip, a torque control catheter should be used when visceral arteries are catheterized from the axilla.

With age, the aorta becomes elongated and tortuous, and the left subclavian artery becomes progressively oriented toward the ascending aorta. Although several methods have been devised to help negotiate the angle that develops between the left subclavian artery and the aorta, the simplest is the use of a manipulator instrument (Figs. 1–12 and 1–19). The catheter is advanced so that its tip lies in the thoracic aorta just distal to the orifice of the left subclavian artery. A manipulator guide wire is then advanced into the catheter until its tip reaches the tip of the catheter. The catheter is bent with the instrument, and the bend is directed posterolaterally toward the patient's left. The instrument is held stationary and the catheter advanced over the manipulator guide wire toward the descending aorta. As the catheter tip enters the descending thoracic aorta, the bend in the manipulator wire is relaxed and the wire again advanced to the tip of the catheter. The wire and the catheter are then advanced together down the thoracic aorta to the abdominal aorta. The same technique can be used to catheterize the abdominal aorta from the right axillary approach.

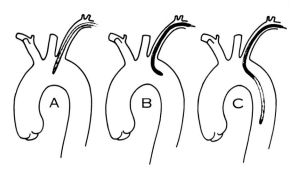

Figure 1–12. Use of the manipulator instrument for catheterization of the abdominal aorta from the left axillary artery in elderly patients.

A. The catheter is advanced from the left axillary artery into the thoracic aorta.

B. A manipulator guide wire is advanced into the catheter so that the tip reaches the tip of the catheter. A bend is made, and the catheter tip is directed posterolaterally.

C. The manipulator instrument is held stationary as the catheter is advanced down the descending thoracic aorta.

Catheterization of Aortic Visceral Branches

The celiac artery arises from the aorta anteriorly at the level of the lower half of the T12 vertebral body or the T12–L1 interspace; the superior mesenteric artery arises anteriorly at the T12–L1 interspace or the upper portion of the L1 vertebral body and the inferior mesenteric artery approximately at the lower L3 vertebral body anteriorly and slightly to the left of the midline. The area on which the image intensifier is to be centered for the catheterization can be easily localized by identifying the last rib (and thereby T12) and then counting down the appropriate number of vertebral bodies. Another localization method requires renal artery catheterization first and then appropriate adjustment of the catheter. The superior mesenteric artery lies anterior and just cephalad to the right renal artery, and the celiac artery lies 0.5 to 2.0 cm further cephalad.

When the intensifier is centered over the artery to be catheterized, the catheter is ro-

tated so that its tip is anterior. If the catheter is rotated in a clockwise direction at the groin, it will appear to the patient's right if the tip is posterior and to the left if the tip is anterior. Conversely, a counterclockwise rotation will make the tip move toward the patient's right if the tip is anterior and to the left, if posterior. This relationship is sometimes difficult for the beginning angiographer to grasp but comes readily with a little experience.

The celiac or superior mesenteric artery may be catheterized either with the tip extended upward or with the catheter turned so that the tip points downward (Fig. 1–13). In most people the celiac artery has a downward direction and the turned position is best, but in obese patients, the celiac artery generally has an upward direction at its origin and is more easily catheterized with an upward pointing catheter tip. The superior mesenteric artery can generally be catheterized with either technique.

When the guide wire is removed from a catheter in the aorta, the catheter tip usually points upward. The tip can generally be turned downward simply by advancing the catheter without the guide wire in place. The tip usually enters a

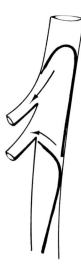

Figure 1–13. Catheterization with the tip in the extended and turned positions. An artery may be entered by advancing the catheter with the tip extended or the catheter may be withdrawn into the artery with the tip in the turned position.

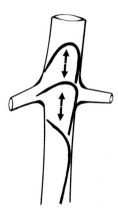

Figure 1–14. Turning the catheter tip in a renal artery. The catheter tip can be either turned or extended by catheterizing a renal artery. This can be done in arteries other than the renal arteries, but the renal is easiest because of its relatively constant location at the Ll-2 interspace and its lateral position in the aorta. When the desired direction of the catheter tip is achieved, the tip is rotated anteriorly and advanced or withdrawn into the celiac or superior mesenteric arteries.

renal, lumbar, celiac or mesenteric artery. Further advancing then turns the tip. On occasion it is difficult to get the catheter tip turned downward, usually because the distal limb is too long for the diameter of the patient's aorta. If this difficulty occurs, one should catheterize a renal artery at the L1–2 interspace, and then continue to advance the catheter up the aorta. The tip will back out of the renal artery in the turned position (Fig. 1–14). If this is not possible, the catheter can be advanced to the aortic arch, where it generally turns into its natural, preshaped configuration. The catheter can then be drawn into the abdominal aorta with the tip in the turned position. To prevent the tip from catching in orifices on the way down, the catheter should be rotated as it is drawn back. Whenever the catheter tip enters an arterial orifice or catches on an atherosclerotic plaque, rotation will cease. The catheter must then be advanced slightly and the rotation and withdrawal procedure continued.

However, if the catheter is in the turned position and it is desirable to have the tip extended, this can generally be accomplished by simply drawing the catheter down. The tip then catches in an arterial

orifice, and continued withdrawal extends the tip (Fig. 1–14). On rare occasions the guide wire must be reintroduced while withdrawing the catheter in order to extend the tip.

If the radius of the distal bend of the catheter or the length of the tip is too great, the tip may point back toward the center of the aorta in the turned position, and the visceral vessels become impossible to enter. Two maneuvers may be used to correct this prior to catheter exchange. First, catheterization can be tried with the tip pointing up. This is generally unsatisfactory since there is not enough anterior angulation at the tip. Second, if the catheter is in the turned position, the tip can be directed against the wall by inserting a guide wire to change the angle of the bend (Fig. 1–15). This often is successful if no atherosclerosis is present. If a fair degree of

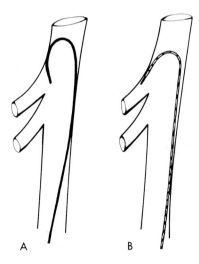

A   B

Figure 1–15. Distal limb of the catheter too long for the diameter of the aorta.

A. When the catheter tip is too long for the patient's aorta, the tip is directed back toward the lumen and introduction of the catheter into the celiac or superior mesenteric arteries becomes impossible. Even turning the catheter in the renal arteries as demonstrated in Figure 1–14 is impossible. Frequently the catheter will have to be exchanged for one with a more suitable distal limb.

B. Prior to exchanging the catheter, however, a guide wire can be introduced to the tip in an attempt to extend the tip of the catheter slightly and direct it toward the wall of the aorta.

atherosclerosis is present, the catheter must be exchanged for one with a more suitable tip. Conversely, in patients with ectatic aortas, the catheter must have a greater radius of curvature and a longer distal limb. In the latter patient this is also important to prevent recoil during the injection. The appropriately shaped catheter is so necessary to the completion of an examination that one must always be willing to exchange catheters.

The inferior mesenteric artery is slightly more difficult to catheterize than either the celiac or superior mesenteric artery because the lower aorta is narrower and often has significant atherosclerotic changes. Also, the orifice of the inferior mesenteric artery is much smaller than that of the celiac and superior mesenteric arteries. With a correctly shaped catheter, however, inferior mesenteric artery catheterization generally can be accomplished.

When the catheter has been placed in the desired artery, it should be seated as far as possible into the artery, and any redundancy along the catheter should be removed. Both of these maneuvers help prevent catheter recoil and subintimal dissection during the injection of contrast medium. A forceful hand injection of saline should be made during fluoroscopic monitoring to see if the catheter position is stable.

Catheterization in the Presence of Atherosclerosis

If the patient does not have atherosclerotic irregularity of the aorta, the catheterization of the abdominal visceral branches is quite easy and takes only several seconds of fluoroscopy time. When atherosclerosis is present, however, a steady, smooth manipulation of the catheter tip may be difficult. The most common problem that the beginning angiographer has when confronted with atherosclerosis is that the catheter tip turns against a plaque and stops, even though rotation is continued at the puncture site. Suddenly the tip releases and flips around the aorta. This can be avoided in two ways. First, short, sawing motions should be used as one slowly rotates the catheter. This helps to avoid catching the tip on plaques. If the catheter tip still catches and stops, it should be rotated in the other direction. Frequently, the catheter tip will then be easier to control. Also, if torque is built up during rotation, the catheter should be rapidly "unwound" when it begins to move.

Occasionally, with severe aortic atherosclerosis, the catheter cannot be readvanced to the desired level when it has been drawn too far caudally because the tip keeps running into plaques. If this occurs, the catheter should not be forced back up or an attempt made to turn the tip in the more narrow, distal aorta. Instead, the guide wire should be reinserted to above the level of interest and the catheter then advanced over the guide wire.

It is extremely important to remember that a guide wire exiting from a catheter does not bend until it is more than 1 cm beyond the catheter tip, even though the guide wire is flexible. Thus, all the force of the guide wire is straight ahead, and if the catheter tip is against an atherosclerotic plaque, the guide wire can easily dissect under the plaque. To avoid this, the catheter should be withdrawn slightly as the guide wire exits. Doing so will help avoid one of the more common, unnecessary complications of angiography.

When atherosclerosis is quite severe and catheterization is extremely difficult, it is useful to inject small test doses of contrast medium as the catheter is being withdrawn in the correct area. When the catheter tip is near the desired orifice, contrast medium enters the artery, and the proper manipulations can be made.

Since celiac occlusion is not uncommon in patients with severe atherosclerosis, it should always be considered when difficulty is encountered in catheterizing this vessel. If the celiac artery cannot be entered or the orifice localized with contrast medium, a superior mesenteric angiogram or lateral aortogram should be performed. This will define the nature of the atherosclerosis around the celiac axis and frequently demonstrate a cause for the inability to catheterize the vessel.

Catheter Exchange

More than one shape of catheter will frequently be necessary to complete an angiographic examination. Catheter exchange is done by reinserting a guide wire, being careful to withdraw the catheter as the guide wire exits through the catheter tip. The guide wire should be placed well beyond the catheter tip so that the end of the guide wire remains in the abdominal aorta when the catheter tip is withdrawn through the skin. This can be accomplished by simultaneous catheter withdrawal and guide wire insertion. The puncture site is compressed with the distal three fingers of the left hand and the guide wire firmly grasped between the index finger and thumb. After the catheter is removed, the guide wire is wiped with a dry gauze pad. The new catheter is then introduced over the guide wire.

Injection of Contrast Medium

Contrast medium should be injected at a rate that approximates as closely as possible the rate of blood flow in the artery being opacified. Injecting too slowly results in incomplete filling of the artery with contrast medium, hemodilution and poor opacification of the vascular bed. Too rapid an injection, on the other hand, results in reflux of contrast medium into the aorta and filling of extraneous aortic branches, particularly the renal arteries, which are bothersome at visceral angiography. Too rapid an injection also results in a higher incidence of recoil of the catheter out of the arterial orifice. The celiac and superior mesenteric arteries have a blood flow of 10 to 15 cc per second in most patients, and the inferior mesenteric artery, 4 to 6 cc per second. If the patient is elderly, small, a child or has significant atherosclerosis, these volumes are less. If the patient has cirrhosis or another disease which causes increased arterial blood flow to the viscera, these rates are greater. We have used an average injection of 10 cc per second for the celiac and superior mesenteric arteries and 5 cc per second for the inferior mesenteric artery. These rates are adjusted according to the clinical status of the patient and the disease being investigated.

Contrast Medium

The tendency in recent years has been to increase the amount of contrast medium used for celiac and mesenteric angiograms. Some time ago, Grayson et al. (1961) demonstrated that contrast medium could have a toxic effect on the bowel wall. The contrast medium that caused most of the problem is no longer available for clinical usage. Since then, much less toxic contrast media have been developed, and none of those currently used are toxic to the organs supplied by the celiac or mesenteric arteries. These organs appear to have a higher threshold of toxicity than the heart, brain or kidneys. Amounts of contrast medium used for single celiac and superior mesenteric artery injections are now in the range of 30 to 60 cc. Even larger doses may be used for demonstration of the venous side of the visceral circulation. In the inferior mesenteric artery, the range is 15 to 20 cc. Because of the lack of apparent toxicity, most angiographers now use 75 to 76 per cent contrast media for all visceral angiography in order to obtain the slightly higher contrast afforded over the 50 to 60 per cent contrast media. Since methylglucamine salts of the contrast media have been shown to be less toxic than sodium salts when used in the brain and kidneys, these are used in the visceral circulation as well.

Although the volumes of individual injections are greater than in the past, attention must still be paid to the total volume used for the entire examination. Total volumes of more than 3 to 4 cc per kilogram should not be used, and particular care should be taken to avoid dehydration in patients with impaired renal function.

Catheter Recoil

Catheter recoil is a rocket phenomenon which occurs during every injection of contrast medium (Olin, 1963). One need only hold a catheter in the air and inject fluid through it at a moderate rate to note how much recoil a small flow causes. In most patients the catheter recoils to the point at which its bend meets the opposite wall of the aorta. At this point the tip should still be in the orifice of the artery being injected so that all the contrast medium enters that vessel. For this reason, the distal limb of the catheter should always be slightly longer than the width of the aorta. Also, the distal limb of the catheter should be straight, with a rather abrupt bend, as shown in Figure 1–3A. A gentle curve extending from the tip will result in frequent recoil. Occasionally the catheter recoils completely out of the artery regardless of the shape, and most of the injection is made into the aorta. A number of things can be done to prevent recoil during subsequent injections. The easiest is to decrease the injection rate. Catheters recoiling at 12 cc per second will probably not recoil at 8 cc per second. This may reduce the quality of the examination, but it is preferable to the quality obtained with recoil. If decreasing the injection rate fails, the catheter must be exchanged. Since the reason for the catheter recoil is too short a distal limb, the new catheter should have a longer one. Also, side holes placed near the catheter tip make the catheter more stable during injection. It is often easiest to combine these and exchange the recoiling catheter for one with side holes and a longer tip.

Side Holes

Most newcomers to the field of angiography believe that the purpose of side holes is to decrease resistance at the catheter tip so that a higher rate of injection can be used. This is true only with catheters with large inner diameters or when the end hole is small relative to the inner diameter of the catheter. In smaller catheters, such as those used for selective angiography, the resistance along the length of the catheter is the primary factor limiting the rate of flow of contrast medium. The real purpose of side holes in small catheters is to increase stability during injection. By redistributing part of the jet in a lateral direction, the jet at the catheter tip is decreased and the rocket effect thereby is diminished.

A catheter without side holes is easier to check to be sure the tip is free in the arterial lumen. If the end hole lies against an atherosclerotic plaque or against the wall of the artery, no flow will return, and the catheter can be adjusted until free flow is obtained before an injection is made. During injection, however, recoil may place the tip against the wall, resulting in a subintimal injection. Properly positioned side holes cause the catheter to have a central

position in the arterial lumen during injection. Because blood flow can be obtained through the side holes even if the tip is obstructed, however, a subintimal injection may occur at the start of injection.

SUPERSELECTIVE CATHETERIZATION TECHNIQUE

The arteries of the visceral organs frequently overlie one another, and assignment of a vascular abnormality to a specific organ may be difficult at celiac or superior mesenteric angiography. For example, the arteries of the stomach are superimposed on those of the left lobe of the liver, the upper pole of the spleen and most of the pancreas. In the mesenteric circulation, several arterial branches to the bowel may be superimposed on one another. To avoid this problem, techniques have been developed to catheterize specific branches of the celiac and mesenteric arteries so that the blood supply to only one organ is injected. In addition to the selective look at the blood vessels in an organ or part of an organ, two other advantages have made superselective techniques an important part of visceral angiography. First, a higher concentration of contrast medium can be obtained when a smaller artery is injected, resulting in more complete filling of all of the branches through the organ. This is particularly important for magnification techniques, since it does not make sense to magnify vessels that are only partially filled with contrast medium. Second, the venous drainage of the organ can be better visualized at superselective angiography, in part because the concentration of contrast medium reaching the veins is greater, but also because the veins are seen without extraneous superimposed veins.

Conventional celiac and superior mesenteric angiograms should always be done prior to the superselective injections. The conventional studies are necessary to have an adequate "road map" of the visceral arteries and their branches. This will facilitate the superselective catheterization procedure, and time will not be wasted looking for branches that have variant origins. Also, superselective angiography is frequently accompanied by arterial spasm which may mimic primary disease, particu-

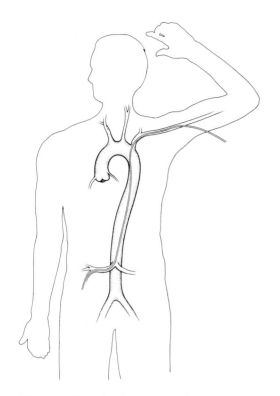

Figure 1–16. Axillary approach to superselective visceral angiography. A torque control catheter with a slight bend at the tip to catch the orifice of the major visceral branches has been introduced. The left axillary artery is preferable to the right because of the better alignment of the left subclavian artery with the descending aorta. The catheter is advanced into the abdominal aorta over a guide wire; the guide wire is removed, the catheter tip directed toward the anterior wall of the aorta and the desired aortic branch entered. The catheter generally passes out of the celiac or superior mesenteric artery into the major arterial branches, particularly in patients with caudally directed celiac arteries. Catheterization of secondary branches of the celiac or superior mesenteric artery may be more difficult, especially in patients with atherosclerosis. Frequently, particularly in older patients, a catheter passed from the left subclavian artery enters the ascending instead of the descending aorta. The problem can be easily overcome by using a manipulator instrument (see Fig. 1–12).

larly invasion by tumor. Finally, in the evaluation of patients with tumors, particularly pancreatic tumors, it is important to obtain a hepatic angiogram and good delineation of the visceral veins.

The original superselective catheterizations were done from the axillary artery approach (Boijsen, 1966). Most of the branches of the celiac and superior mesenteric arteries can be catheterized from this approach (Fig. 1–16). However, the greater incidence of complications from axillary catheterization and the technical difficulty created by the long distance between the puncture site and the artery to be catheterized generally have caused this technique to be abandoned for techniques using the femoral approach. Occasionally the axillary approach is still used in patients who cannot be catheterized from the femoral artery. When it is necessary to use the axillary approach for superselective angiography, a torque control catheter should be employed to make manipulation of the tip easier.

The methods currently in general use for catheterization of branches of the visceral arteries include the catheter exchange method utilizing guide wires and specially shaped catheters (Rösch and Grollman, 1969), manipulator instruments (Almén, 1966; Reuter, 1969) and the coaxial catheter method described by Paul et al. (1965) and improved by Eisenberg (1973).

Catheter Exchange Method

This is the simplest of the three methods for superselective catheterization because it requires no equipment except that generally used for selective angiography. Following a celiac angiogram, the catheter tip is introduced as far as possible toward the major branch to be catheterized, usually the hepatic or the splenic artery (Fig. 1–17). Some contrast medium is injected as the catheter is manipulated, and if this flows to the desired branch, a guide wire will probably also enter that branch. A long guide wire (approximately 140 cm) is then introduced into the catheter and gently advanced through the tip as far into the splenic or hepatic artery as possible. Then, while the guide wire is held stationary, the catheter is slowly withdrawn over the wire until it exits from the puncture site. Occasional fluoroscopic monitoring insures that the tip of the guide wire has not slipped back as the catheter is withdrawn. A new catheter, the tip of which corresponds to the patient's arterial anatomy, is then introduced over the guide wire. It

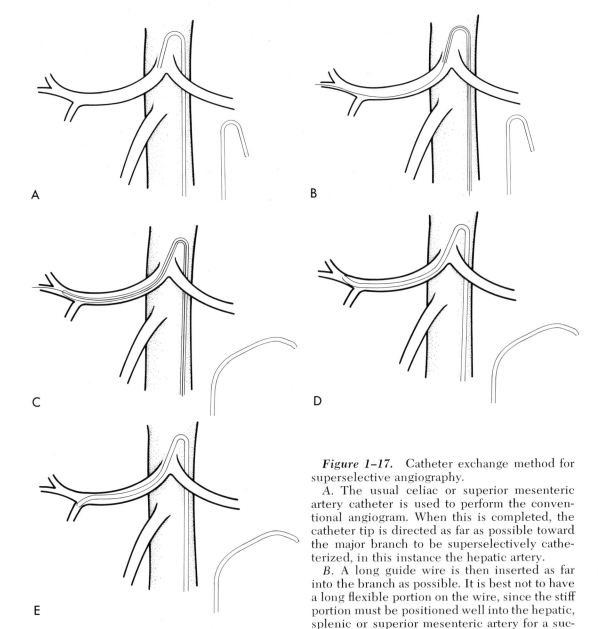

A

B

C

D

E

Figure 1–17. Catheter exchange method for superselective angiography.

A. The usual celiac or superior mesenteric artery catheter is used to perform the conventional angiogram. When this is completed, the catheter tip is directed as far as possible toward the major branch to be superselectively catheterized, in this instance the hepatic artery.

B. A long guide wire is then inserted as far into the branch as possible. It is best not to have a long flexible portion on the wire, since the stiff portion must be positioned well into the hepatic, splenic or superior mesenteric artery for a successful catheter exchange. With the guide wire held stationary against the patient's leg, the conventional catheter is then removed.

C. A superselective catheter (lower right) is then advanced over the guide wire until the tip is at or beyond the secondary branch to be catheterized, in this instance the gastroduodenal artery. Although the superselective catheter shape shown here usually allows catheterization of the gastroduodenal, right or left hepatic, dorsal pancreatic, jejunal or ileal branches, this shape must occasionally be modified to conform more to the patient's anatomy, especially when the arteries are tortuous.

D. The guide wire is then removed.

E. The catheter is rotated and advanced or withdrawn until the tip enters the desired secondary branch.

must be advanced slowly and carefully as it makes the bend from the aorta into the celiac artery and into the hepatic or splenic branches. When the catheter has been advanced the desired distance, the guide wire can be removed and the catheter tip manipulated into the desired secondary branch—the right or left hepatic artery, the gastroduodenal or dorsal pancreatic artery or the left gastric artery. Occasionally, a straight guide wire cannot be advanced through an angulated or tortuous celiac artery, and a C-shaped or a very tight J guide wire may be required. In the catheter exchange method it is also important to use guide wires with a progressive transition in stiffness between the very flexible tip of the wire and the stiff portion of the wire, since wires with abrupt transi-

tion may lift the catheter out of the artery into the aorta as the stiff portion begins to make the bend. The stiff portion of the guide wire must be in the hepatic or splenic artery before the replacement catheter can be advanced. If only the soft portion of the guide wire is in the artery, the superselective catheter will not follow the guide wire but will lift it out of position into the aorta.

The catheter exchange method is relatively easy to perform in patients with a cephalad-directed celiac axis, generally those patients who are obese (Fig. 1–18). It may also succeed in patients with a transverse celiac axis but is rarely useful in patients with caudally directed celiac arteries. This is because the direction of thrust from the femoral artery is upward and can

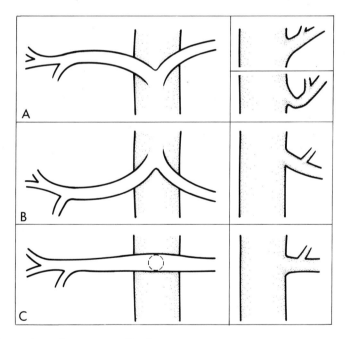

Figure 1–18. General configurations of celiac arteries.
A. In the patient with a cephalad-directed celiac artery superselective angiography is generally easy to perform using the catheter shape shown in Figure 1–17C. In most of these patients, the origin of the celiac artery points in the same general direction as the distal portion, as shown in the lateral view (A, upper right). However, in some patients with a cephalad celiac axis, the initial part of the artery passes caudally under the median arcuate ligament before the major portion of the artery is directed cephalad (A, lower right). In these patients, superselective catheterization may be difficult, depending upon the degree of compression by the median arcuate ligament.
B. In a patient with a caudally directed celiac axis and branches, superselective catheterization is also generally easy and is best performed using a manipulator instrument.
C. In a patient with a transverse celiac artery and branches, superselective catheterization is difficult using either the catheter exchange or manipulator instrument method. It is in this type of configuration that coaxial catheterization may be the preferred method.

even be upward and outward, but only rarely can the thrust be reversed downward without using a manipulator instrument.

For the same reason the catheter exchange method is occasionally useful for superselective study of the superior mesenteric artery. It works best in those patients who have a rather transverse proximal superior mesenteric artery and is less useful when the superior mesenteric artery is sharply angulated caudally.

Manipulator Instruments

Several manipulator instruments are available, ranging from very simple instru-

ments which only bend the catheter, to those built into the catheter, through complex instruments capable of irrigating the area around the guide wire (Fig. 1–19). Whichever is chosen, it is important to be sure that the manipulator guide wire bends the specific catheter to be used; some instruments utilize manipulator guide wires that bend only the manufacturers' catheters. We prefer the simpler instruments because they allow the flexibility of choosing a wide variety of catheters and shapes.

When a manipulator instrument is to be used, the orifice of the celiac or superior mesenteric artery (determined by the position of the conventional catheter) should be centered in the fluoroscopic field and its

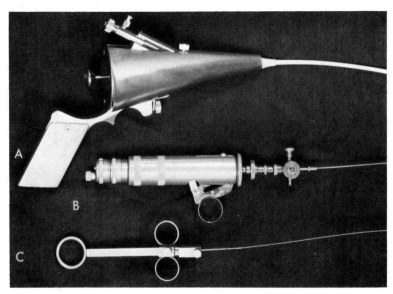

Figure 1–19. Manipulator instruments.

A. The Medi-tech manipulator instrument utilizes four small wires extending through the catheter to the tip. The wires are connected to a "joy stick." Moving the "joy stick" in any direction causes a corresponding bend of the catheter tip in that direction. The rinse apparatus, through which a guide wire can be inserted, is in a direct line with the catheter lumen. The major advantage of the instrument is the possibility for rotating the catheter tip in any direction without changing the position of the instrument. The major disadvantage is the large outer diameter of the catheter supplied with the instrument.

B. The Müller-USCI instrument is a complex mechanism for unidirectionally bending a catheter tip. A rinse apparatus is available with the instrument. The major weakness of the instrument is the relatively weak bending power of the guide wire; it does not bend the polyethylene catheters generally used for visceral angiography. It has most frequently been used with the small thin-walled neuroradiologic polyethylene catheters.

C. The Cook instrument also bends the guide wire in only one direction. The design is simple, and it is available with a number of different sizes of manipulator guide wires. Generally, 0.045-inch diameter guide wires are used for visceral angiography. The instrument has a rinse apparatus available which attaches to the catheter rather than to the instrument itself. The major advantages of the instrument are its simplicity and the strong bending power of the manipulator guide wires. The major disadvantage is the design of the rinse apparatus. For this reason the Cook instrument, although excellent for visceral superselective work, should probably not be used in cardiac or neuroangiography.

location related to a pedicle or other landmark on the upper lumbar spine so that it can be located easily using the stiff manipulator instrument and catheter. When the aortic branch to be catheterized is centered in the field, the table should be locked in position until after the artery is catheterized.

The conventional catheter is exchanged for a new catheter with a shape appropriate for the artery to be superselectively catheterized (Fig. 1–20). The manipulator guide wire is then introduced into the new catheter, and a bend is made with the manipulator instrument. This bend effaces the preformed shape of the catheter and produces a shape suitable for catheterization of the celiac or superior mesenteric artery, which

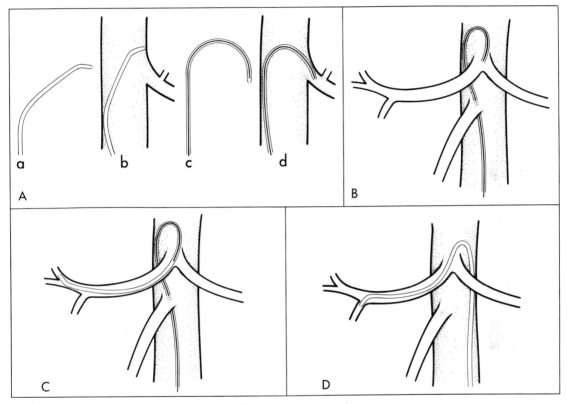

Figure 1–20. Superselective angiography using a manipulator instrument.

A. When the orifice of the aortic branch to be catheterized has been centered in the fluoroscopic field, the conventional catheter is removed and replaced with a superselective catheter (*a*). This is advanced up the aorta until the tip is just cephalad to the aortic branch to be catheterized (*b*). A manipulator guide wire is then advanced to the tip of the catheter. When a bend is placed on the manipulator wire with the instrument handle, the superselective catheter shape is effaced, and the catheter assumes a rounded celiac curve (*c*). The combination of catheter and manipulator wire is then manipulated until the catheter tip is well seated in the celiac or superior mesenteric artery (*d*). If the patient has a cephalad-directed celiac axis, the bend can then be released and the catheter tip directed toward either the hepatic or the splenic artery.

B. If the patient has a caudally directed celiac artery or if the superior mesenteric artery is to be catheterized, the tip of the catheter is directed toward the desired branch. In the celiac artery this generally requires moving the aortic portion of the catheter toward the right aortic wall for hepatic artery catheterization (as shown in the illustration) and toward the left aortic wall for splenic artery catheterization.

C. With the manipulator instrument held stationary, the catheter is fed off into the desired branch. Frequently, as shown, the catheter tip enters the left or right hepatic artery. The catheter may also resume its original shape as it advances, in which case the tip will enter the gastroduodenal artery.

D. The manipulator instrument is then removed, and the catheter is rotated and withdrawn until the tip engages the desired secondary branch.

is then engaged. The catheter and manipulator guide wire are securely positioned in the orifice of the artery, and the catheter is advanced, while the manipulator instrument is held steady and the guide wire taut. The catheter will usually move toward the desired artery. If it meets an obstruction, the wire will back out of the catheter. The wire should then be reinserted and the catheterization repeated in a different phase of inspiration. If the manipulator instrument still backs away from the catheter tip, it should be allowed to do so. As it does, the bend in the manipulator wire advances up the aorta so that there are several centimeters of catheter (tip still in the celiac axis) distal to the bend in the manipulator wire (Fig. 1–21). The catheter and manipulator wire can then be moved up and down in the aorta and celiac artery with the patient in slightly different phases of respiration until the catheter tip slips by the obstruction into the desired branch.

In patients with caudally directed celiac arteries, it is best to align the shaft of the catheter and the manipulator instrument

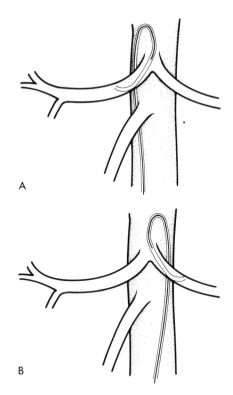

Figure 1–22. Superselective catheterization of caudally directed hepatic and splenic arteries.

A. When the aortic portion of the catheter is placed along the right aortic wall, the tip of the manipulator instrument and the catheter are directed toward the hepatic artery. As the catheter is advanced off the manipulator guide wire, it generally passes into the hepatic artery.

B. Conversely, catheterization of the splenic artery should be done with the aortic portion of the catheter along the left aortic wall. As the catheter is advanced in a "loop the loop" manner, it enters the splenic artery.

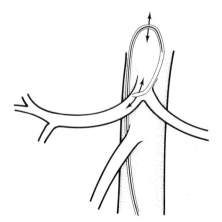

Figure 1–21. Movement of catheter and manipulator guide wire with the manipulator wire proximal to the catheter tip. Occasionally, when the cather is fed off the manipulator wire, as shown in Figure 1–20, the tip of the catheter catches on a small arterial branch or atherosclerotic plaque. Further advancing of the catheter causes the manipulator wire to back away from the catheter tip and to assume a configuration similar to that shown here. When this occurs, the manipulator instrument and catheter can be advanced and pulled back as a unit, using slightly different degrees of rotation until the catheter tip slides by whatever has caused the original impediment.

along the same side of the aorta as the branch to be catheterized. For example, if the hepatic artery is to be catheterized, the catheter should be placed along the right wall of the aorta (Fig. 1–22). The catheter is then advanced off the manipulator wire in a "loop the loop" manner toward the hepatic artery. Conversely, the catheter should be placed along the left wall of the aorta if the splenic artery is to be catheterized. If the celiac artery is directed cephalad, the manipulator wire needs to be bent only slightly, and the catheter tip can be pointed directly toward the desired branch (Fig. 1–23). A transverse celiac artery is the most difficult to superselect because of the several right angle bends in-

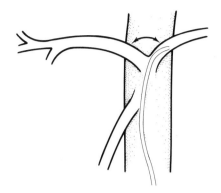

Figure 1–23. In patients with a cephalad-directed celiac artery and branches, the generally used superselective catheter can be advanced into either the hepatic or splenic artery by pointing the tip in the proper direction.

volved (see Fig. 1–18). Frequently, several maneuvers must be attempted with the manipulator instrument in order to catheterize a transverse celiac artery, and much experience is required for consistent success.

The motion of the tip of the catheter and the bend of the manipulator instrument can and should be constantly modified throughout the catheterization. When working from the right groin, the examiner should manipulate the catheter with his left hand while modifying the bend in the manipulator guide wire with his right hand.

The manipulator instrument is most useful in caudally directed celiac arteries and in the superior mesenteric artery, which is generally directed caudally. When the manipulator instrument is used, the manipulator guide wire should never be advanced beyond the catheter tip into the aorta or one of its branches because the manipulator tip is rigid and can damage the intima. For this reason we use a 0.045 manipulator wire while keeping the tip of the catheter tapered to a 0.038 guide wire. Also, when the manipulator instrument is positioned so that it is tip to tip with the catheter, the combination is quite rigid, particularly when a bend has been placed on the manipulator guide wire. For this reason, the combination of guide wire and catheter should be manipulated with great care and should not be advanced or withdrawn against resistance. It is important to learn to position the catheter with the left

hand while using the right hand for other manipulations, such as bending the manipulator guide wire or injecting small amounts of contrast medium through the catheter during manipulation. It is awkward to perform these functions while manipulating the catheter with the right hand. The lengths of the catheter and manipulator guide wires should be kept short. A 60 to 80 cm manipulator guide wire is perfectly adequate for any of the superselective abdominal catheterizations, and a 100 cm or longer wire is unwieldy.

Coaxial Catheterization

Although the techniques for coaxial catheterization were described some time ago, the method was not frequently used for superselective catheterization until Eisenberg (1973) modified the Cope catheter. The coaxial catheter has three parts, a central "torque control" guide wire, a small inner catheter and a larger outer catheter. After the outer catheter has been introduced into the celiac or superior mesenteric artery, the inner catheter and the guide wire are advanced through it into the desired major branch (Fig. 1–24). The soft, curved tip of the guide wire can be directed into either the hepatic or splenic artery by rotating the "torque control" guide wire in the proper direction. The inner catheter can then be advanced over the guide wire, followed by the outer catheter. The guide wire is then manipulated to enter the desired branch of the splenic, hepatic or superior mesenteric artery, and the process is repeated. When the outer catheter is in place in the desired branch, the guide wire and inner catheter are removed and an injection made. For small branches, the injection can be made through the inner catheter. The guide wire can be directed into second and third order branches if desired, and even more selective injections can be obtained.

The superselective catheterization method the angiographer eventually adopts will depend on his experiences with the various procedures. All have advantages and disadvantages, and, in our experience, some work better than others in certain anatomical situations. For example, if a pa-

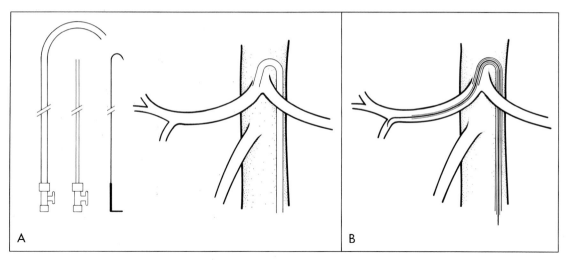

Figure 1–24. Coaxial catheterization method for superselective angiography.

A. The equipment is shown on the left. The larger outer catheter is not tapered at the tip, and the inner catheter just passes through the outer catheter. The torque control guide wire has a curved tip. The core of the guide wire extends to a bent handle which, when rotated, rotates the tip of the catheter as well. Both outer and inner catheters are fitted with grommeted rinse stopcocks so that contrast medium can be injected with the guide wire in place.

To begin the coaxial catheterization, the outer catheter is introduced into the celiac or superior mesenteric artery and the tip directed toward the major branch to be catheterized, as shown on the right.

B. The inner catheter and guide wire are then introduced through the outer catheter into the desired branch. The inner catheter is positioned proximal to the secondary branch to be catheterized, and the torque control guide wire is used to enter that branch. With the torque control guide wire well positioned in the secondary branch, the inner catheter is advanced over the guide wire until it also has a position in the branch to be injected. The guide wire is then withdrawn, and the angiogram is performed through the inner catheter. If large flow rates are desired, the outer catheter can be advanced over the inner catheter until it also has a position in the artery to be injected. The inner catheter can then be withdrawn and the injection made through the outer catheter.

tient has an upward-directed celiac axis, the catheter exchange method works very well; the manipulator instrument seems best in patients with caudally directed celiac axes. Neither of these methods works particularly well in people with transverse celiac arteries, and with these difficult patients the coaxial system may be the best technique. Also, neither the catheter exchange method nor manipulator instrument method is suitable in the catheterization of third order branches. If catheterization of the pancreaticoduodenal arcades or second and third order mesenteric branches is desired, the coaxial method should be used.

The beginning angiographer should not be discouraged if all does not go well at first. Experience is necessary to perform any of the superselective methods with consistent success, and he should keep trying.

Left Gastric Artery Catheterization

The techniques described in the previous section are best suited to catheterization of the right, left and common hepatic arteries, the gastroduodenal artery or pancreaticoduodenal arcades, the dorsal pancreatic artery, the splenic artery, the inferior pancreaticoduodenal artery and the branches of the superior mesenteric artery. Most of these branches are directed caudally or transversely from the celiac or superior mesenteric artery. A slightly different technique and catheter shape are necessary for catheterization of the left gastric artery or of a dorsal pancreatic artery arising from the superior surface of the superior mesenteric artery (see Fig. 4–65).

We most frequently use the catheter exchange method (Fig. 1–25). A straight or

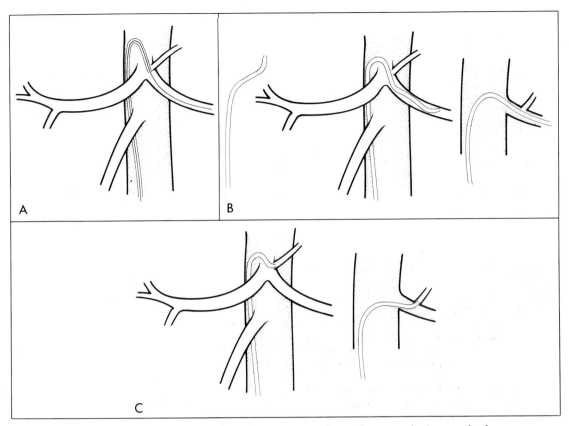

Figure 1–25. Left gastric artery catheterization using the catheter exchange method.

A. The procedure is begun by advancing a guide wire through a conventional celiac catheter as far into the hepatic or splenic artery as possible. It makes no difference which major branch is chosen, as long as the left gastric artery arises from the proximal celiac trunk. If the left gastric artery arises from either the hepatic or splenic artery, then that specific branch must be selected. Holding the guide wire stationary, the conventional catheter is withdrawn, leaving the guide wire in the hepatic or splenic artery.

B. A catheter shaped like that shown on the left is introduced over the guide wire so that its tip is in either the splenic or hepatic artery when the guide wire is subsequently removed.

C. The catheter is slowly withdrawn while small amounts of contrast medium are injected. It is important to keep the catheter tip pointing cephalad. When the tip reaches the orifice of the left gastric artery, contrast medium is seen to enter the vessel. Advancing the catheter should then cause it to enter the left gastric artery.

tight J guide wire is passed through the celiac catheter into the distal hepatic or splenic artery. The celiac catheter is then withdrawn, leaving the guide wire in place, and a specially shaped catheter with a slight "dog leg" at the tip is introduced over the wire. After the guide wire has been removed, the catheter is slowly drawn back with the tip pointing cephalad. A small amount of contrast medium is injected during the withdrawal. When the catheter tip enters the left gastric artery, contrast medium can be seen to fill that vessel. The catheter is then advanced slightly into the orifice, and the angiogram can be performed in the usual manner. Occasionally, the catheter tip will pass the orifice without entering it. Contrast medium enters the left gastric artery when the catheter tip is opposite the orifice, but when the catheter is advanced, it passes into the hepatic or splenic artery. When this occurs, the catheter tip is again withdrawn to a point opposite the left gastric artery orifice, and a straight guide wire is introduced. The guide wire generally enters the artery, and the catheter may be advanced into the left gastric artery over the guide

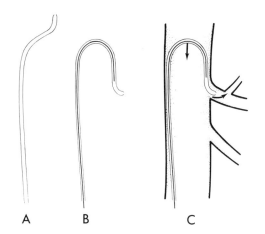

Figure 1–26. Left gastric artery catheterization using the manipulator instrument.

A. The same catheter shape is used as for the catheter exchange method (see Fig. 1–25). The manipulator guide wire is introduced not to the tip, but just to the beginning of the distal bend.

B. When the manipulator wire is bent with the manipulator handle, the catheter assumes the configuration shown, with the tip extended.

C. The combination of manipulator instrument and catheter is then advanced and pulled back as a unit until the celiac orifice is entered. It is then pulled down as the bend on the manipulator instrument is released, and the catheter tip advances along the celiac artery and into the left gastric artery.

A   B   C

wire. This technique is successful in about 80 per cent of patients. When it fails, the manipulator instrument is used.

The technique for catheterizing the left gastric artery using the manipulator instrument is illustrated in Figure 1–26. The same catheter shown in Figure 1–25 is used, and the manipulator guide wire is placed just proximal to the final bend of the catheter. When the instrument is bent, the catheter assumes the appearance shown in Figure 1–26B. The catheter tip is introduced into the celiac artery. As it advances

through the celiac artery, the bend is released slowly, allowing the distal portion of the "dog leg" to extend upward toward the left gastric artery. If the catheter tip enters the artery, as it usually does, it is advanced slightly into the orifice and the angiogram performed. If the catheter tip bypasses the orifice, it is advanced over the manipulator guide wire into the hepatic or splenic artery, and the withdrawal technique described previously is tried. If these manipulations are unsuccessful, the shape of the distal tip must be modified by making a more acute

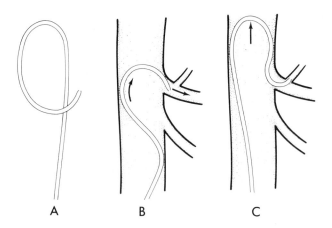

A   B   C

Figure 1–27. Left gastric artery catheterization with the Waltman catheter.

A. The shape of the catheter is shown.

B. When placed in the aorta over a guide wire, the catheter assumes the shape illustrated. The tip is introduced into the celiac or superior mesenteric artery, and the tip is advanced as far as possible into the hepatic, splenic or superior mesenteric artery.

C. As the secondary curve advances, the catheter inverts and assumes the shape shown. If the catheter has initially entered the celiac artery, advancing the loop up the aorta withdraws the tip until it engages the left gastric artery. If the tip has initially entered the superior mesenteric artery, it is drawn back into the aorta and the celiac artery entered. Pulling the loop back down the aorta then causes the tip to enter the left gastric artery orifice.

or longer distal bend, and the process is repeated.

Waltman et al. (1973) devised a technique for left gastric catheterization using a preshaped catheter without a manipulator instrument. The catheter is shown in Figure 1–27A. The catheter is introduced into the abdominal aorta and the tip turned in the renal or superior mesenteric artery. If the tip cannot be turned, a manipulator instrument can be introduced to turn the tip downward. The celiac artery is then catheterized and, as the tip enters the celiac artery, continued withdrawal of the aortic portion of the catheter results in cephalad extension of the tip, which usually enters the left gastric artery.

Injection Factors for Superselective Angiography

In general, the rate of injection for superselective angiograms is slightly greater than the expected blood flow of the artery being injected to ensure complete filling of the vascular bed. For example, several branches of the celiac and superior mesenteric arteries supply the pancreas. The blood flow in most of these arteries can be reversed by an injection into either the gastroduodenal or dorsal pancreatic artery, and the entire vascular supply is demonstrated.

TABLE 1–2.   Injection Factors for Superselective Angiography

ARTERY	INJECTION RATE (cc/sec)	QUANTITY OF CONTRAST MEDIUM (cc)
Hepatic		
General technique	8–10	30–40
Infusion technique	2–4	50
Splenic		
General technique	8–10	30–40
Arterial portography	8–10	60
Left gastric		
General technique	3–5	12–15
Arterial portography	7–8	28–32
Gastroduodenal	6–8	10–16
Dorsal pancreatic	2–5	6–10
Inferior pancreaticoduodenal	4–6	6–10
Jejunal–Ileal	3–5	6–10

Occasionally, the vascular bed of an organ may be flooded with contrast medium in order to improve demonstration of the venous drainage, such as overfilling the left gastric artery to demonstrate esophageal varices. The quantities and injection rates generally used for superselective angiograms are given in Table 1–2. These vary, of course, depending upon the clinical problem being investigated. Some investigators have injected pancreatic arteries with large doses of contrast medium, up to 40 cc at the rate of 10 cc per second, with or without tolazoline (Priscoline) (Eisenberg, 1973; Hawkins et al., 1975). Such an injection provides an excellent capillary phase, and a poorly vascularized pancreatic carcinoma stands out as a filling defect in the pancreatogram.

BIBLIOGRAPHY

Agnew, C. H., Cooley, R. N., Derrick, J., et al.: Technical considerations of selective arteriography. Radiology 74:81, 1960.

Almén, T.: A steering device for selective angiography and some vascular and enzymatic reactions observed in its clinical application. Acta Radiol. (Suppl. 260), 1966.

Amplatz, K.: Rapid film changers. In Abrams, H. L. (ed.): Angiography. 2nd ed. Boston, Little, Brown and Company, 1971.

Amplatz, K.: A simple non-thrombogenic coating. Invest. Radiol. 6:280, 1971.

Antonovic, R., Rösch, J., and Dotter, C. T.: The value of systemic arterial heparinization in transfemoral angiography: a prospective study. Amer. J. Roentgenol. 127:223, 1976.

Barnhard, H. J., and Barnhard, F. M.: The emergency treatment of reactions to contrast media: Updated 1968. Radiology 91:74, 1968.

Bates, B. F., and Bookstein, J. J.: Intercurrent embolization during cerebral angiography: Clinical and experimental observations. Invest. Radiol. 1:107, 1966.

Baum, S.: Catheters and injectors. In Abrams, H. L. (ed.): Angiography. 2nd ed. Boston, Little, Brown and Company, 1971.

Baum, S., and Abrams, H. L.: A J-shaped catheter for retrograde catheterization of tortuous vessels. Radiology 83:436, 1964.

Bernstein, E. F., Greenspan, R. H., and Loken, M. K.: Intravenous aortography: Its clinical application. Arch. Surg. 80:71, 1960.

Björk, L., Enghoff, E., Grenvik, A. et al.: Local circulatory changes following brachial artery catheterization. Vasc. Dis. 2:283, 1965.

Boijsen, E.: Superselective pancreatic angiography. Brit. J. Radiol. 39:481, 1966.

Boijsen, E., and Judkins, M. P.: A hook-tail "closed-end" catheter for percutaneous selective cardioangiography. Radiology 87:872, 1966.

Bouhoutsos, J., and Morris, T.: Femoral artery complications after diagnostic procedures. Brit. Med. J. 3:396, 1973.

Bron, K. M.: Selective visceral and total abdominal arteriography via the left axillary artery in the older age group. Amer. J. Roentgenol. 97:432, 1966.

Christenson, R., Staab, E. V., Burko, H., et al.: Pressure dressings and postarteriographic care of the femoral puncture site. Radiology 119:97, 1976.

Cooley, R. N.: Injection systems in angiography. Amer. J. Roentgenol. 95:785, 1965.

Desilets, D. T., and Hoffman, R.: A new method of percutaneous catheterization. Radiology 85:147, 1965.

Desilets, D. T., Ruttenberg, H. D., and Hoffman, R. B.: Percutaneous catheterization in children. Radiology 87:119, 1966.

dos Santos, R., Lamas, C., and Caldas, P.: Les récents progrès dans la technique de l'artériographie de l'aorte abdominale. Presse Med. 39:574, 1931.

Dotter, C. T., Judkins, M. P., and Frische, L. H.: Safety guidespring for percutaneous cardiovascular catheterization. Amer. J. Roentgenol. 98:957, 1966.

Driscoll, S. H., Grollman, J. H., Ellestedt, M. H., et al.: Single wall arterial puncture with disposable needle. Radiology 113:470, 1974.

Durst, S., Leslie, J., Moore, R., et al.: A comparison of the thrombogenicity of commercially available catheters. Radiology 113:599, 1974.

Eisenberg, H.: Pancreatic angiography. In Hilal, S. K. (ed.): Small Vessel Angiography: Imaging, Morphology, Physiology, and Clinical Applications. St. Louis, C. V. Mosby Company, 1973, pp. 405–433.

Formanek, G., Frech, R. S., and Amplatz, K.: Arterial thrombus formation during clinical percutaneous catheterization. Circulation 41:833, 1970.

Grayson, T., Margulis, A. R., Heinbecker, P., et al.: Effects of intra-arterial injection of Miokon, Hypaque, and Renografin in the small intestine of the dog. Radiology 77:776, 1961.

Haut, G., and Amplatz, K.: Complication rates of transfemoral and transaortic catheterization. Surgery 63:594, 1968.

Hawkins, I. F., Kaude, J. V., and McGregor, A.: Priscoline and epinephrine in selective pancreatic angiography: A comparison study using high pressure injection, Valsalva maneuver and geometric magnification. Radiology 116:311, 1975.

Hugh, A. E.: The distribution and dispersal of contrast medium injected from catheters into vessels: A study using ultra-short exposure radiography. Clin. Radiol. 20:183, 1969.

Jacobsson, B., Paulin, S., and Schlossman, D.: Thromboembolism of leg following percutaneous catheterization of femoral artery for angiography: Symptoms and signs. Acta Radiol. (Diagn.) (Stockh.) 8:97, 1969.

Jacobsson, B., and Schlossman, D.: Angiographic investigation of formation of thrombi on vascular catheters. Radiology 93:355, 1969.

Judkins, M. P., Kidd, H. J., Frische, L. H., et al.: Lumen-following safety J-guide for catheterization of tortuous vessels. Radiology 88:1127, 1967.

Klatte, E. C., Sloan, O. M., and Burko, H.: Selective Teflon arteriographic catheters. Radiology 90:1205, 1968.

Ludin, H.: Aortography fluid dynamics and technical problems. Acta Radiol. (Suppl. 256) (Stockh.), 1966.

Nebesar, R. A., Fleischli, D. J., Pollard, J. J., et al.: Arteriography in infants and children: With emphasis on the Seldinger technique and abdominal diseases. Amer. J. Roentgenol. 106:81, 1969.

Ödman, P.: Percutaneous selective angiography of the coeliac artery. Acta Radiol. (Suppl. 159) (Stockh.), 1958.

Ödman, P.: Percutaneous selective angiography of main branches of aorta: Preliminary report. Acta Radiol. 45:1, 1956.

Ödman, P.: The radiopaque polythene catheter. Acta Radiol. 52:52, 1959.

Olin, T.: Studies in Angiographic Technique. Lund, Sweden, Håkan Ohlssons Boktryckeri, 1963.

Paul, R. E., Jr., Miller, H. H., Kahn, P. C., et al.: Pancreatic angiography with application of subselective angiography of the celiac or superior mesenteric arteries to the diagnosis of carcinoma of the pancreas. New Eng. J. Med. 272:283, 1965.

Redman, H. C., Berg, N. O., and Boijsen, E.: Absence of toxicity of contrast media in the superior mesenteric artery. A pathologic study in rabbits. Invest. Radiol. 2:119, 1967.

Reuter, S. R.: Superselective pancreatic angiography. Radiology 92:74, 1969.

Reuter, S. R., and Atkin, T. W.: High dose left gastric angiography for demonstration of esophageal varices. Radiology 105:573, 1972.

Riley, J. M., Hanafee, W., and Weidner, W.: Left axillary approach to the abdominal aorta. Radiology 84:96, 1965.

Rösch, J., and Grollman, J. H., Jr.: Superselective arteriography in the diagnosis of abdominal pathology: Technical consideration. Radiology 92:1008, 1969.

Rossi, P., and Verdu, C. C.: The floppy wire as an aid in arterial catheterization. Amer. J. Roentgenol. 97:511, 1966.

Seldinger, S. I.: Catheter replacement of the needle in percutaneous arteriography. A new technique. Acta Radiol. 39:368, 1953.

Siegelman, S. S., Caplan, L. H., and Annes, G. P.: Complications of catheter angiography: Study with oscillometry and 'pullout' angiograms. Radiology 91:251, 1968.

Susman, N., and Diboll, W. B., Jr.: Fluid dynamics in the tip of the multiholed angiographic catheter. Radiology 92:843, 1969.

Sweet, D., and Grismer, J. T.: Percutaneous noncatheter retrograde brachial arteriography. Use of the Amplatz needles. Minn. Med. 50:185, 1967.

Verel, D.: A modified Seldinger needle. Clin. Radiol. 24:65, 1973.

Viamonte, M., Jr., and Hobbs, J.: Automatic electric injector: Development to prevent electromechanical hazards of selective angiocardiography. Invest. Radiol. 2:262, 1967.

Wallace, S., Medellin, H., DeJongh, D., et al.: Systemic heparinization for angiography. Amer. J. Roentgenol. 116:204, 1972.

Waltman, A. C., Courey, W. R., Athanasoulis, C. A., et al.: Technique for left gastric artery catheterization. Radiology 109:732, 1973.

Wholey, M. H.: A modified J-shaped guide wire for angiography. Brit. J. Radiol. 41:388, 1968.

VASCULAR ANATOMY

A thorough knowledge of anatomy has always been fundamental to the practice of radiology. Both the performance and interpretation of any radiographic procedure are dependent upon this knowledge, and angiography is no exception. In gastrointestinal angiography, a three-dimensional understanding of both vascular and organ anatomy is necessary. Many variations are found in the branching patterns of the celiac and superior mesenteric arteries. These can be quite confusing until it is recognized that only about half of all people fit the textbook pattern of anatomy. An understanding of the embryologic basis for this variability helps in the evaluation of the many vascular patterns that are encountered.

EMBRYOLOGY

Organogenesis occurs in the human fetus between 2 and 8 weeks after fertilization. During this period, the various organs, including the vascular system, are laid down, and differentiation begins. From the ninth week on, some further differentiation occurs, but the major change is growth of organs and tissues already present.

The primitive vascular supply is dual, with double aortas and both a dorsal and ventral arterial supply to the abdominal viscera. As the organs differentiate, modification of the primitive circulation leads to elimination of much of the double vascular supply. The many variations in visceral

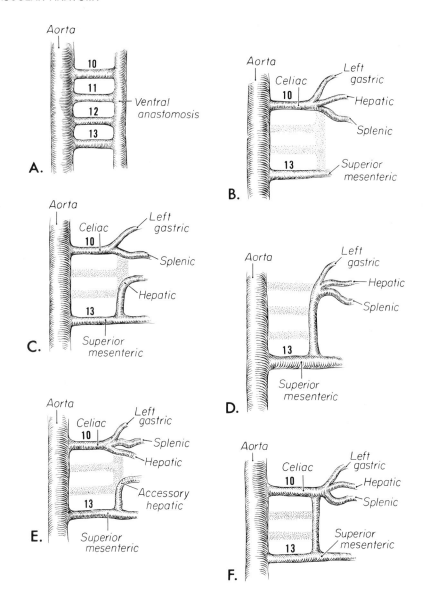

Figure 2-1. Embryologic basis for vascular variations.

A. Primitive vascular supply. The tenth to thirteenth vitelline arteries migrate caudally to the lower thoracic-upper lumbar region. These paired arteries run from the aorta to the ventral anastomotic artery.

B. The usual anatomic arrangement. The ventral anastomosis and the eleventh and twelfth vitelline roots have regressed. The tenth root has become the celiac trunk and the thirteenth, the superior mesenteric artery. This arrangement is found in 55 to 65 per cent of people.

C. Replaced hepatic artery to the superior mesenteric artery. The ventral anastomosis has not entirely regressed, and the hepatic artery utilizes this pathway to form a hepatomesenteric trunk.

D. Common origin of the celiac and superior mesenteric arteries. The tenth, eleventh and twelfth vitelline roots have regressed. The ventral anastomosis has persisted, connecting the celiac artery and its branches to the superior mesenteric artery to form a celiacomesenteric trunk.

E. Partially replaced hepatic artery to the superior mesenteric artery. The eleventh and twelfth roots have regressed. A portion of the ventral anastomosis has persisted to link part of the hepatic artery to the superior mesenteric artery.

F. Arc of Bühler. The eleventh and twelfth roots have regressed but the ventral anastomosis remains patent, and becomes a direct pathway between the celiac and superior mesenteric arteries.

circulation result from the differing degrees of persistence of the dual blood supply, along with variations in the caudal migration of the abdominal organs and rotation of the gut (Arey, 1965; Patten, 1968).

Tandler (1903, 1904) first described the origin and development of the celiac, superior and inferior mesenteric arteries. The paired dorsal aortas give rise to a series of paired vitelline arteries which are the anlage of these three vessels. At 4 weeks the vitelline arteries lie at the lower cervical–thoracic level, and by 7 weeks they have migrated caudally to their final position. They have a ventral longitudinal anastomosis which usually disappears during differentiation. The vitelline arteries fuse, and the tenth pair generally forms a celiac trunk, while the thirteenth pair forms the superior mesenteric artery, and the twenty-first or twenty-second pair forms the inferior mesenteric artery.

The common variations of the celiac and superior mesenteric arteries can be explained by persistence of some or all of the primitive ventral anastomoses of the vitelline arteries and associated variations in the preservation of the tenth and thirteenth vitelline roots (Fig. 2–1). Preservation of the ventral anastomosis between the superior mesenteric artery and the celiac trunk may lead to complete or partial replacement of the celiac trunk and its branches to the superior mesenteric artery, if the tenth vitelline artery regresses. If the tenth vitelline artery does not regress and the ventral anastomosis persists, an arc of Bühler is formed.

The location of some arteries is determined by positional changes of other organs. Thus, the superior mesenteric artery rotates approximately 180 degrees with the rotation of the gut. This generally occurs distal to the origin of the inferior pancreaticoduodenal artery, which arises from the right of the superior mesenteric artery. If rotation occurs higher, the inferior pancreaticoduodenal artery can arise from the left. The two primordial sources of the pancreas from the roof of the duodenum and from the gut floor explain why circulation between the head and the tail of the pancreas is sometimes poorly developed, while that between the duodenum and pancreatic head and between the pancreatic tail and spleen is generally good.

A knowledge of the embryologic basis for vascular anatomy, therefore, makes the many variations understandable and helps in the correct interpretation of gastrointestinal angiograms.

ARTERIAL ANATOMY

Celiac Trunk

The celiac trunk, sometimes called the celiac axis, arises from the ventral surface of the aorta between the lower half of the twelfth thoracic vertebral body and the T12–L1 interspace. It supplies blood to the upper abdominal viscera.

Celiac Artery

The first portion of the celiac trunk (Fig. 2–2), the celiac artery, generally courses caudally for 1 to 2 cm and then runs ventrally. In obese people, the initial course may be ventral or cranioventral. The celiac artery divides into three branches, the left gastric, splenic and common hepatic arteries, in 55 to 65 per cent of patients. The inferior phrenic arteries also arise from the celiac artery, either separately or as a single trunk, in more than 55 per cent of patients. When they arise from the celiac artery, the inferior phrenic arteries are usually the first branches. Occasionally, the dorsal pancreatic artery also arises from the celiac artery. In the remaining population, one or more of these vessels has a replaced origin. This marked variability in the origins of the major celiac arterial branches is extremely important to the angiographer. Both the performance of a complete examination and the correct interpretation of the angiogram depend on a thorough understanding of these multiple variations.

Left Gastric Artery

The left gastric artery is commonly the first major branch of the celiac trunk (Fig. 2–3); it may arise anywhere along the trunk from its origin at the aorta to a trifurcation with the common hepatic and splenic arteries. It occasionally has a common origin with the dorsal pancreatic artery. Rarely, the left gastric artery arises from the aorta

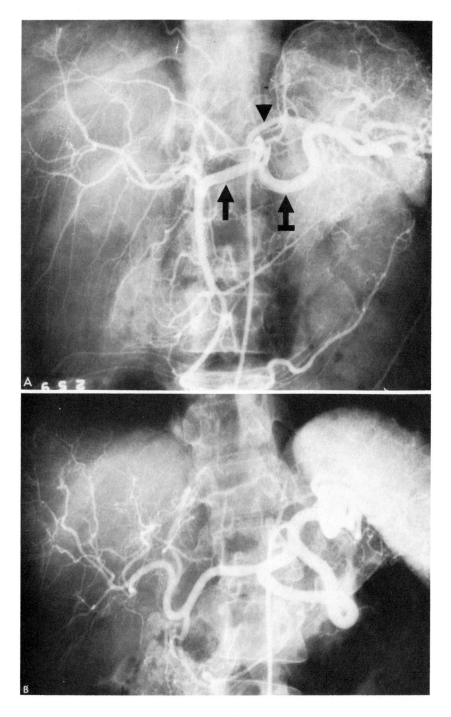

Figure 2-2. Normal celiac trunks in young and elderly patients.

A. Celiac angiogram in a 34 year old woman. The common hepatic (➡), left gastric (▶) and splenic (➡) arteries arise from the celiac trunk. This anatomic pattern occurs in 55 to 65 per cent of the population.

B. Celiac angiogram in a 74 year old woman. The splenic artery is elongated and tortuous, and the branches of the hepatic artery are slightly tortuous compared to those of younger patients.

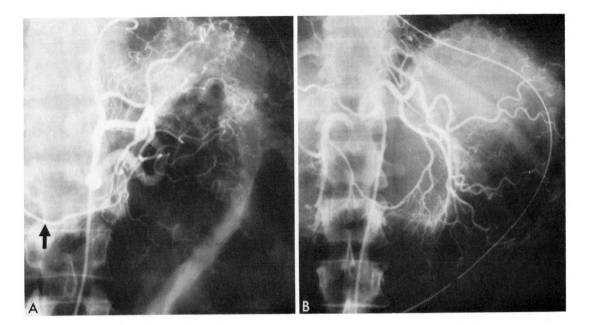

Figure 2–3. Normal left gastric artery.

A. Selective left gastric angiogram in a 46 year old man. The branches of the left gastric artery have a gently undulating course across the stomach to the greater curvature. Contrast medium is forced through the left gastric–right gastric lesser curvature arcade (➡) toward the left hepatic artery.

B. Selective left gastric angiogram in a 38 year old woman. As in A, the arteries have a gently undulating course across the stomach toward the greater curvature. The left hepatic artery is filled by contrast medium refluxing across the lesser curvature arcade.

as a separate branch, from the other branches of the celiac trunk or from a combined celiac–superior mesenteric trunk.

The left gastric artery has a posterior position at its origin and courses ventrally and cranially to reach the anterior wall of the omental bursa. At the cardia of the stomach it generally turns caudally and divides into anterior and posterior branches, each going to its respective gastric surface. The posterior branches usually anastomose with the right gastric artery, though these anastomoses are not often seen during angiography. Both posterior and anterior branches anastomose with right gastroepiploic branches.

The peripheral branches also anastomose widely with short gastric arteries arising from the splenic or the left gastroepiploic arteries and with cardioesophageal branches of the left inferior phrenic artery. They may also anastomose with other esophageal arterial branches.

The degree of distention and position of the stomach modify the angiographic ap-pearance of the left gastric artery more than variations in the branching pattern. Gastric dilatation stretches, straightens and separates the left gastric branches, when compared with the nondistended stomach.

Accessory left gastric arteries (Fig. 2–4) occur relatively frequently, arising from the splenic, common hepatic, celiac and left hepatic arteries, especially from left hepatic arteries which are replaced to the left gastric artery. An accessory left gastric artery supplies either the anterior or posterior surface of the stomach and is of moderate size. At angiography, it is frequently difficult to distinguish an accessory left gastric artery from a superior polar splenic artery on an anteroposterior projection.

In approximately 25 per cent of the population, the left gastric artery gives rise to a replaced hepatic artery (Fig. 2–5). About half of these variations represent complete replacement of the left hepatic artery, and the remainder are partial replacements. One or both of the inferior phrenic arteries occasionally arise from the left gastric arte-

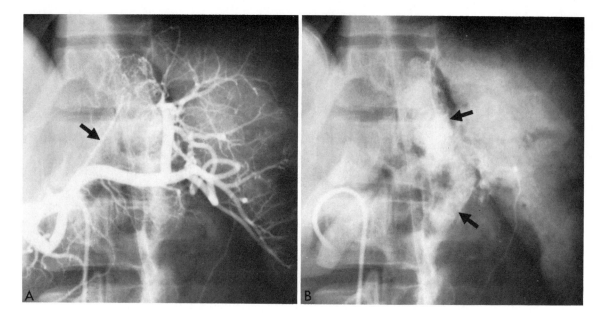

Figure 2-4. Accessory gastric artery. Splenic angiogram in a 46 year old man.

A. Arterial phase. The accessory gastric artery (➡) arises from the proximal third of the splenic artery. Such accessory arteries may supply either the anterior or posterior gastric wall.

B. Venous phase. There is moderately dense accumulation of contrast medium in the gastric mucosa (➡) supplied by the accessory artery. Although accessory gastric arteries and superior polar splenic arteries have a similar appearance in the arterial phase, the two vessels can be differentiated in the venous phase by determining whether or not they supply gastric mucosa or splenic parenchyma.

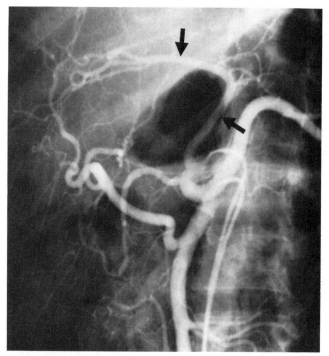

Figure 2-5. Left hepatic artery replaced to the left gastric artery. Simultaneous celiac–superior mesenteric angiogram in a 55 year old woman with pancreatitis. The entire blood supply to the left lobe of the liver arises from the left gastric artery (➡). In this patient, the right hepatic artery is also replaced to the superior mesenteric artery, and the celiac artery gives rise to a small branch of the middle hepatic artery.

Figure 2-6. Normal splenic artery. Celiac angiogram in an 11 year old girl. The splenic artery arises from the celiac artery and follows an undulating course to the left. The pancreatica magna artery (➡) to the pancreas and a superior polar splenic artery (►) are demonstrated.

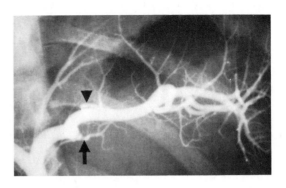

ry. Finally, the left gastric artery generally gives off some cardioesophageal branches early in its course.

Splenic Artery

The splenic artery arises from the celiac artery distal to the origin of the left gastric artery (Fig. 2–6). It may arise from the left, ventral or even the right surface. Its origin is infrequently replaced to the aorta or, rarely, to the superior mesenteric artery (Fig. 2–7). The splenic artery runs to the patient's left, closely associated with the body and tail of the pancreas. In younger patients it is generally short and follows a gently undulating course to the spleen. With age it becomes elongated and tortuous and is one of the first visceral arteries to show changes of atherosclerosis (Fig. 2–8).

Splenic Artery Branches

The splenic artery gives off a variable series of branches to the spleen, pancreas and stomach.

BRANCHES TO THE SPLEEN. The arteries to the spleen itself are varied. The superior and inferior splenic arterial branches sometimes arise from the splenic artery well proximal to the spleen, but generally this division occurs near the splenic hilum (Fig. 2–9). They divide primarily and secondarily into a variable number of terminal branches within the splenic parenchyma. Primary branching usually occurs prior to the entrance of these arteries into the spleen. A branch of the inferior splenic artery generally gives rise to the left gastroepiploic artery. Superior and inferior polar arteries to the spleen are frequently present (Fig. 2–10). The superior polar ar-

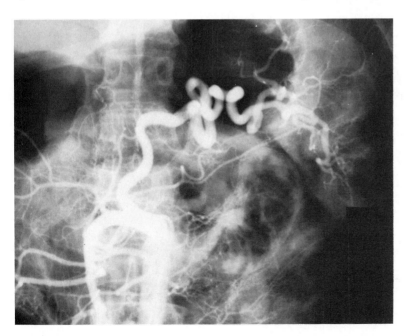

Figure 2-7. Splenic artery replaced to the superior mesenteric artery. Superior mesenteric angiogram in a 35 year old man. The splenic artery arises from the left superior surface of the superior mesenteric artery. This is an unusual anatomic variation.

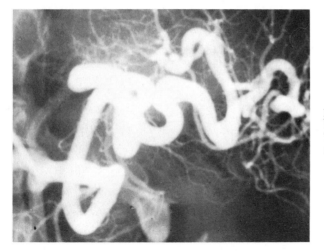

Figure 2-8. Splenic angiogram in a 72 year old woman. With age, the splenic artery becomes markedly elongated and tortuous. The splenic artery is generally the first artery to show atherosclerotic changes.

Figure 2-9. Arterial branches to the spleen. Splenic angiogram in a 33 year old woman. The superior splenic artery (⇨) supplies the majority of the splenic parenchyma. A smaller inferior splenic artery goes to the midportion of the spleen. Both superior and inferior splenic polar arteries are present (▷). The left gastroepiploic artery arises from the inferior polar splenic artery. The pancreatica magna artery is well demonstrated, arising from the midportion of the splenic artery.

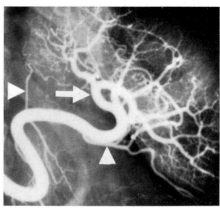

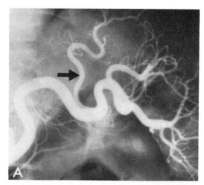

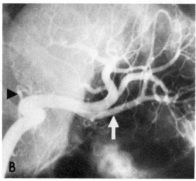

Figure 2-10. Polar splenic arteries.

A. Celiac angiogram in a 31 year old man. A large superior polar splenic artery (➡) is present. In this patient, it arises near the splenic hilum and should not be confused with an accessory left gastric artery.

B. Splenic angiogram in a 38 year old man with pancreatitis. An inferior polar splenic artery (⇨) is present. Also seen is a small accessory left gastric artery (▶) which must not be confused with a superior polar splenic artery.

tery occurs in about 65 per cent of patients and inferior polar arteries exist in about 82 per cent (Michels, 1955). These vessels usually arise from the splenic artery well proximal to its primary division. The superior polar artery, however, may arise from the celiac axis itself or from the primary superior or inferior splenic artery branches. Differentiation of a superior polar splenic artery from an accessory left gastric artery may be difficult.

BRANCHES TO THE PANCREAS. The dorsal pancreatic artery arises from the proximal portion of the splenic artery in about 40 per cent of people (Fig. 2–11). This artery goes to the dorsal surface of the pancreas, contributing a branch to the uncinate process. It usually gives rise to the transverse pancreatic artery that runs through the tail of the pancreas (Fig. 2–12). An anastomotic branch passing to the right generally communicates with branches of the anterior or posterior pancreaticoduodenal arcades. The dorsal pancreatic artery may also communicate directly with the superior mesenteric artery.

Many small pancreatic arteries arise from the splenic artery throughout its course. The pancreatica magna artery is the largest of these (Fig. 2–13). It usually arises in the midportion of the splenic artery and divides after a brief course into several branches which anastomose with the transverse pancreatic and other small pancreatic arteries. The caudal pancreatic artery arises from the distal splenic artery or left gastroepiploic artery. Frequently there are several caudal pancreatic arteries. The branches of the caudal pancreatic artery anastomose widely with the transverse pancreatic artery, branches of the pancreatica magna artery and other pancreatic rami.

BRANCHES TO THE STOMACH. Short gastric arteries arise from the splenic artery and its primary branches. The left gastroepiploic artery usually arises just proximal to the primary division of the splenic artery; however, it may arise from the inferior splenic artery or its branches (Fig. 2–14). The left gastroepiploic artery anastomoses directly with the right gastroepiploic artery through small branches in about 90 per cent of people.

Common Hepatic Artery

The third major branch of the celiac artery is the common hepatic artery (Fig. 2–

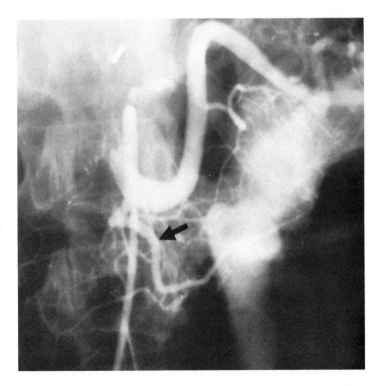

Figure 2–11. Origin of the dorsal pancreatic artery from the splenic artery. Splenic angiogram in a 55 year old man. The dorsal pancreatic artery (➡) arises from the proximal splenic artery, an origin found in about 40 per cent of people.

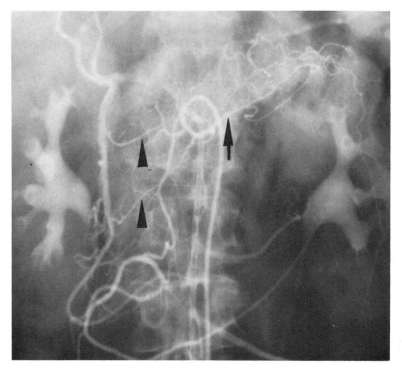

Figure 2–12. Dorsal pancreatic artery. Selective dorsal pancreatic angiogram in a 30 year old woman. The transverse pancreatic artery (➡), anastomotic branches and both the posterior and anterior pancreaticoduodenal arcades (▶) are filled.

Figure 2–13. Pancreatica magna artery. Splenic angiogram in a 24 year old woman. The pancreatica magna artery (⟹) arises from the midsplenic artery. Other smaller pancreatic rami are also present. A superior polar splenic artery arises from the cephalad surface of the splenic artery.

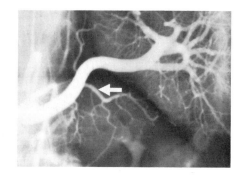

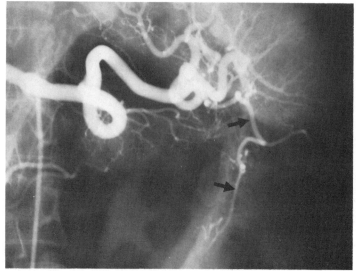

Figure 2–14. Left gastroepiploic artery. Celiac angiogram in a 51 year old man. The left gastroepiploic artery (➡) arises from the inferior splenic artery, passing along the greater curvature of the stomach to meet the right gastroepiploic artery in 90 per cent of people.

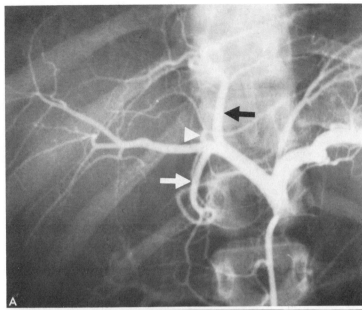

Figure 2–15A. Common hepatic artery. Celiac angiogram in a 9 year old boy. The gastroduodenal artery (⟹) arises distal to the left hepatic artery(➡), and the middle hepatic artery (▷) arises just distal to the gastroduodenal artery. The right hepatic artery is the terminal branch of the common hepatic artery.

Figure 2–15B. Replaced common hepatic artery. Replacement of the entire hepatic blood flow to the superior mesenteric artery. Superior mesenteric angiogram in a 63 year old man with moderately severe cirrhosis. When this unusual variation occurs, the gastroduodenal artery generally arises from the replaced common hepatic artery.

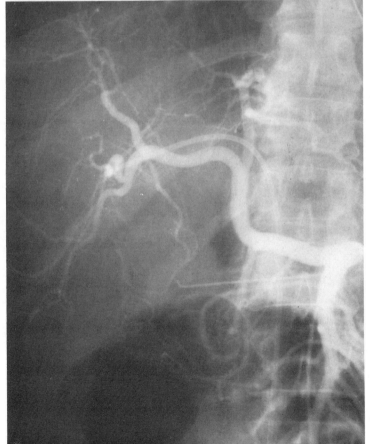

15). It is generally slightly smaller than the splenic artery and courses to the right and anteriorly, giving off the gastroduodenal artery, and sometimes the dorsal pancreatic artery. Following the origin of the gastroduodenal artery, the hepatic trunk is referred to as the proper hepatic artery. This artery is usually short and divides into the right, left and, occasionally, middle hepatic arteries. This blood supply occurs in about half the population. In the remainder, one or more of the hepatic artery branches have a partially or totally replaced origin. The proper hepatic artery also frequently gives rise to the right gastric artery. Rarely, the entire hepatic blood supply is replaced to the superior mesenteric artery (Fig. 2–15B).

RIGHT HEPATIC ARTERY. The right hepatic artery generally gives rise to the cystic artery early in its course (Fig. 2–16), and then supplies the right lobe of the liver with several branches to the superior and inferior aspects of each hepatic segment. The terminal branches supply single pyramidal lobules. In about 45 per cent of people the right hepatic artery gives rise to the middle hepatic artery. The right hepatic artery has a completely replaced origin from the superior mesenteric artery in about 14 per cent of persons (Fig. 2–17), and an accessory right hepatic artery arises from the superior mesenteric artery in about 8 per cent.

LEFT HEPATIC ARTERY. The left hepatic artery generally divides into two main branches, going to the inferior and superior aspects of the lateral segment of the left lobe of the liver (Fig. 2–18). The left hepatic artery also gives rise to about 45 per cent of middle hepatic arteries. The left hepatic artery has a partially or totally replaced origin from the left gastric artery in about 25 per cent of patients (Fig. 2–19).

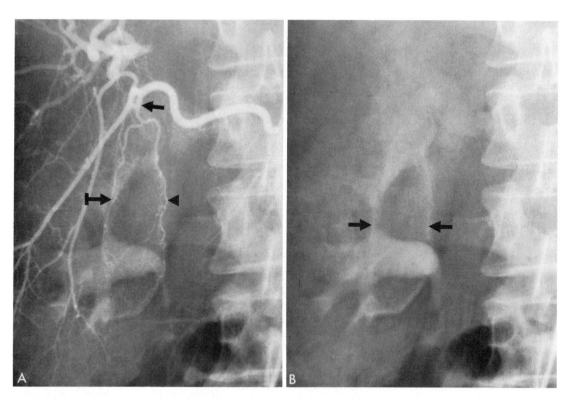

Figure 2–16. Cystic artery. Superior mesenteric angiogram in a 39 year old woman.
A. Arterial phase. The cystic artery (➡) arises from the right hepatic artery, which has an origin replaced to the superior mesenteric artery. The cystic artery then divides into deep (▶) and superficial (➡) branches, which pass around the gallbladder. Branches of the deep and superficial branches have gently undulating courses across the gallbladder.
B. Venous phase. Accumulation of contrast medium is seen in the gallbladder wall (➡).

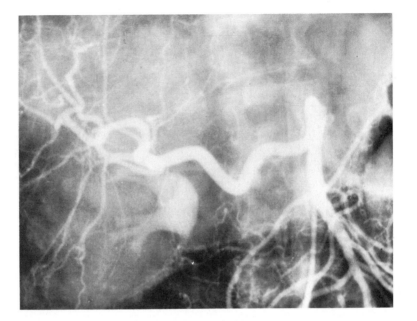

Figure 2-17. Replaced right hepatic artery from the superior mesenteric artery. Superior mesenteric angiogram in a 47 year old man. Complete right hepatic artery replacement occurs in 14 per cent of people; partial replacement occurs in about 8 per cent.

MIDDLE HEPATIC ARTERY. The middle hepatic artery generally arises from either the right or left hepatic artery. In about 10 per cent of people it originates directly from the proper hepatic artery (Fig. 2-19). It supplies the main circulation to the quadrate lobe of the liver and may also supply the caudate lobe and gallbladder.

While the arteries to the liver are end arteries, multiple collateral arteries are present between the hepatic arterial branches in the hilum of the liver and sometimes more peripherally (Fig. 2-20). These collaterals are most often demonstrated at angiography when some part of the circulation to the liver is compromised.

RIGHT GASTRIC ARTERY. The right gastric artery is seen infrequently at angiography unless it is providing collateral blood supply to the left gastric artery (Fig. 2-21; also see Fig. 2-3). It is a small vessel which arises from the proper hepatic artery shortly after the origin of the gastroduodenal artery. It may also arise from the proximal left hepatic artery, especially when the right hepatic circulation is replaced to the superior mesenteric artery.

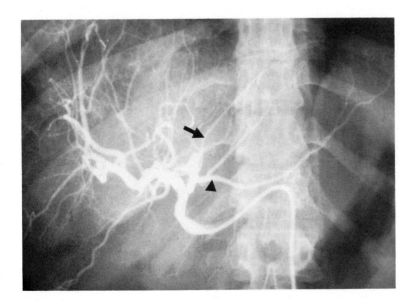

Figure 2-18. Left hepatic artery. Proper hepatic angiogram in a 37 year old woman. The proper hepatic artery divides into right and left hepatic arteries. The left hepatic artery arises from the anterosuperior surface of the proper hepatic artery and divides into superior (▶) and inferior (➡) branches.

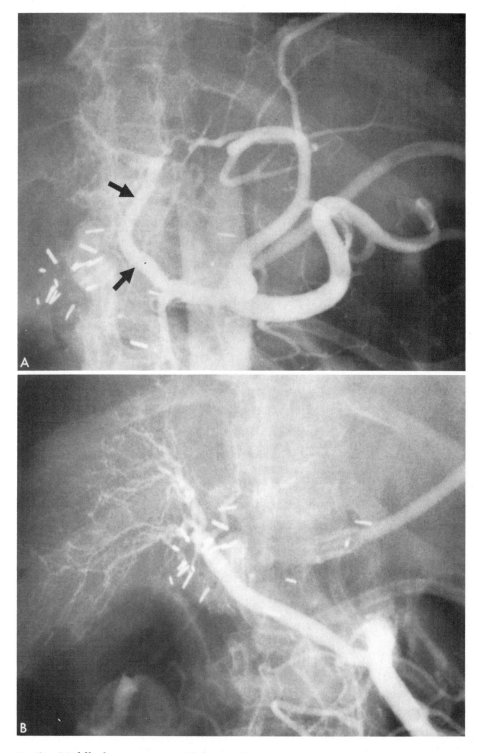

Figure 2-19. Middle hepatic artery. Celiac and superior mesenteric angiograms in a 54 year old man with severe cirrhosis and a portacaval shunt.

A. Celiac angiogram. The left hepatic artery is replaced to the left gastric artery, and the middle hepatic artery (➡) and gastroduodenal arteries arise from the celiac hepatic artery.

B. Superior mesenteric angiogram. The right hepatic artery is replaced to the superior mesenteric artery.

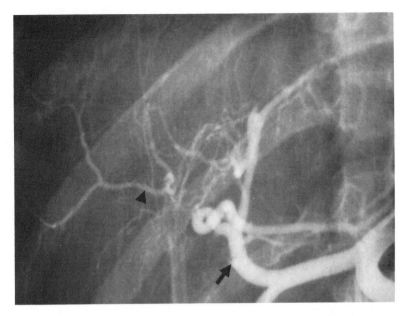

Figure 2-20. Collateral arteries in the hilum of the liver. Celiac angiogram in a 65 year old man with traumatic occlusion of the right hepatic artery. The right hepatic artery is occluded at its origin (➡), and multiple small collateral arteries from the left hepatic artery bridge the occluded segment, supplying blood flow to the distal right hepatic artery (▶).

The right gastric artery supplies the pylorus and distal posterior surface of the stomach and generally anastomoses with the posterior branches of the left gastric artery.

GASTRODUODENAL ARTERY. The gastroduodenal artery arises from the common hepatic artery in about 75 per cent of people (Fig. 2-22). In most of the remainder, the hepatic circulation is anomalous, and the gastroduodenal artery then arises from that portion of the hepatic circulation coming from the celiac artery. It rarely arises directly from the celiac or superior mesenteric artery (Fig. 2-23) or from a totally replaced hepatic trunk. The gastroduodenal artery almost always arises before the division of the common hepatic artery into hepatic branches.

The branches of the gastroduodenal artery are quite variable, and their nomenclature is confusing. These branches are important in the evaluation of pancreatic, duodenal and antral disease, and their anatomy must be understood. Three constant branches are present: the posterior and anterior pancreaticoduodenal arcades and the right gastroepiploic artery.

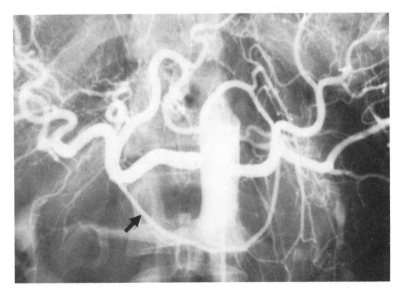

Figure 2-21. Right gastric artery. Celiac angiogram in a 63 year old man. A moderate amount of contrast medium has refluxed into the aorta. The right gastric artery (➡) arises from the left hepatic artery and passes along the lesser curvature of the stomach, anastomosing with the left gastric artery. The right gastric artery is more dilated in this patient than is usually seen, implying some stenosis at the origin of the left gastric artery.

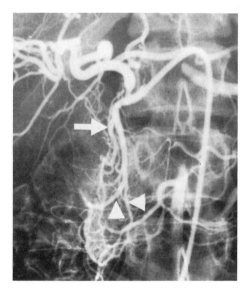

Figure 2-22. Gastroduodenal artery. Gastroduodenal angiogram in a 33 year old woman. Contrast medium refluxes through the posterior (⇨) and anterior (▷) pancreaticoduodenal arcades to fill the inferior pancreaticoduodenal artery and the proximal superior mesenteric artery. The many anastomotic arteries in the head of the pancreas are demonstrated. The right gastroepiploic artery is only very faintly seen.

Posterior Pancreaticoduodenal Arcade. The posterior pancreaticoduodenal arcade arises 1 to 2 cm from the origin of the gastroduodenal artery. This artery is also called the retroduodenal or posterior superior pancreaticoduodenal artery. It anastomoses distally with the superior mesenteric or inferior pancreaticoduodenal artery and gives branches to the duodenum and the head of the pancreas (Fig. 2–24). The duodenal branches pass to the right, while the pancreatic branches pass to the left. The pancreatic branches anastomose freely with other arteries in the head of the pancreas, including branches of the anterior pancreaticoduodenal arcade and the dorsal pancreatic artery. The posterior pancreaticoduodenal arcade may have several origins, and, although its proximal origin is usually from the gastroduodenal artery, it may arise from the common or right hepatic artery or may be absent. Frequently, the arcades are multiple; both posterior and anterior arcades may have three or four branches.

Anterior Pancreaticoduodenal Arcade. The anterior pancreaticoduodenal arcade (also called the superior pancreaticoduodenal or the anterior inferior pancreaticoduodenal artery) is the second constant branch of the gastroduodenal artery and is

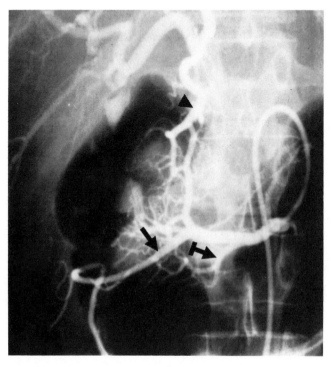

Figure 2-23. Gastroduodenal artery replaced to the superior mesenteric artery. Selective gastroduodenal angiogram in a 40 year old woman with chronic pancreatitis. The catheter has been passed through the superior mesenteric artery and introduced selectively into the gastroduodenal artery. When this variation occurs, the initial portion of the gastroepiploic artery (➡) tends to be directed laterally instead of caudally. Also, the posterior pancreaticoduodenal arcade (►) usually has a direct origin from the hepatic artery, while the anterior pancreaticoduodenal arcade (➡) arises from the gastroduodenal artery.

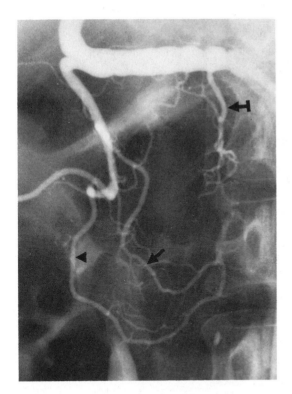

Figure 2-24. Posterior and anterior pancreaticoduodenal arcades. Common hepatic angiogram in a 55 year old man. The posterior pancreaticoduodenal arcade (➡) arises proximally from the first portion of the gastroduodenal artery and distally from the inferior pancreaticoduodenal artery. The anterior pancreaticoduodenal arcade (▶) arises from the distal gastroduodenal artery with the gastroepiploic artery. Distally the anterior arcade anastomoses with the inferior pancreaticoduodenal artery and frequently anastomoses with the first jejunal artery. In this patient the dorsal pancreatic artery (➡) arises from the common hepatic artery.

a terminal branch, along with the right gastroepiploic artery (Fig. 2-24). The anterior pancreaticoduodenal arcade frequently gives off a pyloric branch early in its course and then runs down and through the ventral aspect of the head of the pancreas to anastomose with the superior mesenteric or the inferior pancreaticoduodenal artery. The anterior pancreaticoduodenal arcade may also have several origins. Generally, branches of the posterior arcade anastomose with those of the anterior arcade. Frequently it also has anastomoses with the dorsal pancreatic and transverse pancreatic

arteries. Anastomoses with the middle colic artery occur occasionally.

Right Gastroepiploic Artery. The third branch of the gastroduodenal artery is the right gastroepiploic artery (Fig. 2-25) which follows an undulating course along the greater curvature of the stomach to anastomose with the smaller left gastroepiploic artery from the splenic artery in about 90 per cent of people. Early in its course, the right gastroepiploic artery gives off an ascending pyloric branch to the pylorus and first part of the duodenum. This artery may be difficult to distinguish from pancreatic branches. Multiple ascending gastric branches anastomose with descending branches of the right and left gastric arteries. Omental and anterior epiploic branches run caudally, anastomosing with each other and with posterior epiploic arteries.

Other Arteries. Other, less constant branches of the gastroduodenal artery include the right gastric artery, the transverse pancreatic artery, an accessory cystic artery and the supraduodenal artery, which is usually a branch of the posterior pancreaticoduodenal arcade. Thus, it is easy to see that the vascular anatomy around the head of the pancreas is variable and that each angiogram must be evaluated with these variations in mind.

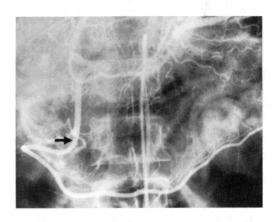

Figure 2-25. Right gastroepiploic artery. Combined celiac–superior mesenteric angiogram in a 37 year old man. Late arterial phase. The gastroduodenal artery divides into the anterior pancreaticoduodenal arcade and the right gastroepiploic artery (➡), which supplies the greater curvature of the stomach with many branches. Branches of the right and left gastric arteries are also present.

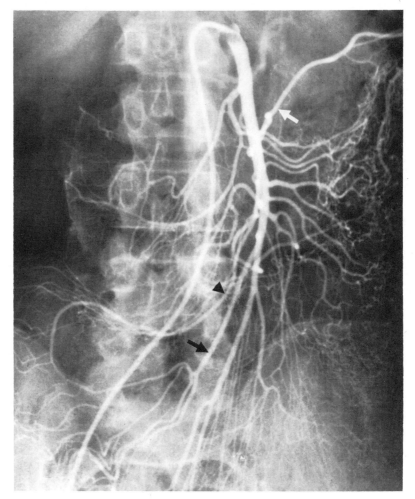

Figure 2–26. Superior mesenteric artery. Superior mesenteric angiogram in a 45 year old woman. The first branch to the right is an accessory middle colic artery which also gives off a right colic branch. The inferior pancreaticoduodenal artery is not opacified. The middle colic artery ($\Longrightarrow$) arises from the right, but immediately runs to the left. Many jejunal and ileal arteries arise from the left of the superior mesenteric artery. A right colic artery ($\blacktriangleright$) and the ileocolic artery ($\longrightarrow$) arise from the right in association with the most distal ileal arteries.

Superior Mesenteric Artery

The superior mesenteric artery arises from the ventral surface of the aorta 2 mm to 2 cm below the celiac trunk at approximately the level of the T12–L1 interspace or the upper portion of the first lumbar vertebral body (Fig. 2–26). It runs caudally behind the pancreas, entering the root of the mesentery at the inferior border of the pancreatic neck. It then passes ventral to the fourth portion of the duodenum and

continues caudally, giving rise to pancreatic, jejunal, ileal and colic branches.

Inferior Pancreaticoduodenal Artery

The first constant branch of the superior mesenteric artery is the inferior pancreaticoduodenal artery, which generally arises as a single branch from the right of the superior mesenteric artery (Fig. 2–27). However, it may arise from the left or as a branch of the first or second jejunal artery. It runs to the right and anastomoses with

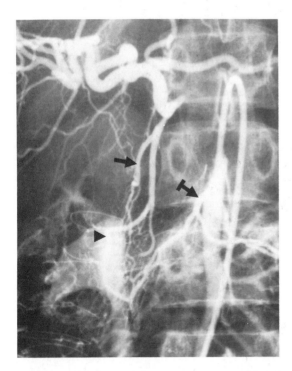

Figure 2-27. Inferior pancreaticoduodenal artery. Selective inferior pancreaticoduodenal angiogram in a 33 year old woman with chronic pancreatitis (same patient as in Figure 2-22). Contrast medium refluxes through the anterior (►) and posterior (➡) pancreaticoduodenal arcades to the gastroduodenal and hepatic arteries. In this patient the inferior pancreaticoduodenal artery (➡) has a common origin with the first jejunal artery.

the anterior and posterior pancreaticoduodenal arcades from the gastroduodenal artery. The inferior pancreaticoduodenal artery may be double or may arise from a replaced hepatic artery from the superior mesenteric artery.

Jejunal and Ileal Arteries

The jejunal and ileal branches of the superior mesenteric artery arise from its left side and vary in number from 10 to 20 (Fig. 2-28). Several branches may arise together as a jejunal or ileal trunk. These arteries send off lateral branches in the mesentery which anastomose with adjacent branches, forming a series of arcades sometimes four or five deep. The distal arcades run along the mesenteric border of the bowel and give off the straight vasa recta to the bowel itself. There are many vasa recta, and each

generally gives off a posterior and anterior division to the bowel. The bowel, therefore, has a large vascular bed with many anastomoses available to maintain adequate blood supply. A jejunal trunk rarely has a replaced origin from the celiac artery (Fig. 2-29).

Middle Colic Artery

The middle colic artery usually arises from the anterior right surface of the superior mesenteric artery slightly distal to the origin of the inferior pancreaticoduodenal artery (Fig. 2-30). It divides into right and left branches which course along the mesenteric border of the colon, anastomosing with branches of the right and left colic

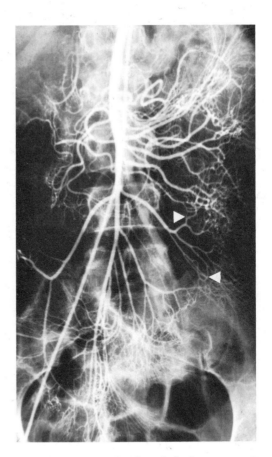

Figure 2-28. Jejunal and ileal arteries. Superior mesenteric angiogram in a 31 year old woman. The superior mesenteric artery gives off a series of left-sided branches to the jejunum and ileum. These have communicating arcades (▷) and terminate in the fine vasa recta to the wall of the small bowel.

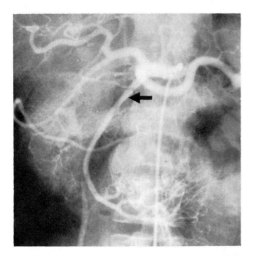

Figure 2–29. Replaced jejunal arteries from the celiac artery. Celiac angiogram in a 33 year old man. A jejunal trunk (➡) arises from the celiac artery. The venous drainage of the jejunum paralleled the arterial supply in this unusual variation.

Figure 2–30. Middle colic artery.

A. Superior mesenteric angiogram in a 74 year old man. The middle colic artery (➡) arises from the right side of the superior mesenteric artery. It divides into right and left branches to the transverse colon. The right branch usually anastomoses with an ascending branch of the right colic artery, and the left branch, with an ascending branch of the left colic artery.

B. Selective middle colic angiogram in a 48 year old man. The division of the middle colic artery into right and left branches can be better visualized on the selective study. These branches, in turn, anastomose with branches of the right and left colic arteries.

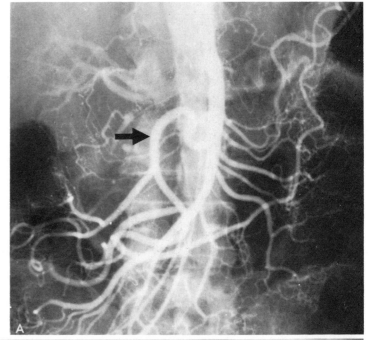

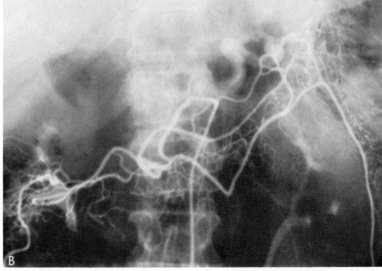

arteries respectively. There may be more than one middle colic artery; it may give off the dorsal pancreatic artery; it occasionally arises from the celiac artery.

Right Colic Artery

The right colic artery (Fig. 2–31) arises from the right of the superior mesenteric artery distal to the middle colic artery. The right colic artery divides into ascending and descending branches which give off numerous straight vasa recta to the upper ascending colon and the proximal transverse colon. The descending branch anastomoses with the ascending branch of the ileocolic artery, and the ascending branch anastomoses, sometimes poorly, with the right branch of the middle colic artery. The right colic artery may be double, absent or a branch of either the middle colic or ileocolic artery.

Ileocolic Artery

The ileocolic artery (Fig. 2–31) courses down and to the right after arising as a terminal branch of the superior mesenteric artery. It divides into an ascending branch, which anastomoses with the descending branch of the right colic artery, and a descending branch. The descending branch supplies the anterior and posterior aspects of the cecum and the appendix and gives off a fourth branch to the distal ileum which anastomoses with the terminal superior mesenteric arterial branch.

Other Arteries

Occasionally arteries have replaced origins from the superior mesenteric artery. The dorsal pancreatic artery arises from the superior mesenteric artery in about 14 per

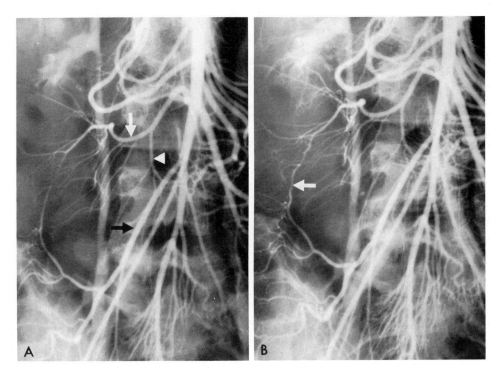

Figure 2–31. Right colic and ileocolic arteries. Superior mesenteric angiogram in a 24 year old woman.

A. Early arterial phase. The right colic artery arises from the right of the superior mesenteric artery and divides into an ascending branch (▷) and a descending branch (⇒) which anastomoses with an ascending branch of the ileocolic artery (➡).

B. Later arterial phase. The anastomosis between the right colic and ileocolic arteries is filled (⇒). The distal ileocolic branches to the cecum and ascending colon are also opacified. The last ileal artery usually has an anastomosis with the ileocolic artery.

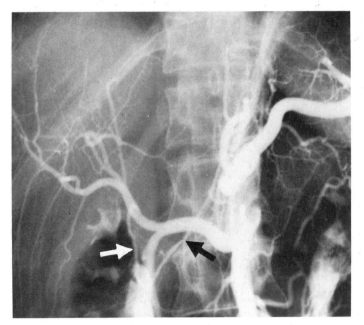

Figure 2-32. Complete common hepatic artery replacement to the superior mesenteric artery with a celiac splenic–left gastric trunk. Combined celiac–superior mesenteric angiogram in a 22 year old woman. The entire hepatic arterial supply and the gastroduodenal artery are replaced to the superior mesenteric artery. The right gastric artery (➡) arises from the proper hepatic artery and anastomoses with the left gastric artery arising from the splenic–left gastric trunk.

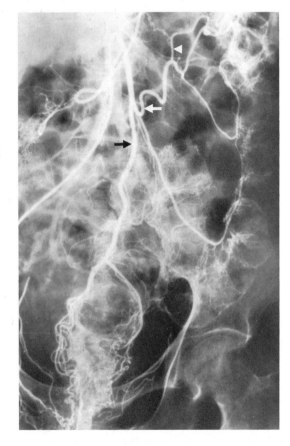

Figure 2-33. Inferior mesenteric artery. Inferior mesenteric angiogram in a 47 year old man. The inferior mesenteric artery runs caudally for about 5 cm and then gives off the left colic artery (⇨) and a sigmoid arterial trunk, which sends off several branches to the sigmoid colon. The superior hemorrhoidal artery (➡) is the terminal branch. It supplies the distal sigmoid colon and the rectum and anastomoses with pelvic branches of the internal iliac arteries. The marginal artery of Drummond along the mesenteric border of the colon is well demonstrated. The arch of Riolan (▷) is not prominent in this patient.

cent of people. A totally or partially replaced right hepatic artery arises from the superior mesenteric artery in about 22 per cent. The entire hepatic arterial supply occasionally is replaced to the superior mesenteric artery (Fig. 2–32). Less frequently, the transverse pancreatic artery may arise directly from the superior mesenteric artery.

Inferior Mesenteric Artery

The inferior mesenteric artery arises from the anterior surface of the aorta at the level of the third lumbar vertebral body or the L3–4 interspace (Fig. 2–33). It courses caudally and to the left for 1 to 5 cm before giving off two or more branches. The left colic artery, the first major branch, has an ascending branch that anastomoses with the middle colic artery through arcades in the mesentery and also through a marginal artery. It supplies the descending colon through multiple straight vasa recta. The left colic artery may give off one or more descending colic branches, or these may arise directly from the inferior mesenteric artery. The more distal of these branches are the sigmoid arteries. The inferior mesenteric artery terminates as the superior hemorrhoidal artery. The distal sigmoid branches anastomose with the superior hemorrhoidal artery, but this anastomosis is incomplete in about 5 per cent of patients.

There is much confusion about the various branches of the inferior mesenteric artery, primarily due to a widely varied nomenclature. The arcade of Drummond is an anastomotic, marginal colonic artery which runs along the mesenteric surface of the colon and gives off the vasa recta to the bowel. This artery generally anastomoses with the marginal artery from the middle colic artery, forming an arcade. The arch of Riolan is a left colic arterial branch which runs cephalad in the mesentery to anastomose with the middle colic artery near the splenic flexure. This artery often becomes the primary collateral pathway in occlusion of the inferior mesenteric artery.

ARTERIAL SUPPLY TO SPECIFIC ORGANS

In order to adequately evaluate a specific diagnostic problem, it is necessary not only to understand the vascular anatomy and its variations, but also to know what arteries must be injected to study a given organ completely. Therefore, a brief summary of the arterial supply to the organs of the gastrointestinal tract follows.

Liver

In 55 to 65 per cent of the population, the entire hepatic arterial supply is demonstrated by a common hepatic artery injection; in the remainder, one of several variations is present. The left hepatic artery arises from the left gastric artery in about 25 per cent of people (Fig. 2–34). Half of these variations are partial replacements. The right hepatic artery has a completely replaced origin from the superior mesenteric artery in about 14 per cent of people and a partially replaced origin in 8 per cent (Fig. 2–35). Rarely, the right hepatic artery arises directly from the aorta. The left hepatic artery occasionally arises from the aorta or the superior mesenteric artery, and the entire hepatic artery may be replaced to the superior mesenteric artery (see Fig. 2–32). When complete demonstration of the liver is required, these variations must be considered.

Gallbladder

The gallbladder is supplied by the cystic artery (Fig. 2–36), which is single in 75 per cent of people and double or multiple in the remainder. The cystic artery, or arteries, arises from the right hepatic artery regardless of its origin in about 90 per cent of the population, though the second or deep cystic artery may arise from the right hepatic artery deep in the hepatic hilum. It may also arise from the common, middle or left hepatic artery, the gastroduodenal artery (see Fig. 2–35) or its branches or directly from the aorta. The cystic artery has deep and superficial divisions which send off multiple fine branches across the anterior and posterior surfaces of the gallbladder.

Spleen

The spleen receives its blood supply from the splenic artery. Multiple spleens and accessory spleens also receive their

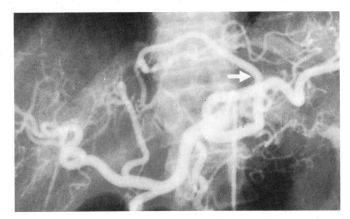

Figure 2–34. Replaced left hepatic artery. Celiac angiogram in a 64 year old man. The left hepatic artery (⟹) rises entirely from the left gastric artery. A discrete middle hepatic artery is present.

Figure 2–35. Partially replaced right hepatic artery. Combined celiac–superior mesenteric angiogram in a 42 year old man with pancreatitis. An accessory right hepatic artery (⟹) arises from the superior mesenteric artery. The remainder of the hepatic circulation has a standard origin. The cystic artery (►) is replaced to the gastroduodenal artery, an uncommon variation.

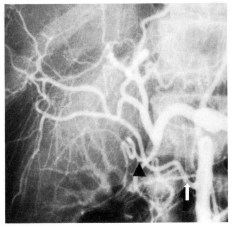

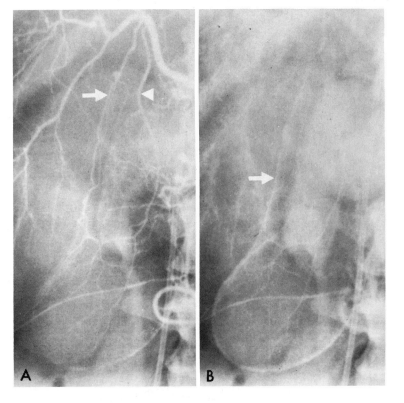

Figure 2–36. Double cystic arteries. Celiac angiogram in a 43 year old woman.

A. Arterial phase. The deep (▷) and superficial (⟹) cystic arteries arise separately from the right hepatic artery.

B. Parenchymal phase. Contrast medium accumulation outlines the gallbladder wall (⟹).

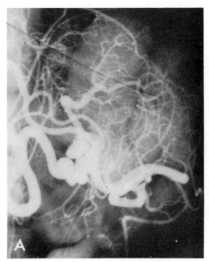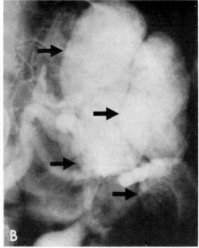

Figure 2-37.   Multiple spleens. Celiac angiogram in a 43 year old man.
A. Arterial phase. The intrasplenic arterial branches have an atypical branching pattern.
B. Venous phase. Four separate spleens can be delineated (➡), each with a draining vein.
(Courtesy of Dr. Lawrence Campbell.)

blood supply from branches of the splenic artery (Fig. 2–37).

Stomach

The entire gastric blood supply comes from branches of the celiac trunk in the average patient (Fig. 2–38). The arteries that are usually demonstrated at angiography include the left gastric artery, the right gastric artery arising from the proper or left hepatic artery, the right gastroepiploic artery from a terminal branch of the gastroduodenal artery and the left gastroepiploic artery from the distal splenic artery. Injection of the celiac artery will generally opacify all these arteries. Superselective left gastric and gastroduodenal angiograms may be necessary in specific patients.

Pancreas

The arterial supply to the pancreas arises from both the celiac and superior mesenteric arteries (Fig. 2–39). The arterial supply is quite variable, and superselective angiography is necessary to evaluate the intrapancreatic arteries adequately. Superselective gastroduodenal and splenic angio-

grams will usually demonstrate the entire pancreatic circulation. Occasionally the dorsal pancreatic or inferior pancreaticoduodenal artery will have to be studied to complete the examination.

Small Bowel

The small bowel receives its blood supply almost exclusively from the jejunal and ileal branches of the superior mesenteric artery. The first jejunal artery frequently anastomoses with the duodenal branches of the posterior pancreaticoduodenal arcade proximally, and the last ileal branch anastomoses with branches of the ileocolic artery distally. Superior mesenteric or superselective angiography of any given branch is therefore adequate to study the small bowel completely.

Colon

The blood supply to the colon usually comes entirely from the superior and inferior mesenteric arteries (Fig. 2–40). The middle colic artery occasionally arises from the celiac artery in association with the dorsal pancreatic artery. Therefore, celiac

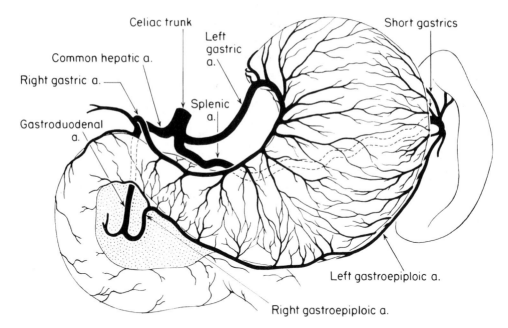

Figure 2–38. Line drawing of arterial supply to the stomach. The arteries to the stomach are enlarged for emphasis. The left gastroepiploic and right gastric arteries are frequently not identified at angiography unless they are serving as a collateral pathway.

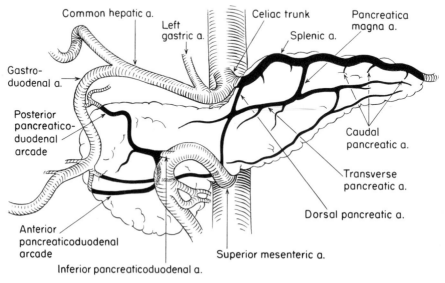

Figure 2–39. Line drawing of arterial supply to the pancreas. The pancreatic branches are enlarged for emphasis. In this example, the dorsal pancreatic artery arises from the splenic artery and gives off the transverse pancreatic artery. It receives an anastomotic branch from the anterior pancreaticoduodenal arcade. The relationships of the pancreatic arteries are variable and must be evaluated in each patient.

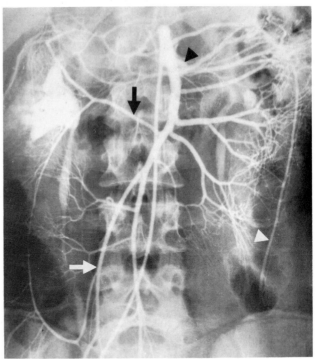

Figure 2-40. Colonic arterial supply. Superior mesenteric angiogram in a 16 year old girl. The ileocolic (⇒), right colic (➡) and middle colic (►) arteries are well opacified. The ascending branch of the left colic artery (▷) is also demonstrated. The anastomoses between these various arteries are all patent in this patient.

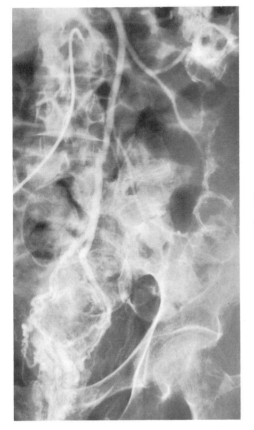

Figure 2-41. Inferior mesenteric vein. Venous phase of an inferior mesenteric angiogram in a 47 year old man. The inferior mesenteric vein drains the left and sigmoid colons and the rectum and enters the splenic vein prior to its junction with the superior mesenteric vein.

angiography or superselective dorsal pancreatic angiography will sometimes be necessary to evaluate the vascular supply of the colon completely.

VENOUS ANATOMY

The venous anatomy of the gastrointestinal tract is less complicated than the arterial anatomy, but it is also variable and is seldom completely demonstrated at angiography. However, a thorough knowledge of venous anatomy and drainage patterns is important for a complete interpretation of angiograms.

The veins of the gastrointestinal tract drain into the portal venous system. The left and sigmoid colons are drained by branches of the inferior mesenteric vein (Fig. 2–41). These veins parallel the inferior mesenteric artery branches to a large extent. A marginal vein along the colon generally receives the colonic venous branches. Anastomotic venous arcades are present in the mesentery. The inferior mesenteric vein enters the splenic vein to the left of its junction with the superior mesenteric vein. The superior mesenteric vein drains the cecum, right and transverse colons and all the jejunum and ileum (Fig. 2–42). These veins also parallel the arterial supply with anastomoses connecting adjacent veins along the margin of the bowel and in the mesentery. The superior mesenteric vein joins the splenic vein to form the portal vein (Fig. 2–43). The veins draining the pancreas enter either the portal or the superior mesenteric vein. The right gastroepiploic vein drains the greater curvature of the stomach and generally enters the portal vein directly. The veins from the lesser curvature and pylorus form the coronary vein which drains into the splenic or portal vein (Fig. 2–44).

The portal vein enters the liver hilum and

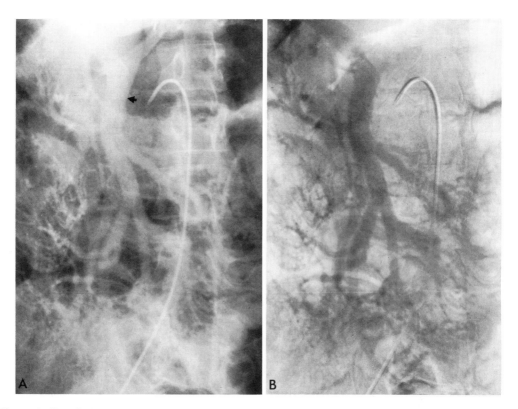

Figure 2–42. Superior mesenteric veins.

A. Venous phase of a superior mesenteric angiogram in a 35 year old woman. Veins from the ileum, jejunum and colon unite to form the superior mesenteric vein (➡), which flows into the portal vein near the upper left-hand corner of the picture.

B. Subtraction technique. The jejunal veins over the spine can be better seen.

Legend continued on the following page.

divides into right and left branches (Fig. 2–45). The right branch usually divides into the anterior and posterior segmental veins, which further subdivide. The left portal vein is generally smaller than the right and follows a longer, straight course before dividing into medial and lateral segmental veins which further subdivide. The portal veins normally empty toward the periphery of the liver and are oriented toward the liver hilum.

The hepatic veins are rarely seen at angiography, unless they are injected directly (Fig. 2–46). They lie between the hepatic segments. There are generally right, middle and left hepatic veins, all of which drain obliquely cranially and centrally to enter the inferior vena cava. All three may enter as a single trunk, but more commonly the right hepatic vein enters separately, and the middle and left veins form a common trunk. Several smaller hepatic veins draining the caudate lobe and portions of the right lobe generally enter the inferior vena cava separately. Anasto-

moses between these veins are usually present.

Differentiation of hepatic and portal veins is usually not difficult. The direction of emptying is the most useful identifying characteristic; the portal veins drain peripherally, and the hepatic veins drain toward the right atrium. The portal veins are oriented toward the liver hilum, and the hepatic veins toward the right atrium. Finally, the portal vein radicles are somewhat coarser than those of the hepatic veins, and the portal branches arise at more of a right angle than hepatic vein branches, which have an acute branching angle.

The portal venous system has several potential anastomoses with the systemic venous system (Edwards, 1951; Johns and Blackwell, 1962; Ruzicka, 1969). The veins of Retzius form a retroperitoneal plexus with communications between colic, splenic, duodenal and pancreatic veins, and the inferior vena cava through phrenic and azygos veins. A normally patent collateral pathway exists between the gastric and

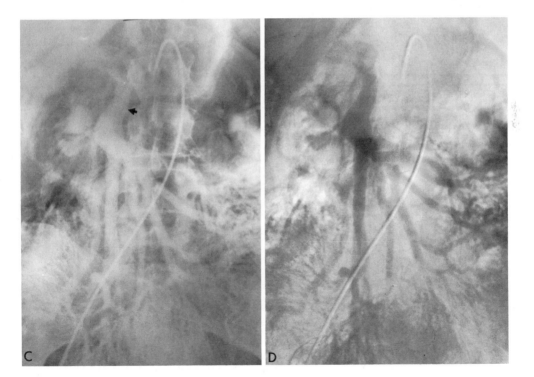

Figure 2–42. *Continued.*

C. Venous phase of a superior mesenteric angiogram in a 48 year old woman. Jejunal, ileal and colonic veins unite to form the superior mesenteric vein (➡). This, in turn, flows into the portal vein.

D. Subtraction technique. The veins overlying the spine are better seen.

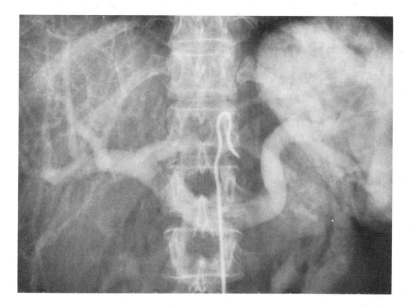

Figure 2-43. Splenic and portal veins. Venous phase of a high-dose celiac angiogram in a 35 year old woman. The splenic vein passes dorsal to the head of the pancreas and joins the superior mesenteric vein at the level of the spine to form the portal vein. The main right and left portal vein branches are well visualized. However, the peripheral portal vein radicles through the right lobe of the liver are better visualized than those on the left because of layering of the contrast medium.

splenic veins and the left renal veins through inferior phrenic or retroperitoneal veins. Additional communications generally exist between the splenic vein and omental and posterior epiploic veins. In the presence of portal hypertension, the umbilical vein from the left portal vein may recanalize and anastomose with the anterior abdominal wall veins running inferiorly to join the systemic venous system. Blood in the inferior mesenteric vein often flows in a retrograde direction to anastomose with the hemorrhoidal veins of the systemic circulation in the pelvis.

Figure 2-44. Gastric veins. Venous phase of a selective left gastric angiogram in a 38 year old woman. Veins draining the gastric mucosa join to form the left gastric vein (➡), which drains into the superior surface of the portal vein.

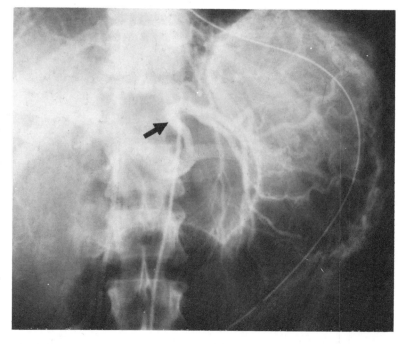

Figure 2–45. Right and left portal veins. Venous phase of a celiac angiogram in a 60 year old woman. Both the right (➡) and left (►) main portal vein radicles are well visualized. Most branches of the right portal vein are apparent, while the left portal vein radicles are poorly visualized. This discrepancy is caused by the preferential layering of the contrast medium toward the more posteriorly situated right portal vein branches.

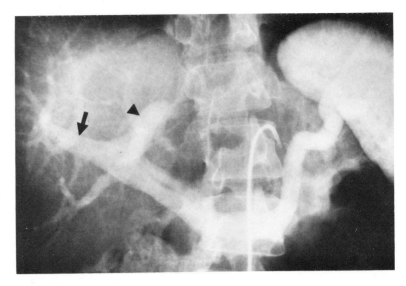

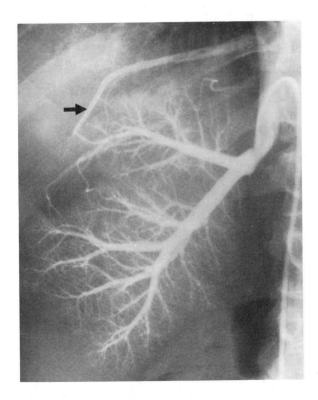

Figure 2–46. Normal right hepatic veins. Hepatic venogram in a 24 year old woman. The right hepatic vein courses medially and cranially to enter the inferior vena cava. Both the main hepatic vein and its branches taper gently. Most of the branches enter at an acute angle. An anastomosis (➡) to an accessory right hepatic vein is filled.

THE ARCADE ARRANGEMENT OF VISCERAL VESSELS

From this description of vascular anatomy, it is apparent that almost every visceral organ has two or more sources of blood supply and venous drainage. The blood supply is frequently arranged in arcades, each end of a given arcade arising from or draining a major visceral artery or vein. Thus, ready-made pathways are available whenever vascular occlusions occur. Their effectiveness accounts for the frequent lack of symptoms encountered in patients with extensive visceral atherosclerosis, and an understanding of these arcades is essential to the interpretation of angiograms in the presence of vascular disease.

Left Gastric–Right Gastric

The left gastric–right gastric arterial arcade connects the celiac artery with the distal hepatic artery and is an important collateral pathway in patients with common hepatic or left gastric artery occlusion. This arcade does not have a venous counterpart.

Left Gastroepiploic–Right Gastroepiploic

The left gastroepiploic–right gastroepiploic arcade connects the common hepatic and splenic arteries and becomes an important source of collateral blood flow to the spleen or liver in patients with splenic or hepatic artery occlusion. On the venous side, this arcade is an important pathway between the splenic vein and portal vein in patients with splenic vein occlusion.

Pancreas

Pancreaticoduodenal arcades connect the superior mesenteric and celiac arteries via the gastroduodenal artery. The arc of Bühler, if present, also accomplishes this connection. These pancreatic arcades are among the most important and most utilized anastomotic channels in the abdomen since they become the main collateral pathways in patients with celiac or superior mesenteric artery occlusion.

Superior Mesenteric Artery–Inferior Mesenteric Artery

The arcades between the superior mesenteric artery and the inferior mesenteric artery occur through the marginal artery of Drummond and the arch of Riolan. Such connections are commonly seen in clinical angiography because of the frequency of inferior mesenteric artery occlusion in the elderly population. They are also important collateral pathways in superior mesenteric artery occlusion.

Celiac Artery–Systemic and Inferior Mesenteric Artery–Systemic

Although not arcades in the usual sense, the anastomoses between the celiac artery and systemic vessels, such as bronchial, esophageal and intercostal arteries, and those between the inferior mesenteric artery and the internal iliac artery branches are important collateral pathways to the abdominal viscera if all the major visceral arteries are occluded.

NORMAL VARIATIONS IN THE ANGIOGRAPHIC APPEARANCE OF THE LIVER AND SPLEEN

An understanding of the variations in the position and shape of the liver and spleen is important in the interpretation of abdominal angiograms.

Liver

The liver lies in the right upper quadrant immediately beneath the diaphragm and against the right lateral abdominal wall. The right lobe may extend caudally in a Riedel's lobe but usually lies entirely above the right costal margin. The inferior

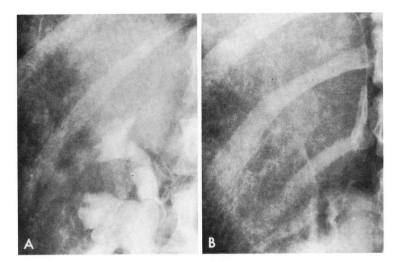

Figure 2-47. Normal variants of the hepatogram.
A. Celiac angiogram, hepatogram phase, in a 31 year old man. The hepatogram is coarsely mottled. Both percutaneous liver biopsy and an operative wedge biopsy were normal.
B. Common hepatic angiogram in 39 year old woman. The hepatogram is mottled, having a salt-and-pepper appearance. Operative wedge biopsy was normal.

liver edge is often not well visualized at angiography. The porta hepatis normally lies to the right of the spine and runs obliquely from left to right toward the lateral costophrenic angle. The left lobe is more variable in shape and position than the right. Though it generally extends to the left of the spine, it may be poorly demonstrated during angiography. On the other hand, it may reach the left abdominal wall. In such patients, the left lobe can cause a mass defect on the fundus of the stomach and may displace the spleen posteriorly and inferiorly. The estimation of liver volume, especially of the left lobe, is very difficult to determine by angiography.

The hepatogram or parenchymal phase is consistent throughout the normal liver, although the pattern varies from patient to patient, especially with superselective angiography (Fig. 2-47). The most frequent pattern is homogeneous and even. The entire liver becomes more dense in the parenchymal phase. However, the accumulation may be diffusely mottled, giving a speckled or a salt-and-pepper appearance. An even coarser pattern which may simulate hematogenous metastases is sometimes present. Fortunately, these latter patterns are rare, since they may result in false positive diagnoses.

The hepatic veins are not often seen during angiography in normal livers. Occasionally they are demonstrated during superselective hepatic artery injections. The portal venous phase generally begins about 6 to 10 seconds after contrast medium is injected into the celiac, splenic or superior mesenteric artery. Earlier visualization raises the possibility of an arteriovenous shunt. Lack of portal vein visualization may be due either to hemodilution or pooling of the contrast medium in a large spleen.

Spleen

The spleen is a posterior structure and does not necessarily lie against the dome of the diaphragm, as visualized on angiograms. The orientation of the spleen is generally vertical or oblique but may be almost horizontal. It may be long and narrow, or ovoid. The lateral margin frequently has discrete fetal lobulations. These are sharply defined during the parenchymal phase. Accessory spleens are present in about 10 per cent of patients and are best seen during the parenchymal and venous phases (Fig. 2-48). Rarely, several small spleens are present.

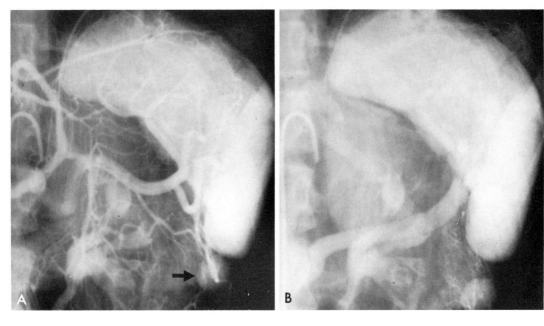

Figure 2–48. Accessory spleen. Celiac angiogram in a 22 year old woman.
A. Late arterial phase. Splenic arterial branches supply a 1 cm in diameter accessory spleen (➡).
B. Venous phase. The accessory spleen has contrast accumulation similar to the spleen itself. Draining veins are not seen in this patient, but are often present.

The parenchymal phase varies from patient to patient but is normally uniform throughout the spleen. The accumulation may be homogeneous or slightly speckled. The density of the accumulation is generally greater when the splenic artery is injected than when the celiac artery is injected. The density of the parenchymal phase depends upon both the volume of contrast medium injected and the volume of splenic parenchyma present.

The splenic vein is generally seen 6 to 8 seconds after contrast medium injection, though it may be seen earlier in superselective splenic artery injections. Filling of the splenic vein in the first 1 to 3 seconds of contrast medium injection indicates an arteriovenous shunt.

BIBLIOGRAPHY

Arey, L. B.: Developmental Anatomy: A textbook and laboratory manual of embryology. 7th ed. Philadelphia, W. B. Saunders Company, 1965.

Basmajian, J. V.: The main arteries of the large intestine. Surg. Gynec. Obstet., 101:585, 1955.

Bradley, R. L.: Surgical anatomy of the gastroduodenal artery. Int. Surg., 58:393, 1973.

Chuang, V. P.: The aberrant gallbladder: angiographic and radioisotopic considerations. Amer. J. Roentgenol. 127:417, 1976.

Doehner, G. A.: The hepatic venous system; its normal roentgen anatomy. Radiology 90:1119, 1968.

Edwards, E. A.: Functional anatomy of the portasystemic communications. Arch. Intern. Med. 88:137, 1951.

Fontaine, R., Pietri, J., Tongio, J., and Negrieros, L.: Étude angiographique des variations anatomiques des artères hépatiques basée sur 402 examens spécialisés. Angiology 21 110, 1970.

Gabriele, O. F.: Arterial supply to the lung via the celiac axis. Amer. J. Roentgenol., 109:522, 1970.

Haertel, M., and Beusch, H. R.: Der angiographische Normalanatomie der Miltz. Fortschr. Geb. Roentgenstr. Nuklearmed. 120:653, 1974.

Hardy, K. J.: The hepatic veins. Aust. N.Z.J. Surg. 42:11, 1972.

Ingalls, N. W.: A contribution to the embryology of the liver and vascular system in man. Anat. Rec. 2:338, 1908.

Johns, T. N. P., and Blackwell, B. E.: Collateral pathways in portal hypertension. Ann. Surg. 155:838, 1962.

Kahn, P., and Abrams, H. L.: Inferior mesenteric arterial patterns. Radiology 82:429, 1964.

Loeffler, L.: Factors determining necrosis or survival of liver tissue after ligation of hepatic artery. Arch. Path. 21:496, 1936.

Mann, J. D., Wakim, K. G., and Baggenstoss, A. H.: The vasculature of the human liver: A study by the injection-cast method. Proc. Mayo Clin. 28:227, 1953.

McBurney, R. P., Howard, H., Bicks, R. O., et al.: Ischemia and gangrene of the colon following abdominal aortic resection. Amer. Surg. 36:205, 1970.

Menuck, L., and Coel, M.: Vascular impressions of the gut secondary to chronic vascular occlusive disease. Amer. J. Roentgenol. 126:970, 1976.

Michels, N. A.: Blood Supply and Anatomy of the Upper Abdominal Organs. Philadelphia, J. B. Lippincott Company, 1955.

Michels, N. A.: Newer anatomy of the liver and its variant blood supply and collateral circulation. Amer. J. Surg. 112:337, 1966.

Michels, N. A., Siddharth, P., Kornblith, P., et al.: The variant blood supply to the small and large intestines: its import in regional resections. J. Int. Coll. Surg. 39:127, 1963.

Monafo, W. W., Jr., Ternberg, J. L., and Kempson, R.: Accidental ligation of the hepatic artery. Arch. Surg. 92:634, 1966.

Moskowitz, M., Zimmerman, H., and Felson, B.: The meandering mesenteric artery of the colon. Amer. J. Roentgenol. 92:1088, 1964.

Pattern, B. M.: Human Embryology. New York, McGraw-Hill Book Company, 1968.

Quénu, L.: Sur la disposition vasculaire des branches coliques de la mésentérique supérieure chez le foetus humain. C. R. Ass. Anat. 39:84, 1952.

Quénu, L.: Sur la vascularisation comparée des anses grêles l'adulte et chez le foetus humain. C. R. Ass. Anat. 39:89, 1952.

Rappaport, A. M.: Anatomic considerations. In Schiff, L. (ed.): Diseases of the Liver. 4th ed. Philadelphia, J. B. Lippincott Company, 1975.

Redman, H. C., and Reuter, S. R.: Angiographic demonstration of surgically important vascular variations. Surg. Gynec. Obstet. 129:33, 1969.

Redman, H. C., and Reuter, S. R.: Arterial collaterals in the liver hilus. Radiology 94:575, 1970.

Reuter, S. R.: Superselective pancreatic angiography. Radiology 92:74, 1969.

Rodgers, J. B.: Infarction of the gastric remnant following subtotal gastrectomy. Arch. Surg. 92:917, 1966.

Rösch, J.: Roentgenology of the Spleen and Pancreas. Springfield, Illinois, Charles C Thomas, Publisher, 1967.

Ruzicka, F. F., Jr., and Rossi, P.: Arterial portography: Patterns of venous flow. Radiology 92:777, 1969.

Smith, R. F., and Szilagyi, D. E.: Ischemia of the colon as a complication in the surgery of the abdominal aorta. Arch. Surg. 80:806, 1960.

Sondheimer, F. K., and Steinberg, I.: Gastrointestinal manifestations of abdominal aortic aneurysms. Amer. J. Roentgenol. 92:1110, 1964.

Spalteholz, W., and Spanner, R.: Atlas of Human Anatomy. Philadelphia, F. A. Davis Company, 1967.

Sundgren, R.: Selective angiography of the left gastric artery. Acta Radiol. (Suppl. 299) (Stockholm), 1970.

Suzuki, T., Imamura, M., Kawabe, K., and Honjo, I.: Selective demonstration of the variant hepatic artery. Surg. Gynecol. Obstet. 135:209, 1972.

Tandler, J.: Über die varietäten der arteria coeliaca und deren entwicklung. Anat. Hefte 25:472, 1904.

Tandler, J.: Zur Entwickelungsgeschichte der menschlichen Darmarterien. Anat. Hefte 23:187, 1903.

Wieke, L., Spangler, H. R., Firbas, W., et al.: Length of the splenic artery in angiograms. Acta Anat. (Basel) 86:123, 1973.

Yeo, R., and Powell, K.: Avascular gastric necrosis. A complication of partial gastrectomy following interruption of the splenic artery or its branches. Brit. J. Surg. 54:707, 1967.

Chapter 3

VASCULAR DISEASES

Atherosclerosis is commonly encountered during gastrointestinal angiography and has several forms which may mimic the arterial changes of neoplasm and inflammatory disease. Therefore, a knowledge of the arterial alterations caused by atherosclerosis is important. Other less common vascular diseases, including aneurysms of all etiologies, abdominal angina, polyarteritis nodosa, drug toxicity, embolic phenomena and venous thrombosis, can be encountered or diagnosed at angiography. Vascular trauma is included in Chapter 5; angiomas and hemangiomas in Chapter 4; arteriovenous malformations, arteriovenous fistulas and hereditary hemorrhagic telangiectasias in Chapter 6; and ischemic colitis in Chapter 7.

ATHEROSCLEROSIS

Atherosclerotic changes in the visceral arteries can be detected by microscopic examination as early as the third decade. They are not commonly encountered dur-

ing angiography until the fifth decade or later, except in the presence of metabolic diseases. In general, major vessel atherosclerosis is present before the onset of smaller vessel disease (Reiner et al., 1963). Atherosclerosis may cause plaque deposition, with or without luminal narrowing and occlusion, or may produce progressive vascular dilatation and aneurysms. Since aortic atherosclerosis is significant in some gastrointestinal diseases and is frequently a minor impediment in the performance of a selective angiogram, it is discussed first.

Aortic Atherosclerosis

The most frequently encountered form of aortic atherosclerosis is the deposition of many irregular plaques in the aortic wall. This usually occurs distal to the renal arteries and is not associated with change in lumen size (Fig. 3–1). This type of atherosclerosis has little significance in gastrointestinal angiography, except for the

66

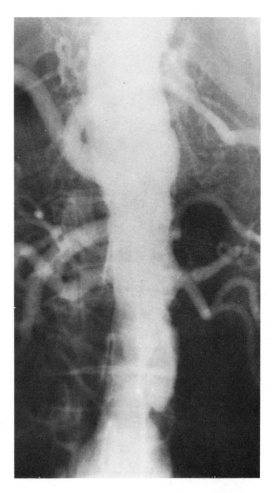

Figure 3–1. Atherosclerosis of the abdominal aorta. Lumbar aortogram in a 71 year old man. The aorta is elongated, and the walls are moderately irregular distal to the origin of the renal arteries. The tortuosity, elongation and multiple atherosclerotic plaques make selective catheterizations difficult.

technical difficulties it causes during catheterization because of stenosis of vessel origins or catheter hangup on the many irregular plaques.

Atherosclerosis with plaque formation may lead to progressive narrowing of the abdominal aorta (Fig. 3–2) and occasionally to occlusion (Fig. 3–3). The actual occlusion is usually secondary to thrombosis (Bron, 1966). Although such occlusions usually occur initially at or just above the aortic bifurcation, the thrombus generally propagates proximally, stopping just distal to the renal artery orifices (Fig. 3–4A and B). The inferior mesenteric artery is occluded in the process. Rarely, a large embolus may lodge at the aortic bifurcation (Fig. 3–4C and D). The celiac, superior mesenteric and inferior mesenteric arteries, along with the intercostal and lumbar arteries, provide collateral circulation to the iliac and femoral arteries (Fig. 3–4E and F). The celiac

artery supplies many small collateral arteries in the paravertebral region and also provides collateral flow through the anterior epiploic arteries. The paravertebral collaterals can simulate a mass lesion impressing the duodenal loop and can mimic or obscure small carcinomas or inflammatory changes in the pancreas. The superior and inferior mesenteric arteries utilize the collateral pathway through the middle colic, left colic and superior hemorrhoidal arteries to the internal iliac and femoral arteries (Fig. 3–5). Some patients with aortic occlusion are asymptomatic, but most have peripheral claudication, and some have abdominal angina. Most patients have no palpable femoral pulses, but a weak pulse is present in a surprising number. Generally, such patients are examined for peripheral vascular disease by translumbar aortography. Selective visceral angiograms must be done from a left axillary approach.

Text continued on page 72

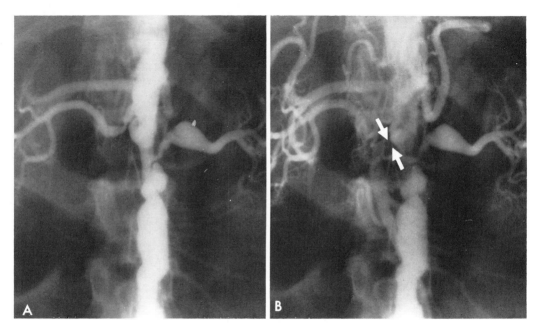

Figure 3–2. Atherosclerosis of the lumbar aorta causing marked irregularity and narrowing. Lumbar aortogram in a 48 year old woman with a 30 year history of hypertension.

A, Early arterial phase. The lumbar aorta is markedly irregular and is severely narrowed at the level of the L2-3 interspace. There are severe stenoses at the origins of both renal arteries with a prominent poststenotic dilatation on the left.

B. Later arterial phase. The proximal portion of the superior mesenteric artery (⟹) is compromised by the extensive atherosclerosis.

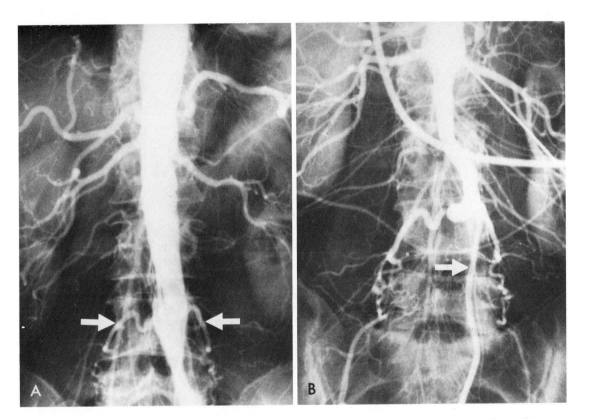

Figure 3-3. Aortic occlusion. Aortography in a 57 year old woman with symptoms of claudication.

A. Transfemoral aortogram. The right common iliac artery is occluded at its origin, and dilated fourth lumbar arteries (⟹) provide collateral blood flow to the peripheral arteries. The distal abdominal aorta is slightly irregular and narrowed. Splenic artery stenosis is present.

B. Translumbar aortogram performed 11 months later because of increased claudication and absent femoral pulses. The aorta is now occluded distal to the inferior mesenteric artery and is markedly narrowed distal to the renal arteries. The dilated superior hemorrhoidal artery (⟹) provides distal collateral blood flow.

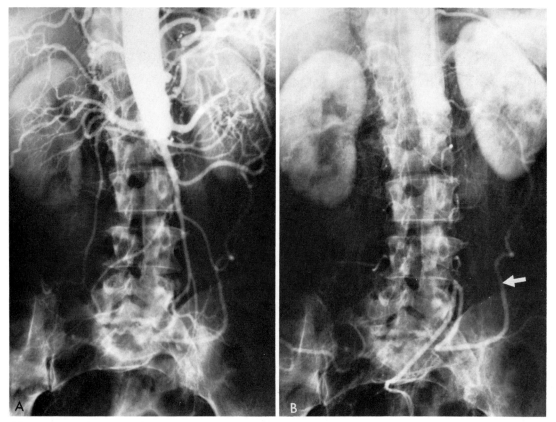

Figure 3–4. Aortic occlusion.

A and B. Aortic occlusion below the renal arteries. Lumbar aortogram in a 55 year old man with progressive claudication.

A. The celiac, superior mesenteric and renal arteries are patent.

B. Collateral blood flow via the middle colic artery and marginal artery of Drummond (⟹) supplies the inferior mesenteric artery distribution. This blood flow also passes to the extremities via the superior hemorrhoidal arteries to the internal iliac arteries.

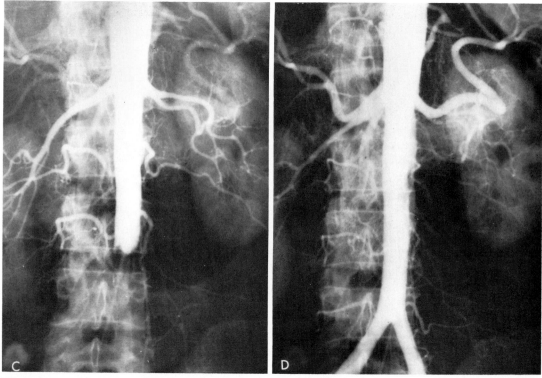

Figure 3–4. See legend on opposite page.

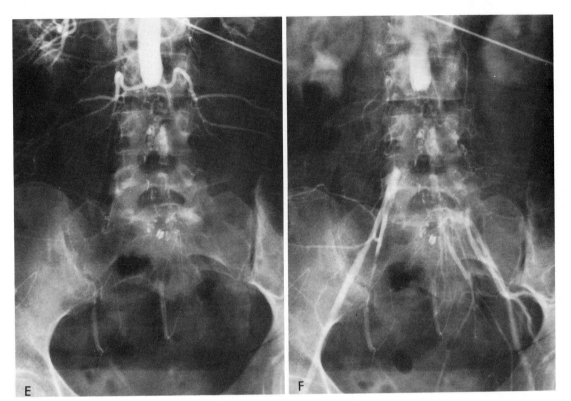

Figure 3–4. *E* and *F*. Lumbar artery collateral circulation in aortic occlusion. Translumbar aortogram in a 65 year old man with chronic claudication.

E. Early arterial phase. The aorta is occluded between the renal arteries and the bifurcation. The third lumbar arteries are markedly dilated.

F. Late arterial phase. The blood supply to both legs is reconstituted via the lumbar, gluteal and internal iliac arteries to the external iliac arteries. The collateral blood flow in this patient was adequate to produce femoral artery pulses.

Figure 3–4. *C* and *D*. Embolic occlusion of the abdominal aorta. Lumbar aortogram in a 61 year old woman with sudden loss of blood flow to the lower extremities.

C. An irregular embolus fills the aortic lumen at approximately the level of the aortic bifurcation. The renal arteries are well demonstrated, but the superior mesenteric artery is poorly visualized. An embolectomy was performed, and clot was also removed from the superior mesenteric artery.

D. Postoperative aortogram. The distal abdominal aorta has a normal appearance. The renal and celiac arteries are well demonstrated, but only the initial portion of the superior mesenteric artery is seen. The patient developed severe abdominal pain, and on reexploration the entire small bowel was ischemic.

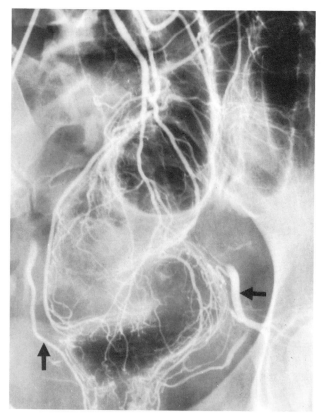

Figure 3–5. Pelvic collaterals from the inferior mesenteric circulation. Inferior mesenteric angiogram in a 42 year old man with claudication. The rectal branches of the superior hemorrhoidal artery fill pelvic branches (➡) of the internal iliac arteries, providing collateral blood supply to the pelvis and legs. (Courtesy of Dr. Leo Sheiner.)

Occlusive Disease at the Origins of the Celiac, Superior Mesenteric and Inferior Mesenteric Arteries

Atherosclerotic stenoses of the origins of the celiac and superior mesenteric arteries are usually caused by plaque deposition in the aorta at the vessel orifice. This type of narrowing is generally circumferential and is frequently present in older patients (Fig. 3–6). If the stenosis is severe enough to cause turbulent blood flow, there may be poststenotic dilatation. If the stenosis significantly lowers the distal blood pressure, collateral circulation develops from a non-stenosed artery to the stenosed artery. The gastroduodenal artery and arteries of the pancreas are the primary collateral pathway in stenoses of the celiac and superior mesenteric arteries. The posterior and anterior pancreaticoduodenal arcades dilate and elongate (Fig. 3–7). The dorsal pancreatic artery may also be a major source of collateral blood flow (Fig. 3–8). Less frequently,

the transverse pancreatic and pancreatica magna arteries become collateral pathways.

The inferior mesenteric artery is the most commonly occluded aortic visceral branch. The collateral blood supply to this artery comes primarily from the superior mesenteric artery through the middle colic–left colic arterial anastomoses. Collaterals to the superior hemorrhoidal artery also come from the pelvic branches of the internal iliac artery (see Fig. 3–5). Since the origin of the inferior mesenteric artery is often difficult to demonstrate on anteroposterior or lateral aortograms, visualization of collateral arteries is often the most satisfactory way to document occlusion. Not infrequently, two or all three major arteries are involved by atherosclerosis and will have some narrowing or occlusion (Fig. 3–9). When this occurs, one vessel sometimes carries the majority of the blood supply to the viscera, with the development of very prominent collateral channels to the other two arteries (Fig. 3–10). Such patients may have no abdominal complaints or may have

Text continued on page 77.

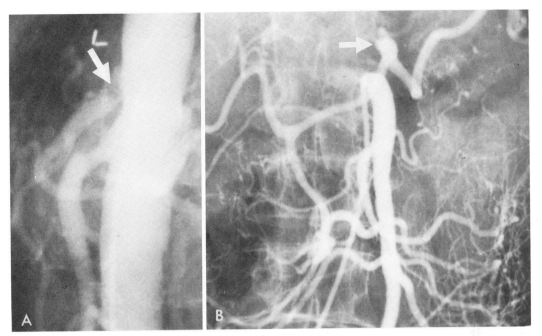

Figure 3-6. Celiac artery stenosis. Angiography in a 79 year old man with gastric carcinoma.

A. Lumbar aortogram in the lateral projection. The celiac artery is severely stenotic primarily from above (⟹), and there is about a 20 per cent circumferential stenosis of the superior mesenteric artery.

B. Superior mesenteric angiogram. The pancreatic arcades and the gastroduodenal artery provide the primary collateral pathway to the celiac trunk, which is entirely filled by this injection. The celiac artery (⟹) has the beaked appearance often seen in severe stenosis or occlusion.

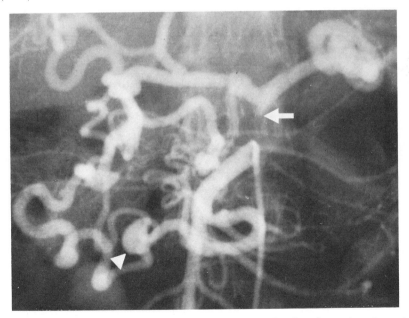

Figure 3-7. Collateral circulation through the pancreaticoduodenal arcades. Superior mesenteric angiogram in a 59 year old woman with abdominal pain. The posterior and anterior pancreaticoduodenal arcades are markedly dilated, and blood flows through these arteries to the gastroduodenal artery and to the entire celiac distribution. There is an aneurysm (▷) on the anterior pancreaticoduodenal arcade and some collateral blood flow through the dorsal pancreatic artery. The typical beak of a severely stenotic celiac artery (⟹) is present.

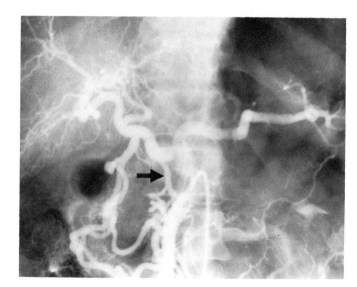

Figure 3-8. Collateral circulation through the dorsal pancreatic artery in celiac stenosis. Superior mesenteric angiogram in a 40 year old man with pancreatitis. Dilated pancreaticoduodenal arcades and a dilated dorsal pancreatic artery (➡) provide collateral blood supply to the entire celiac artery distribution. The celiac artery has a 95 per cent stenosis at its origin.

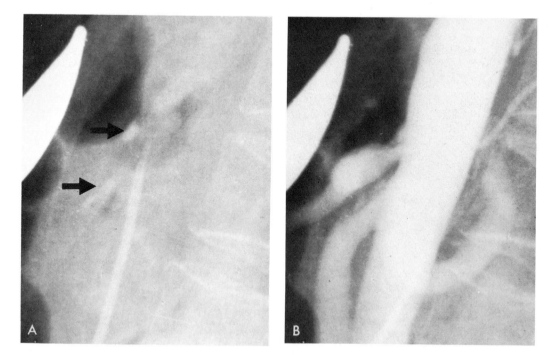

Figure 3-9. Atherosclerotic stenoses of the celiac and superior mesenteric arteries. Lumbar aortogram in a 68 year old woman with abdominal pain and bruit.

A. Preliminary film. Two linear vascular calcifications (➡) are demonstrated.

B. Lumbar aortogram in the lateral projection. The two calcifications are in the walls of the celiac and superior mesenteric arteries. The celiac stenosis is about 60 per cent, and a poststenotic dilatation is present.

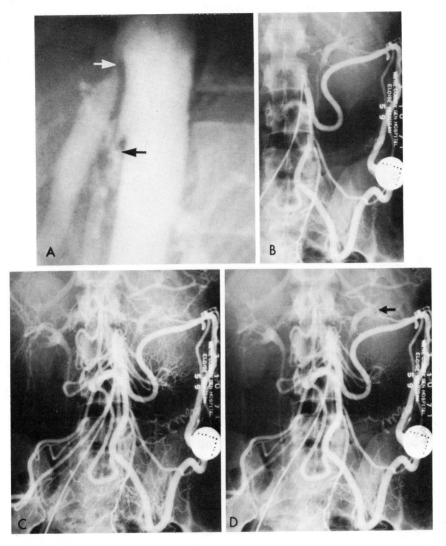

Figure 3-10. Superior mesenteric artery occlusion associated with a severe celiac stenosis in a 44 year old woman with hypertension.

A. Lateral lumbar aortogram. The celiac artery (⟹) is markedly stenotic, and the superior mesenteric artery is occluded (➡).

B. Inferior mesenteric angiogram. The left colic artery and the marginal artery of Drummond are dilated.

C. Slightly later arterial film. The superior mesenteric artery and its branches are filled by collateral flow through the middle colic artery. Early collateral circulation to the celiac artery is seen.

D. Still later arterial film. The hepatic arteries are filling through the pancreaticoduodenal arcades. The splenic artery receives unusual collaterals from the left colic artery (➡).

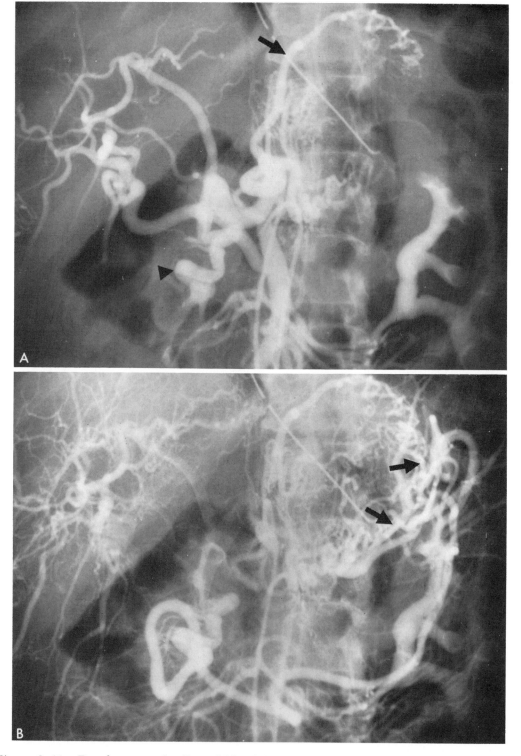

Figure 3–11. Development of collateral blood flow to the spleen following splenic artery occlusion. Simultaneous celiac–superior mesenteric angiogram in a 57 year old man with operative ligation of the splenic artery. The spleen was not removed.

A. Early arterial phase. The left gastric (➡) and gastroduodenal (▶) arteries are dilated.

B. The dilated left gastric artery supplies collateral blood flow to the distal splenic artery via many short gastric branches (➡). The gastroepiploic arteries are also dilated.

Figure 3–11 continued on opposite page.

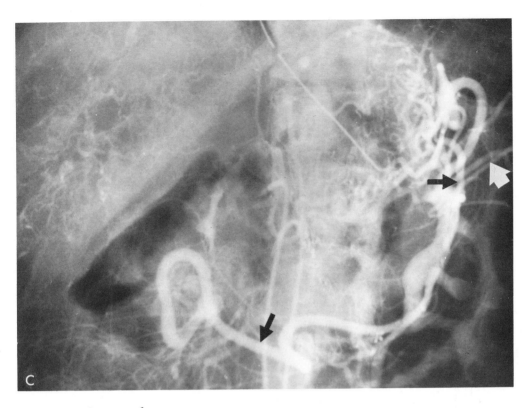

Figure 3-11. Continued.
C. The dilated right and left gastroepiploic arteries (➡) supply collateral blood flow to the distal splenic artery. The intrasplenic artery branches (⇨) can be seen.

symptoms of abdominal angina. When all three vessels are occluded, phrenic, lumbar and pelvic arterial collaterals are prominent (Matz and Kahn, 1968).

Occlusive Disease of Visceral Artery Branches

Stenoses of visceral artery branches are common in older patients. Stenosis or occlusion of the origin of any of the three major branches of the celiac artery produces specific collateral patterns. Splenic artery stenosis causes collaterals to develop through the tail of the pancreas, the gastroepiploic arteries and over the left and short gastric arteries (Fig. 3-11). Stenosis of the common hepatic artery leads to collateral flow through the posterior and anterior pancreaticoduodenal arcades and the gastroduodenal artery (Fig. 3-12). Stenoses or occlusions may also occur at the origins of

any of the superior mesenteric artery branches (Fig. 3-13). While diffuse atherosclerotic changes of these arteries are common in older patients, occlusions of branches are less frequent. When occlusions do occur, the many arcades of the superior mesenteric artery supply collateral circulation (Fig. 3-14).

Diffuse Small Artery Atherosclerosis

Diffuse atherosclerosis of the more peripheral visceral vessels is occasionally present, especially in patients with diabetes (Fig. 3-15). All the arteries are diffusely involved, and even the smallest have luminal irregularities. Collateral circulation is not a prominent feature in such patients. Perhaps because of the sclerosis, no artery is able to respond to blood need by dilatation. The spectrum of abnormali-

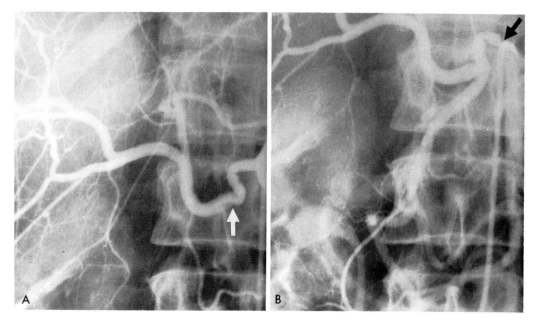

Figure 3–12. Hepatic artery stenosis with collateral blood flow through the pancreaticoduodenal arcades. Angiography in a 34 year old woman with nonspecific abdominal pain.

A. Celiac angiogram. The common hepatic artery is smaller than the proper hepatic artery and has an irregular contour. A negative flow defect (⟹) is seen, caused by nonopacified blood from the gastroduodenal artery.

B. Superior mesenteric angiogram. The hepatic circulation is well filled through dilated, elongated posterior and anterior pancreaticoduodenal arcades. The common hepatic artery stenosis is seen (➡).

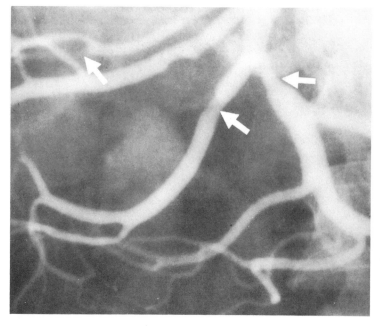

Figure 3–13. Superior mesenteric branch atherosclerosis with ectasia and plaques. Superior mesenteric angiogram in a 74 year old man with melanoma. The ileal arteries are ectatic and have many plaques (⟹) and some occlusions.

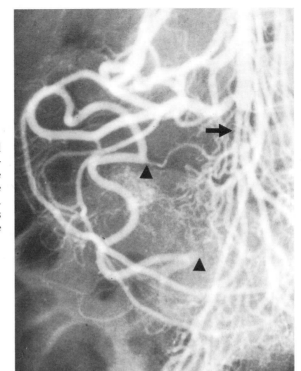

Figure 3-14. Superior mesenteric arterial branch occlusions. Superior mesenteric angiogram in a 74 year old woman with diffuse atherosclerosis. Several ileal arteries are narrowed or occluded near their origins (➡). Peripheral superior mesenteric artery arcades are dilated and supply blood flow to the occluded arteries (▶).

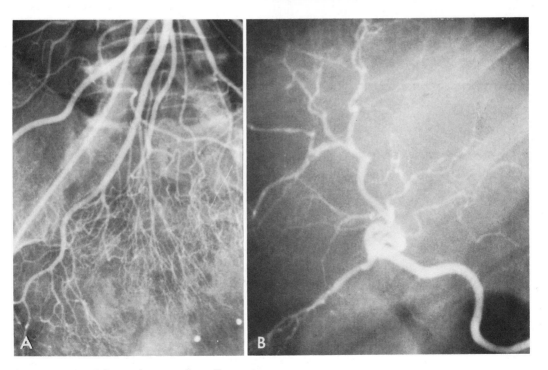

Figure 3-15. Atherosclerosis of small arteries.

A. Superior mesenteric angiogram in a 74 year old man with diabetes and chronic gastrointestinal bleeding. The vasa recta and distal ileal arteries are irregular and somewhat tortuous. Overall vascularity seems increased.

B. Hepatic angiogram in an 89 year old woman with pancreatic carcinoma. The hepatic artery branches are irregular and have many small aneurysms. Autopsy revealed diffuse atherosclerosis.

ties includes luminal irregularity without compromise of the lumen, irregular narrowing with dilatation or simply dilatation. These small atherosclerotic arteries may appear hypervascular, especially in the small bowel and colon.

Ectatic Atherosclerosis

The arterial changes caused by atherosclerosis discussed so far have been stenotic or occlusive. Atherosclerosis may also lead to arterial dilatation or elongation without definite aneurysm formation. This occurs commonly in the aorta and in the brachiocephalic and iliac arteries (Fig. 3–16). Ectasia is generally accompanied by plaque deposition so that the vessel lumen is irregular. Blood flow is usually slow, and the film series must be prolonged if peripheral arterial detail is to be obtained. The elongation can cause rotation of the abdominal aorta, distorting or displacing the origins of the celiac and superior mesenteric arteries. Selective catheterization is made difficult by the rotation, dilatation and tortuosity of the aorta. A catheter with appropriate iliac and aortic curves may have to be used for selective catheterization in these patients. Such a catheter can be shaped during the

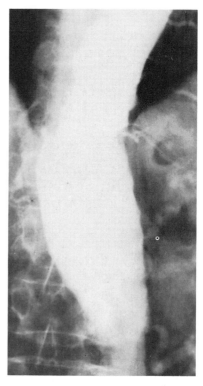

Figure 3–16. Ectasia of the thoracolumbar aorta. Aortogram in a 78 year old man. The aorta is dilated and has an irregular lumen. Blood flow is very slow. At operation, performed because of suspected rupture, the entire aorta was ectatic, and a clot-filled aneurysm just above the bifurcation showed evidence of leakage.

Figure 3–17. Atherosclerotic elongation of the splenic artery. Splenic angiogram in a 70 year old man with abdominal pain. The splenic artery is tortuous and elongated. The proximal splenic artery is narrow and irregular because of plaque deposition (⟹).

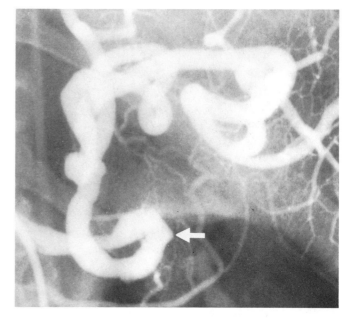

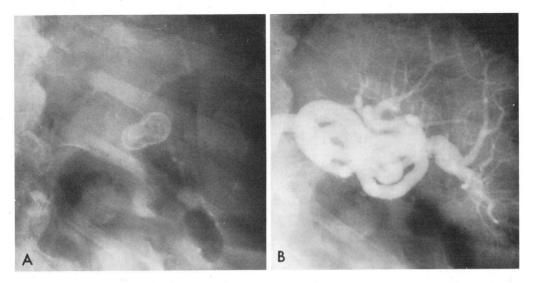

Figure 3–18. Splenic artery calcification. Splenic angiogram in an 82 year old woman with suspected pancreatic carcinoma.
   A. Preliminary film of the left upper quadrant shows curvilinear calcifications.
   B. Splenic angiogram. The splenic artery is markedly elongated and tortuous. The calcifications seen on the preliminary film are in loops of artery rather than in an aneurysm.

study and substituted for the initial one. The distal limb of the catheter should be longer than average to decrease catheter recoil during injection. The use of a torque control type of catheter is also frequently helpful, both in positioning and for stability during injection.

The major branches of the aorta can also undergo atherosclerotic dilatation and elongation. The splenic artery classically elongates with increasing age and may become quite tortuous (Fig. 3–17). Calcification may occur in its walls, simulating an aneurysm on plain films (Fig. 3–18). The superior mesenteric artery and its central branches may also become ectatic.

ANEURYSMS

Atherosclerotic Aneurysms

Atherosclerosis may cause aneurysms of the abdominal aorta (Fig. 3–19). These usually occur distal to the renal arteries but sometimes involve much of the thoracolumbar aorta (Fig. 3–20). If there is mural thrombus, the intercostal and lumbar arteries are generally occluded. In an occasional patient the mural thrombosis can fill

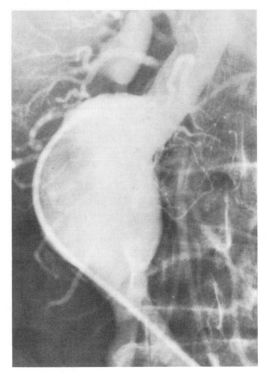

Figure 3–19. Aortic aneurysm below the renal artery origins. Lumbar aortogram in an 81 year old man. There is a large fusiform aneurysm of the distal abdominal aorta distal to the origins of the renal arteries. The catheter could not be advanced proximal to the aneurysm.

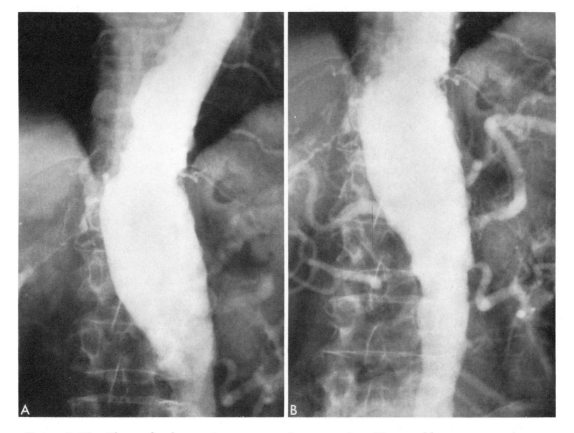

Figure 3-20. Thoracolumbar aortic aneurysm. Aortogram in a 66 year old man.
A. Thoracic aortogram. The thoracic portion of the aorta is ectatic, and irregular thrombus is present along both walls.
B. Lumbar aortogram. The upper lumbar aorta is dilated in a fusiform manner, and a moderate amount of thrombus is present along the walls of the aneurysm. The upper lumbar arteries are not seen. The distal abdominal aorta is irregular but normal in caliber.

part of the aneurysm, and the remaining lumen can appear to have a normal diameter. The nonvisualization of lumbar or intercostal arteries, however, should lead to the diagnosis of aneurysm. The inferior mesenteric artery is usually involved in these aneurysms and is frequently occluded. Collateral blood supply to the descending and sigmoid colons comes from the superior mesenteric artery through the middle-left colic artery anastomoses of the arch of Riolan or the marginal artery. Ultrasound should be used as the primary diagnostic procedure in a suspected aortic aneurysm, since the method has a high accuracy with no associated morbidity. Angiography need only be employed when the ultrasound demonstrates that the aneurysm extends above the renal arteries, and excision is planned.

Dissecting Aneurysms

Dissecting aneurysms almost always arise in the thoracic aorta, except when secondary to trauma, and they generally cause thoracic symptoms before reaching the lumbar aorta. Dissections may be caused by atherosclerosis, but the majority occur in patients with hypertension and cystic medial necrosis or in patients with Marfan's syndrome. Frequently a dissecting aneurysm cuts off circulation to some of the abdominal viscera, and occasionally this causes the initial symptoms. The classical appearance of a lumbar aortic dissecting aneurysm is a narrowed lumen with amputation of some major branches (Fig. 3-21A and B). These arteries may be occluded or may arise from the false lumen. They can

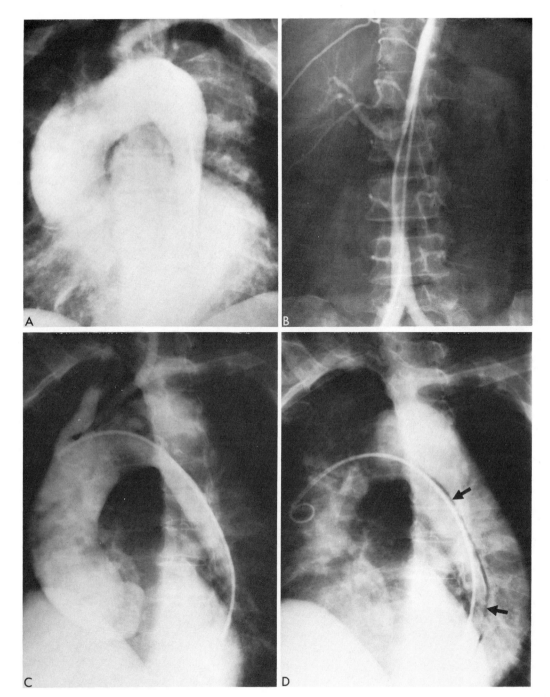

Figure 3-21. Dissecting aneurysms.

A and *B*. Dissecting aneurysm in a 61 year old woman with sudden onset of chest pain.

A. Thoracic aortogram. The dissection begins just beyond the origin of the left subclavian artery, and the true lumen becomes progressively narrowed as the aorta approaches the diaphragm.

B. Lumbar aortogram. The true lumen remains narrowed throughout the abdominal aorta. The right intercostal, lumbar and renal arteries arise from the true lumen. The celiac, superior mesenteric, inferior mesenteric, left renal, intercostal and upper left lumbar arteries arise from the false lumen and are not seen. The dissection terminates just above the aortic bifurcation.

C and *D*. Dissecting aneurysm. Thoracic aortogram in a 66 year old man with sudden onset of chest pain.

C. Early arterial phase. The dissection originates just distal to the left subclavian artery. A communication between the true and false lumina can be observed at the point of origin. During injection the catheter usually straightens and moves to the greater curvature of the aorta. Here, it moves only to the elevated intima.

D. Late arterial phase. Both the true and faluse lumina are filled with contrast medium, delineating the elevated intima (➡).

sometimes be demonstrated if the contrast medium is injected high enough to fill the false lumen and blood flow in the false lumen is adequate to allow such visualization. Also, if contrast medium enters the false lumen, the elevated intima separating the true and false lumina may be demonstrated (Fig. 3–21C and D).

If the femoral pulses are not compromised, suspected dissections can be studied by catheterization from a femoral artery. In the presence of diminished or absent femoral pulses, however, the axillary approach must be used. Catheterization of the false channel is not catastrophic, but manipulation of the guide wires and catheters in these patients should be performed gently, with constant fluoroscopic observation. The thoracic aorta should be studied in the lateral and right posterior oblique positions; the lumbar aorta can be studied in the anteroposterior projection.

Celiac and Superior Mesenteric Artery Aneurysms

Atherosclerotic aneurysms of the celiac (Fig. 3–22) and superior mesenteric (Fig. 3–23) arteries are rare, but should be considered in any patient with a pulsatile epigastric mass, especially when associated with epigastric pain (Naiken et al., 1962). These aneurysms may calcify (Weidner et al., 1970), cause bruits and rupture, and

they markedly distort the origin of the artery, making selective catheterization both difficult and risky. Although it has been stated that aneurysms of both vessels are more likely to be syphilitic or mycotic than atherosclerotic (McClelland and Duke, 1966; Thompson et al., 1965), most lesions seen today are of atherosclerotic origin.

Splenic Artery Aneurysms

Atherosclerotic aneurysms may occur along the main splenic artery or on its branches within the spleen. Those found on the main artery are usually atherosclerotic, although splenic artery aneurysms are not uncommon in patients with chronic pancreatitis (Fig. 3–24). In pancreatitis, the repeated bathing of the artery by pancreatic enzymes during acute attacks may weaken the wall, causing aneurysm formation. Splenic artery aneurysms occur two to three times more frequently in females than in males, and noncalcified splenic artery aneurysms may rupture spontaneously, especially during pregnancy. Calcified aneurysms are much less likely to rupture. Splenic artery aneurysms have been implicated in splenic infarction, either because of embolization or propagation of clot distal to the aneurysm.

Aneurysms on branches of the splenic artery are most frequently seen in patients with splenomegaly and portal hypertension

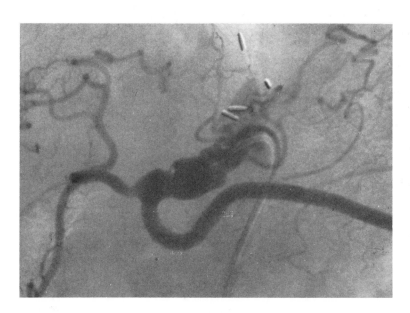

Figure 3–22. Atherosclerotic celiac artery aneurysm. Celiac angiogram in a 62 year old man with suspected pancreatic carcinoma. The celiac artery is aneurysmal throughout its course. The lumen is markedly irregular because of ulcerating atherosclerotic plaques. None of the celiac artery branches are affected by the aneurysm.

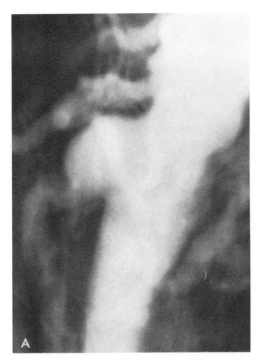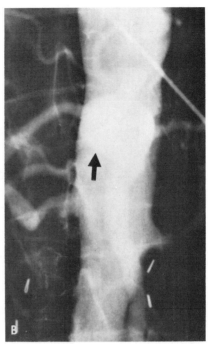

Figure 3-23. Superior mesenteric artery aneurysm. Translumbar aortogram in a 54 year old man with diffuse atherosclerosis.

A. Lateral projection. A saccular 2.5 by 3 cm aneurysm at the origin of the superior mesenteric artery is filled.

B. Anteroposterior projection. The aneurysm (➡) is superimposed on the abdominal aorta. Bilateral renal artery stenoses are present. (Courtesy of Dr. Roger Rian.)

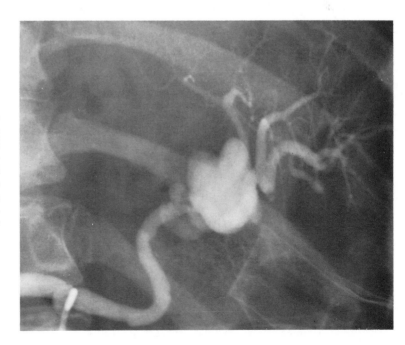

Figure 3-24. Splenic artery aneurysm. Celiac angiogram in a 28 year old man with chronic pancreatitis. An irregular bilobed aneurysm arises from the distal splenic artery. The aneurysm retained the contrast medium after the artery emptied.

(see Fig. 3–33), although they may occur in patients with splenomegaly alone. Other, less common, causes of aneurysms on splenic artery branches are atherosclerosis and polyarteritis nodosa.

Hepatic Artery Aneurysms

Hepatic artery aneurysms of atherosclerotic etiology (Fig. 3–25A and B) are un-common. Fewer than 200 have been reported in the world literature; however, they may be a source of right upper quadrant pain and bleeding. About 80 per cent are extrahepatic; the remainder are intraparenchymal and cannot be identified easily during surgery. These aneurysms can rupture, causing an abdominal catastrophe, but are most frequently found incidentally at surgery. An increasing cause of hepatic

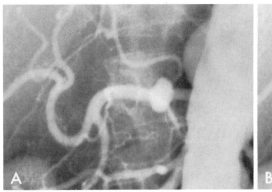 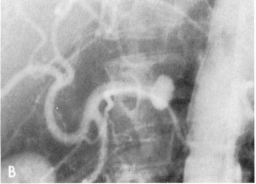

Figure 3–25. Common hepatic artery aneurysms.

A and *B*. Lumbar aortogram performed for hypertension in a 60 year old man.

A. Early arterial phase. A saccular aneurysm arises from the common hepatic artery about 1 cm distal to its origin from the celiac artery.

B. Late arterial film. The aneurysm remains well filled with contrast medium, and the hepatic arteries distal to the aneurysm empty somewhat more slowly than the other branches of the celiac artery.

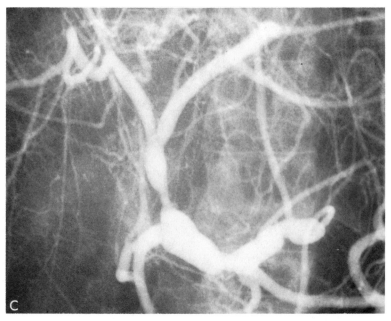

Figure 3–25. *C.* Celiac angiogram in a 64 year old woman following 7 days of infusion of chemotherapeutic agents through a catheter in the proper hepatic artery. A fusiform aneurysm is present on the common hepatic artery, and the proximal proper hepatic artery is narrowed. Such changes are common following prolonged placement of arterial catheters.

artery aneurysms is prolonged catheter placement in the hepatic artery for the infusion of chemotherapeutic drugs in patients with hepatic tumors (Fig. 3–25C).

Smaller Branch Aneurysms

Atherosclerotic aneurysms occur on the smaller branches of the celiac, superior mesenteric and inferior mesenteric arteries. Most frequently these aneurysms are incidental findings at angiography (Fig. 3–26. They have been described on the right gastroepiploic artery, the left gastric artery, jejunal, ileal and colic arteries and on a pancreatic arcade (see Fig. 3–7). The increasing use of visceral angiography will undoubtedly lead to the discovery of aneurysms on all visceral arteries. Many are of atherosclerotic origin, but occasion-

ally they are caused by trauma or infection. Aneurysms can be congenital, and these generally occur at arterial bifurcations.

Aneurysms on branches of the mesenteric arteries may rupture into the mesentery, causing a mesenteric hematoma, or, if the aneurysms are situated on marginal arteries, they may rupture into the lumen of the bowel, causing massive gastrointestinal bleeding. The angiographic appearance of aneurysms on marginal arteries to the colon, however, is almost indistinguishable from that of slowly bleeding diverticula. Since bleeding diverticular are much more common than marginal artery aneurysms, the former diagnosis should be favored when a rounded collection of contrast medium is seen on the colonic marginal artery in a patient with active lower gastrointestinal bleeding.

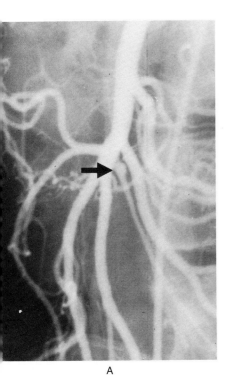
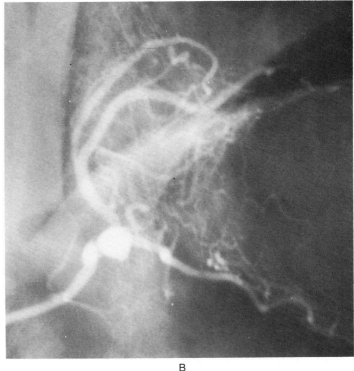

A   B

Figure 3–26. Aneurysms on small visceral arteries.

A. Jejunal artery aneurysm. Superior mesenteric angiogram in a 49 year old woman with abdominal trauma. A 4 mm aneurysm (➡) is present near the origin of the third jejunal artery.

B. Left gastric artery aneurysm. Left gastric angiogram in a 52 year old man with upper gastrointestinal bleeding. A 10 mm aneurysm is present on the distal portion of the main left gastric artery.

Mycotic Aneurysms

Mycotic aneurysms have become uncommon with the increased use of antibiotics, but such lesions can be fatal if not diagnosed and appropriately treated. These aneurysms cause a progressive destruction of the arterial wall with ultimate rupture. Usually only diseased arteries become involved, since the normal intima is highly resistant to infection. Multiple mycotic aneurysms are not uncommon and have a hematogenous distribution. At angiography, these aneurysms cannot be distinguished from those of other causes, but aneurysms of the first portion of the celiac artery and the superior mesenteric artery are frequently mycotic. Mycotic aneurysms are generally saccular, but this is not a diagnostic feature. The rapid development of an aneurysm in a febrile patient should suggest a mycotic origin.

SYNDROMES ASSOCIATED WITH VISCERAL VASCULAR OCCLUSIVE DISEASE

Although visceral occlusive changes are common and generally cause no symptoms, some patients with occlusive disease become symptomatic. Two syndromes, abdominal angina and median arcuate ligament compression, are fairly well established.

Abdominal Angina

Abdominal angina is a controversial syndrome consisting of postprandial abdominal pain associated with weight loss, anorexia, diarrhea, malabsorption and occasional nausea and vomiting. An abdominal bruit may be present. This syndrome is believed by some to be a precursor of acute mesenteric infarction. Significant stenosis or occlusion of two or more of the celiac, superior mesenteric and inferior mesenteric arteries was initially thought to be necessary to cause this syndrome, but more recently, celiac artery stenosis alone has been considered sufficient. The symptoms are believed to be a manifestation of gastrointestinal ischemia brought on by the increased demand on the splanchnic circulation by digestion. Precisely what portion of the viscera gives rise to pain is not known.

Stenosis of one or more of these three arteries is frequent, occurring in at least one of every six abdominal angiograms. Most of these patients do not have abdominal angina, though some may have nonspecific abdominal pain. Indeed, some individuals have complete occlusion of two or all three of these arteries without any abdominal symptoms. Why some patients are symptomatic while others with similar angiographic findings are not is one of the puzzling aspects of the syndrome of abdominal angina. The varying ability of each individual to develop a collateral circulation may be a factor. Because of varied embryologic development, anastomoses between these three vascular beds differ. Vascular ligation during previous surgery may also limit the potential for development of collaterals. The number and size of collaterals are also not indications of clinical significance. Abdominal angina, however, should always be considered in the angiographic evaluation of a patient with obscure abdominal pain in whom no other disease can be found.

Several types of vascular stenosis can lead to abdominal angina. Atherosclerosis can cause stenosis or occlusion of the origins of all three vessels by plaque deposition. These stenoses are generally circumferential in nature and occur at the vessel origins. Aortic atherosclerosis or other systemic atherosclerosis is usually present. Lateral aortography demonstrates the stenoses well, and anteroposterior selective injection of the nonstenotic arteries will show the collateral arterial supply (see Fig. 3–10).

Uncommon causes of abdominal angina have been described. Aneurysms of the superior mesenteric and hepatic arteries have been implicated. Fibromuscular hyperplasia of the celiac artery (Fig. 3–27) and congenital celiac artery occlusion have also been reported. Adhesions from surgery or inflammatory disease or an encasing neoplasm (Fig. 3–28) that produces vascular stenoses can also cause abdominal angina.

A lateral aortogram should be performed first. The filming sequence for the lateral study should cover the arterial phase and

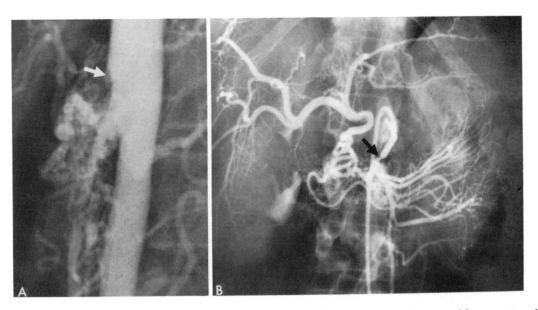

Figure 3–27. Fibromuscular hyperplasia of the visceral arteries in a 40 year old woman with abdominal angina. An anteroposterior lumbar aortogram revealed bilateral renal artery changes characteristic of fibromuscular hyperplasia.

A. Lateral lumbar aortogram. The celiac artery is occluded, (⟹) and the superior mesenteric artery is narrowed. Several collateral arteries are present anterior to the aorta, communicating between the superior mesenteric and hepatic arteries.

B. Superior mesenteric angiogram. There is irregular narrowing of the proximal portion of the superior mesenteric artery (➡). Collateral blood flow has developed from the superior mesenteric artery to the hepatic artery over dilated pancreaticoduodenal arcades and the gastroduodenal artery.

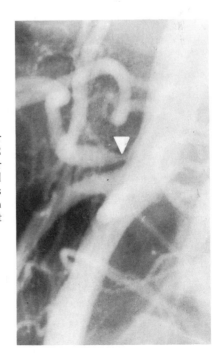

Figure 3–28. Lymphosarcoma encircling the lumbar aorta and the celiac artery. Lateral lumbar aortogram in a 42 year old man being evaluated for abdominal pain. The lumbar aorta is displaced ventrally and narrowed by a retroperitoneal mass. The celiac artery has about 75 per cent stenosis at its origin (▷). At exploration, lymphosarcoma in the lymph nodes of the retroperitoneum encircled the aorta and the root of the celiac artery.

can be limited to two films per second for 2 to 4 seconds. The catheter should be placed so that the side holes are at the level of the celiac artery, and contrast medium should be injected at about 20 cc per second for 2 seconds. The need for an anteroposterior aortogram and any selective studies will depend upon the lateral aortogram. Selective angiograms should be performed when the lateral aortogram is normal, in an attempt to find a cause for the patient's symptoms. When vascular stenoses are demonstrated on the lateral aortogram, selective angiograms may be indicated to exclude other causes of abdominal pain.

Median Arcuate Ligament Compression Syndrome

The median arcuate ligament of the diaphragm can compress the celiac artery. Such compression is usually associated with an epigastric bruit which may vary in intensity during respiration and is most often heard in young women. The lateral aortogram shows a characteristic concave impression on the cranial surface of the celiac artery just beyond its origin (Fig. 3–29). If the aortogram is performed in both full inspiration and full expiration, the degree of stenosis usually changes, generally increasing with expiration and decreasing or disappearing with inspiration (Fig. 3–30). The median arcuate ligament compression syndrome is controversial. Some authors doubt its existence, and, among those who accept the syndrome, at least two schools of thought exist about the etiology of symptoms. One group believes that vascular ischemia of some part of the splanchnic bed is responsible. The second group postulates a neural origin for the symptoms. In any case, the angiographic appearance of median arcuate ligament compression is consistent and is rarely mimicked by atherosclerosis.

It is often possible to catheterize the celiac artery in these patients, particularly if the attempt is made during deep inspiration. Since the catheter tip lies beyond the stenosis, no abnormalities may be seen on such an angiographic series. Injection of the superior mesenteric artery, however, generally shows filling of some or all of the celiac distribution through dilated, elongated pancreaticoduodenal arcades.

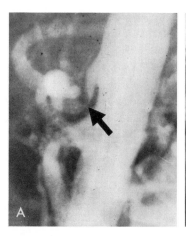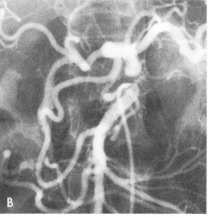

Figure 3–29. Superior mesenteric to celiac artery collaterals in median arcuate ligament compression of the celiac artery. Angiography in a 34 year old woman with abdominal pain.

A. Lateral lumbar aortogram. The celiac artery is nearly completely occluded by a typical rounded superior impression (➡) of the median arcuate ligament.

B. Superior mesenteric angiogram. Both the pancreaticoduodenal arcades and the dorsal pancreatic artery are elongated and dilated. The entire celiac trunk is filled through these collateral channels.

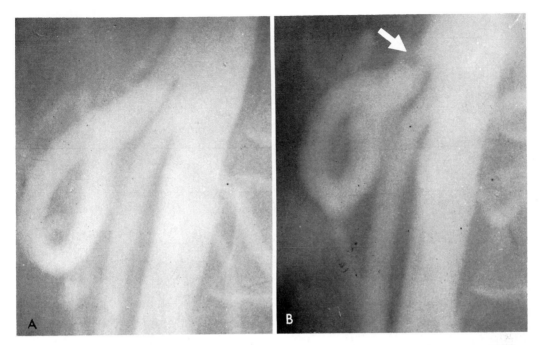

Figure 3–30. Median arcuate ligament compression of the celiac artery with respiratory variation in degree of compression. Lumbar aortogram in a 21 year old woman with abdominal bruit.

A. Full inspiration. The origin of the celiac artery is smooth and there is no stenosis.

B. Full expiration. The origin of the celiac artery now has about a 40 per cent stenosis ($\implies$) caused by median arcuate ligament compression from above. (From Reuter, S. R.: Accentuation of celiac compression by the median arcuate ligament of the diaphragm during deep expiration. Radiology 98:561, 1971.)

POLYARTERITIS NODOSA

Polyarteritis nodosa is a rather poorly understood disease characterized by progressive necrotizing arteritis of the medium and small arteries. The symptom complex of an individual patient depends on the organs involved. The gastrointestinal tract is involved in 51 per cent of patients and the liver in 66 per cent (Capps and Klein, 1970). The kidneys have an 80 per cent rate of involvement. Areas which are easily biopsied, such as skin and skeletal muscle, are involved in only 20 and 30 per cent of patients, respectively.

The typical angiographic findings in polyarteritis nodosa include multiple fusiform or saccular aneurysms associated with irregular caliber of the medium and small arteries (Fig. 3–31). The number of arteries in the involved organ may also be decreased. The aneurysms may rupture, causing hemorrhage into the perirenal, retroperitoneal or intraperitoneal spaces, which may be fatal.

In polyarteritis nodosa, angiography may be used as a diagnostic test for assessment of the extent of pathologic involvement or to locate the site of acute bleeding. Such studies should include aortography and renal angiography to evaluate the retroperitoneum, as well as selective injections of the celiac, superior mesenteric and inferior mesenteric arteries.

Only polyarteritis produces an angiographic appearance of extensive small aneurysm formation with associated vascular irregularity. Citron et al. (1970) have reported necrotizing angiitis in young people following multiple drug abuse (Fig. 3–32). The pathologic and angiographic appearances are the same as in polyarteritis nodosa.

Multiple aneurysms are seen in several other diseases. In portal hypertension, many intrasplenic aneurysms have been reported at arterial bifurcations (Fig. 3–33), and intrasplenic aneurysms have been seen after splenoportography (Boijsen and Efsing, 1967). These aneurysms are not as-

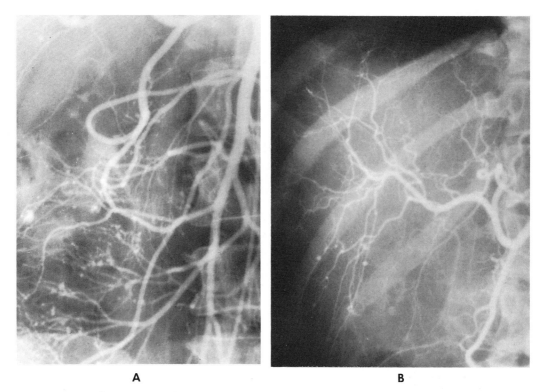

A **B**

Figure 3–31. Polyarteritis nodosa.

A. Superior mesenteric angiogram in a 26 year old woman with polyarteritis nodosa. Several small aneurysms are demonstrated on the mesenteric artery branches. Renal and peripheral artery aneurysms were also present in this patient. (Courtesy of Dr. Joseph J. Bookstein).

B. Celiac angiogram in a 15 year old boy with polyarteritis nodosa. Several small aneurysms are present on branches of the right hepatic artery.

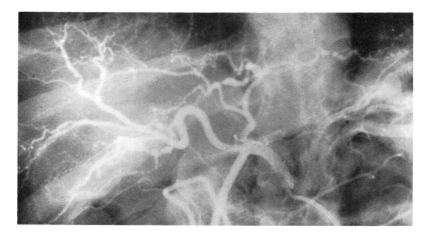

Figure 3–32. Necrotizing angiitis. Celiac angiogram in a 24 year old woman who had been injecting methedrine and cocaine intravenously for about 4 months. The liver is small. All intrahepatic arteries are beaded and irregular. The cystic and left hepatic arteries are most severely involved, and some branches are occluded. The pancreatic and renal arteries were also involved. Liver biopsy showed necrotizing angiitis.

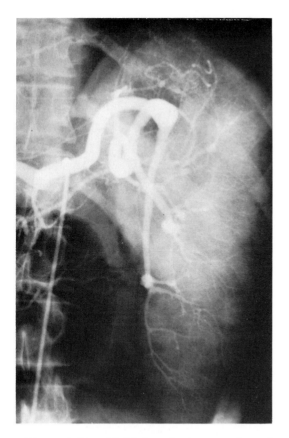

Figure 3–33. Multiple splenic artery branch aneurysms associated with portal hypertension. Celiac angiogram in a 34 year old woman with cirrhosis and portal hypertension. The spleen is markedly enlarged. Several aneurysms are seen throughout the spleen, occurring predominantly at splenic artery branchings.

sociated with lesions in other organs and should not be confused with polyarteritis nodosa. Occasionally, severe, diffuse atherosclerosis may suggest the changes of polyarteritis nodosa (Fig. 3–34), but ath-

erosclerotic involvement of major arteries will help establish the correct diagnosis.

MISCELLANEOUS VASCULAR ABNORMALITIES

Embolic Phenomena

Emboli from various sources, such as valve prostheses, angiographic catheter clots, rheumatic heart lesions and ulcerated atherosclerotic plaques, occasionally are demonstrated at angiography. The angiogram generally shows abrupt, rounded cutoffs of major vessels (Fig. 3–35) and pruning of peripheral arteries (Fig. 3–36). Arteries proximal to the emboli may show marked constriction (Pollard and Nebesar, 1968), and blood flow may be irregularly slowed. Collateral circulation is sometimes present. The parenchymal accumulation of contrast medium may be decreased peripheral to the emboli compared to areas with normal circulation (Fig. 3–37). Emboli may be solitary or multiple. Angiograms performed weeks after the acute stage may show recanalization of the obstructed arteries. The new channels are irregular in caliber and may have a somewhat tortuous course.

Nonocclusive Mesenteric Ischemia

Blood flow to the bowel can be markedly decreased in the absence of morphologic narrowing of the mesenteric arteries. The decreased blood flow occurs because of physiologic redistribution of blood in pa-

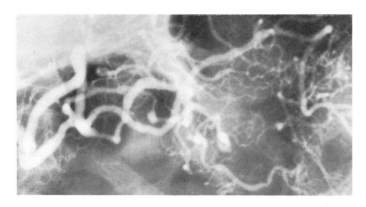

Figure 3–34. Diffuse visceral atherosclerosis. Splenic angiogram in a 72 year old man with diffuse systemic atherosclerosis, including the coronary and peripheral arteries. The splenic artery divides early, and the branches have multiple irregularities with stenoses and aneurysms. Similar atherosclerotic changes were present in the remainder of the celiac and superior mesenteric artery branches.

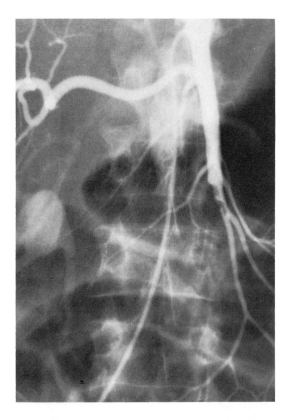

Figure 3–35. Superior mesenteric artery embolism. Arterial phase of a superior mesenteric angiogram in a 53 year old woman with mitral heart disease and atrial fibrillation. A bilobed embolus occludes the midportion of the superior mesenteric artery, after it has given off the jejunal branches. No blood supply is seen to the distal ileum.

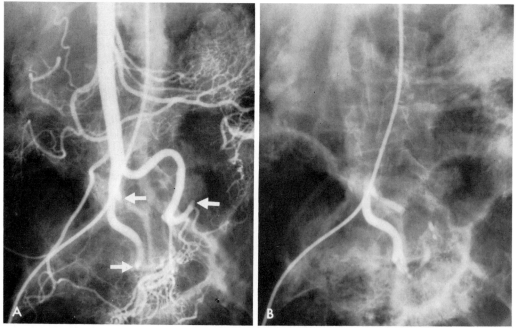

Figure 3–36. Multiple emboli to the superior mesenteric artery. Superior mesenteric angiogram in a 79 year old woman with atrial fibrillation who presented with symptoms of malabsorption.

A. Arterial phase. Several ileal branches are occluded ($\Rightarrow$) proximally. The involved small bowel is supplied through mesenteric anastomoses.

B. Venous phase. Contrast medium remains in the obstructed arteries while the superior mesenteric veins from the remainder of the small bowel begin to fill. (Courtesy of Dr. Philip A. Hoskins.)

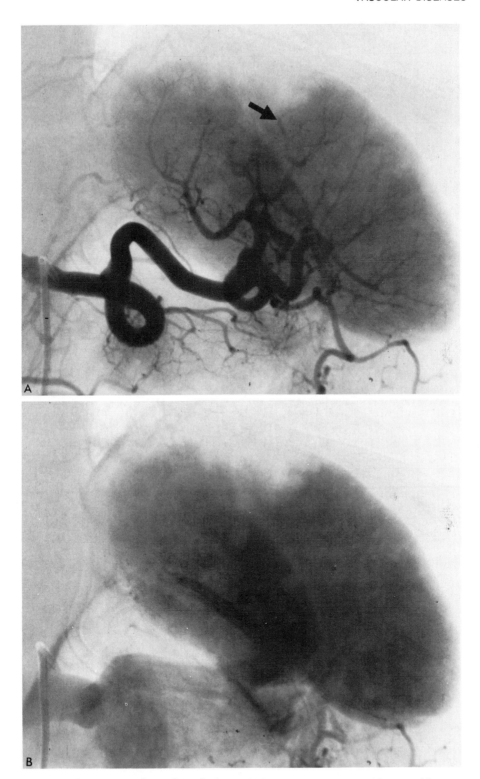

Figure 3–37. Splenic artery branch embolism. Celiac angiogram in a 28 year old woman.

A. Arterial phase. Subtraction technique. A wedge-shaped defect can be seen in the periphery of the upper pole of the spleen. One of the splenic artery branches is occluded (➡).

B. Venous phase. Subtraction technique. The wedge-shaped defect stands out against the homogeneous contrast opacification through the spleen.

tients with hypovolemic shock or digitalis toxicity. Nonocclusive mesenteric ischemia is probably the most common cause of small bowel infarction.

In patients with hypovolemic shock or digitalis toxicity, there is an intense vaso-constriction of the mesenteric arteries. This vasoconstriction is frequently seen in patients undergoing angiography because of massive gastrointestinal bleeding. In patients with hemorrhagic shock, the vasoconstriction reverses when the bleeding

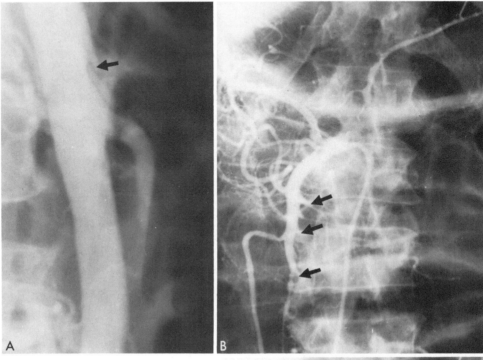

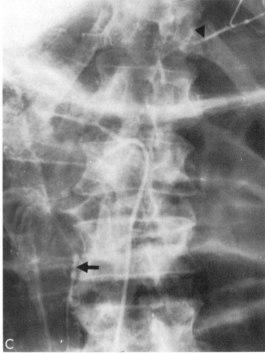

Figure 3–38. Severe nonocclusive mesenteric ischemia. Aortogram and superior mesenteric angiogram in a 68 year old man with severe abdominal pain.

A. Aortogram. The celiac artery (➡) is stenosed, and the midportion of the superior mesenteric artery is markedly narrowed.

B. Arterial phase of a superior mesenteric angiogram. There is abrupt narrowing of the jejunal and ileal branches of the superior mesenteric artery shortly after their origin (➡), and the terminal portion of the superior mesenteric artery has a beaded appearance. The right hepatic artery is replaced to the superior mesenteric artery, and collateral blood flow through the pancreas supplies a narrowed splenic artery distal to the area of celiac stenosis.

C. Venous phase. Contrast accumulation in the right colon is moderately increased, but the blood flow in the superior mesenteric and splenic arteries is markedly slowed. The beaded terminal portions of the superior mesenteric artery (➡) and the distal splenic artery (▶) are still filled with contrast medium.

has ceased and the blood volume returns toward normal. In such patients, bowel necrosis does not occur. However, if the cause of the vasoconstriction is not removed, persistent vasoconstriction can lead to bowel necrosis.

Nonocclusive mesenteric ischemia seems to be a more severe process in the small bowel than in the colon. In the colon, the entity leads to the development of ischemic colitis (described under the section on colitis in Chapter 7) and, rarely, to bowel necrosis. In the small bowel, however, persistent nonocclusive mesenteric ischemia commonly results in death. Unfortunately, as with occlusive intestinal ischemia, the symptoms are not specific, and the problem is not recognized clinically until bowel necrosis develops.

The angiographic appearance of nonocclusive small bowel ischemia is intense constriction of the superior mesenteric ar-

tery and its branches. In the early stages, the vasoconstriction appears similar to that seen in hypovolemic shock. The superior mesenteric artery and its branches are narrowed, and blood flow is slowed. As the vasoconstriction persists, localized narrowings appear at the origins of major branches of the superior mesenteric arteries, and the branches develop a beaded appearance, with narrowed segments of the superior mesenteric artery branches alternating with segments of normal lumen (Fig. 3–38).

Recently, Siegelman et al. (1974) have reversed the vasoconstriction by the injection of papaverine into the superior mesenteric artery. These investigators first use an infusion of 3 mg of papaverine per minute into the superior mesenteric artery for 20 minutes followed by a final bolus of 30 mg. If the mesenteric vasoconstriction is reversed by this test infusion (Fig. 3–39), they continue an infusion of 0.75 mg of

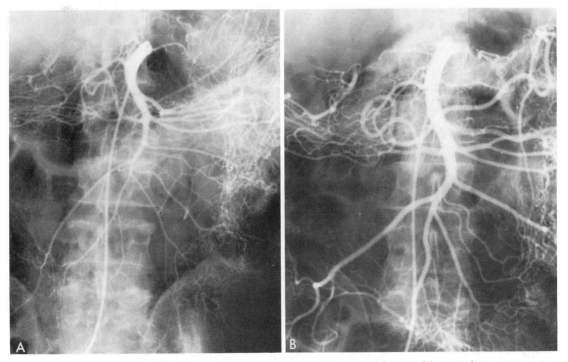

Figure 3–39. Reversal of nonocclusive mesenteric ischemia with vasodilator infusion. Superior mesenteric angiogram in a 62 year old man with hypovolemic shock.

A. Arterial phase of a superior mesenteric angiogram done while the patient was in shock. The superior mesenteric artery and all of its branches are markedly narrowed, and the blood flow is slowed.

B. Superior mesenteric angiogram following the infusion of Priscoline (similar in effect to papaverine at a rate of 3 mg per minute for 20 minutes. The superior mesenteric artery and its branches now have a normal caliber and a normal rate of blood flow.

papaverine per minute for an additional 16 to 20 hours. If the vasoconstriction and beaded appearance of the arteries persist even after the test infusion, they consider that infarction has occurred and that the vasoconstriction is irreversible. It is essential, of course, to diagnose and correct the conditions that have led to the mesenteric arterial vasoconstriction while the infusion of the vasodilator is taking place.

Drug Toxicity

Ergotism can cause irregular narrowing of the mesenteric and hepatic arteries (Fig. 3–40), which have areas of marked narrowing alternating with areas of normal caliber. The involved segments may be long and smooth or short and somewhat irregular. The findings in ergotism are much more common in the peripheral circulation.

These vascular changes will revert to normal as the drug toxicity regresses.

Intraarterial barbiturates will cause severe vascular spasm. Methysergide occasionally causes severe retroperitoneal fibrosis and can cause arterial as well as venous stenosis.

Pseudoxanthoma Elasticum

Pseudoxanthoma elasticum is an hereditary disease causing widespread degeneration of elastic fibers. Early calcification of the arterial intima and media often occurs. Peripheral vascular occlusions due to intimal proliferation and gastrointestinal hemorrhage are also part of the disease. Angiography has demonstrated angiomatous malformations, aneurysms of small arteries and irregular arterial narrowings (Fig. 3–41) (Bardsley et al., 1969).

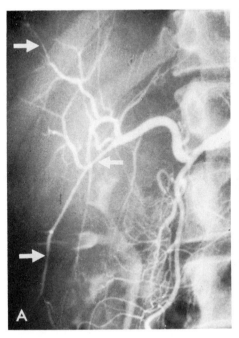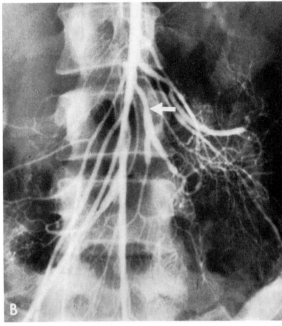

Figure 3–40. Arterial changes of ergotism. Angiography in a 33 year old woman with ergotism.
A. Hepatic angiogram. Intrahepatic arteries have intermittent, smooth narrowings (⟹).
B. Superior mesenteric angiogram. Smooth arterial dilatations and narrowings (⟹) are present. (Courtesy of Dr. Joseph J. Bookstein.)

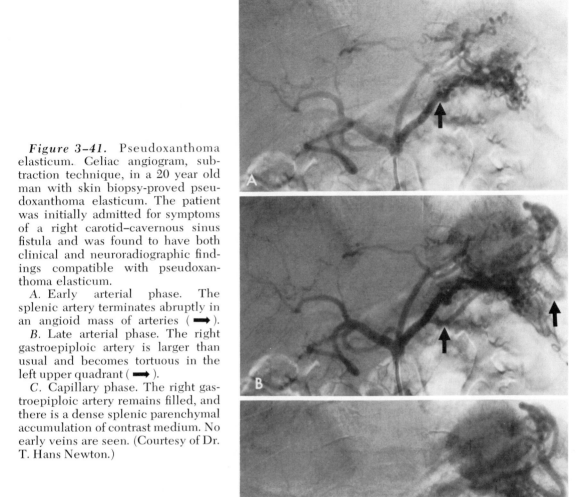

Figure 3–41. Pseudoxanthoma elasticum. Celiac angiogram, subtraction technique, in a 20 year old man with skin biopsy-proved pseudoxanthoma elasticum. The patient was initially admitted for symptoms of a right carotid–cavernous sinus fistula and was found to have both clinical and neuroradiographic findings compatible with pseudoxanthoma elasticum.

A. Early arterial phase. The splenic artery terminates abruptly in an angioid mass of arteries (➡).

B. Late arterial phase. The right gastroepiploic artery is larger than usual and becomes tortuous in the left upper quadrant (➡).

C. Capillary phase. The right gastroepiploic artery remains filled, and there is a dense splenic parenchymal accumulation of contrast medium. No early veins are seen. (Courtesy of Dr. T. Hans Newton.)

Takayasu's Arteritis

Takayasu's arteritis was thought initially to involve only the thoracic aorta and its major branches, but further observations of this disease have shown that the abdominal aorta and its branches may also be involved (Fig. 3–42). The disease is a primary arteritis of unknown etiology, more frequently seen in women. Stenosis and occlusion, as well as dilatation and aneurysm formation, may occur (Hachiya, 1970). In general, the course is progressive for a period of years; the disease then becomes inactive or quiescent. The superior mesenteric artery is more frequently involved than either the celiac or inferior mesenteric artery (Gotsman et al., 1967). Stenosis is more common than dilatation, and prominent collateral circulation may be present. Symptoms similar to abdominal angina have been described in one patient with celiac involvement. Death secondary to

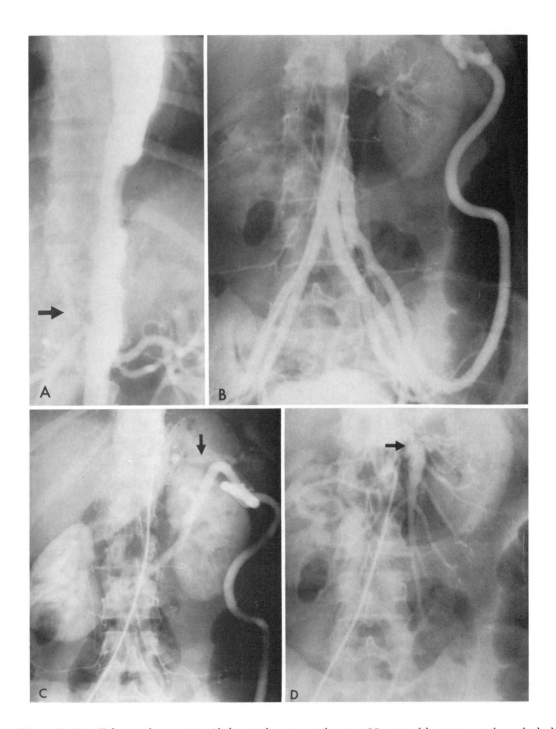

Figure 3-42. Takayasu's arteritis. Abdominal aortography in a 30 year old woman with occluded subclavian arteries, hypertension and an epigastric bruit. Thoracic aortography demonstrated bilateral subclavian artery occlusion.

A. The distal thoracic and proximal lumbar aorta is markedly irregular in contour. The celiac and superior mesenteric arteries are occluded. Stenoses are present at the origin of both renal arteries. The right inferior adrenal artery (➡) is enlarged and probably provides collateral circulation to the celiac artery.

B. The inferior mesenteric artery and the marginal artery of Drummond are markedly enlarged.

C. The middle colic artery supplies collateral circulation directly to the splenic artery (➡). The celiac artery fills in a retrograde manner.

D. The superior mesenteric artery is reconstituted at its origin (➡) by the middle colic artery. Its peripheral branches are intact. (Courtesy of Dr. Morton Glickman.)

100

ischemic rupture of the bowel has also been described. Marked involvement of the abdominal aorta with long segment coarctation is not uncommon. In such patients, the origins of the visceral vessels may be compromised by intimal proliferation. Abdominal aortic occlusion may also occur with collateral circulation developing in a fashion similar to that seen with atherosclerotic occlusion.

Nonspecific Arteritis

Nonspecific visceral arteritis is occasionally encountered during angiography. In our experience, such patients may have symptoms of pancreatic neoplasm. Angiography demonstrates arterial irregularities, occlusions and, sometimes, collateral blood flow (Fig. 3–43). The arterial changes can be similar to encasement by neoplasm. Arterial involvement in several organs will help in making the correct diagnosis.

VENOUS VASCULAR DISEASE

Venous abnormalities can occasionally be demonstrated at visceral angiography. Normally, the superior mesenteric venous branches appear simultaneously or clockwise from jejunal to ileal to colonic intestinal segments. Early, late or absent venous drainage from a specific area should be noted. Venous contours are generally smooth but often indistinct. The most reliable method available for enhancing venous visualization is pharmacoangiography. Various drugs used for this purpose are discussed in Chapter 10. The subtraction technique is also important in the visualization of venous abnormalities.

Portal vein thrombosis can generally be demonstrated by angiography. A long, large injection of contrast medium into either the splenic or superior mesenteric artery at 10 to 14 cc per second for 4 to 6 seconds, accompanied by a prolonged film series of 25 seconds or more, will usually demonstrate

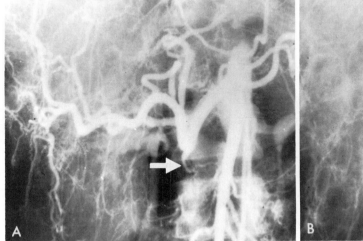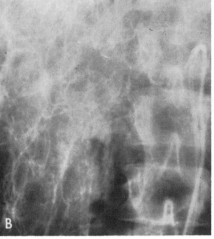

Figure 3–43. Small vessel arteritis. Combined celiac–superior mesenteric angiogram in a 34 year old woman with marked weight loss and abdominal pain. At autopsy, a diffuse nonspecific arteritis of the medium and small arteries was found.

A. Arterial phase. The gastroduodenal artery (⟹) is diminutive, and the right gastroepiploic artery is occluded. The intrahepatic arteries are irregular, some are occluded and many small collateral arteries are filled.

B. Parenchymal phase. The intrahepatic arteries empty slowly and unevenly. The parenchymal accumulation of contrast medium in the liver is irregular.

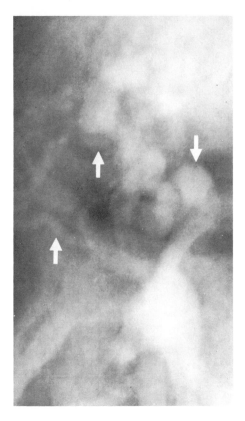

Figure 3–44. Occluded portal vein. Superior mesenteric angiogram in a 76 year old woman with recurrent upper gastrointestinal hemorrhage. Venous phase. The superior mesenteric vein drains into a wormian collection of collateral veins (⇨) in the liver hilum. No portal vein is seen. At exploration, portal cavernomatous transformation was found, probably caused by omphalitis. (From Redman, H. C., and Reuter, S. R.: Angiographic demonstration of surgically important vascular variations. Surg. Gynec. Obstet. *129*:33, 1969. By permission of Surgery, Gynecology & Obstetrics.)

the absence of a true portal vein and will show the wormian collection of collateral veins which replace it (Fig. 3–44). Collateral veins may also drain to systemic veins. The portal–systemic collateral veins that develop in portal vein thrombosis and he-

patic vein thrombosis are discussed in Chapter 8.

Splenic vein occlusion is generally caused by pancreatic disease, either carcinoma or pancreatitis. The blood from the spleen bypasses the obstruction over the

Figure 3–45. Occluded splenic vein. Splenoportogram in a 54 year old man with gastric varices. A pseudocyst in the tail of the pancreas had been drained 2 years earlier. The contrast medium drains from the injected pool in the splenic pulp via short gastric veins communicating through gastric varices to the left gastric vein and the portal vein, bypassing the splenic vein occlusion. No contrast medium is seen in the splenic vein.

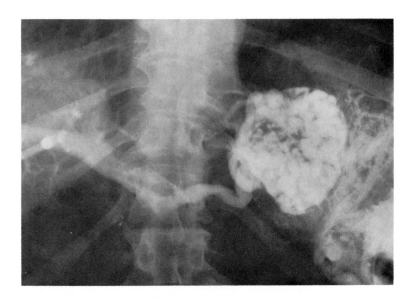

left and right gastroepiploic veins (see Fig. 4–67), the short gastric and left gastric veins (Fig. 3–45) and the arch of Barkow.

BIBLIOGRAPHY

Aakhus, T., and Brabrand, G.: Angiography in acute superior mesenteric arterial insufficiency. Acta Radiol. (Stockh.) 6:1, 1967.

Alvares, F., Parsonnet, V., and Brief, D. K.: Mycotic aneurysm of the superior mesenteric artery. Amer. J. Surg. 111:237, 1966.

Bardsley, J. L., and Koehler, P. R.: Pseudoxanthoma elasticum: angiographic manifestations in abdominal vessels. Radiology 93:559, 1969.

Baum, S., Greenstein, R. H., Nusbaum, M., et al.: Diagnosis of ruptured, noncalcified splenic artery aneurysm by selective celiac arteriography. Arch. Surg. 91:1026, 1965.

Baum, S., Nusbaum, M., Blakemore, W. S., et al.: The preoperative radiographic demonstration of intra-abdominal bleeding from undetermined sites by percutaneous selective celiac and superior mesenteric arteriography. Surgery 58:797, 1965.

Baum, S., Stein, G. N., and Baue, A.: Extrinsic pressure defects on the duodenal loop in mesenteric occlusive disease. Radiology 85:866, 1965.

Berger, R. L., and Byrne, J. J.: Intestinal gangrene associated with heart disease. Surg. Gynec. Obstet. 112:529, 1961.

Bergner, L. H., and Bentivegna, S. S.: Aneurysms of the splenic artery. Ann. Surg. 166:767, 1967.

Bertho, E., Ratte, J., Jean, J., et al.: Iatrogenic ergotism. Angiology 20:455, 1967.

Boijsen, E., Göthlin, J., Hallböök, T., et al.: Preoperative angiographic diagnosis of bleeding aneurysms of abdominal visceral arteries. Radiology 93:781, 1969.

Boijsen, E., and Efsing, H.-O.: Aneurysm of the splenic artery. Acta Radiol. (Diagn.) (Stockh.) 8:29, 1969.

Boijsen, E., and Efsing, H.-O.: Intrasplenic arterial aneurysms following splenoportal phlebography. Acta Radiol. 6:487, 1967.

Boijsen, E., and Larini, G. P.: Aortic hypoplasia combined with coarctation of the thoracic and lumbar aorta. J. Canad. Ass. Radiol. 17:81, 1966.

Boijsen, E., and Olin, T.: Zöliakographie und Angiographie der Arteria Mesenterica Superior. Ergebn. Med. Strahlenforsch. 1:112, 1964.

Boley, S. J., Krieger, H., Schultz, L., et al.: Experimental aspects of peripheral vascular occlusion of the intestine. Surg. Gynec. Obstet. 121:789, 1965.

Bosniak, M. A., and Phanthumachinda, P.: Value of arteriography in the study of hepatic disease. Amer. J. Surg. 112:348, 1966.

Bradley, R. L.: Gastric hemorrhage due to ruptured aneurysm. Amer. J. Surg. 108:431, 1964.

Bramwit, D. N., and Hummel, W. C.: The superior and inferior mesenteric veins as collateral channels in inferior vena cava obstruction. Radiology 92:90, 1969.

Brewster, D. C., Retana, A., Waltman, A. C., et al.: Angiography in the management of aneurysms of the abdominal aorta: Its value and safety. New Eng. J. Med. 292:822, 1975.

Brill, D. R., Bolasny, B., and Vix, V. A.: Colonic varices. Amer. J. Dig. Dis. 14:801, 1969.

Brolin, I., and Paulin, S.: Abnormal communications between splanchnic vessels. Acta Radiol. (Diagn.) (Stockh.) 2:460, 1964.

Bron, K. M.: Thrombotic occlusion of the abdominal aorta: Associated visceral artery lesions and collateral circulation. Amer. J. Roentgenol. 96:887, 1966.

Bron, K. M., and Gajaraj, A.: Demonstration of hepatic aneurysms in polyarteritis nodosa by arteriography. New Eng. J. Med. 282:1024, 1970.

Bron, K. M., and Redman, H. C.: Splanchnic artery stenosis and occlusion. Radiology 92:323, 1969.

Bron, K. M., Strott, C. A., and Shapiro, A. P.: The diagnostic value of angiographic observations in polyarteritis nodosa. Arch. Intern. Med. 116:450, 1965.

Capps, J. H., and Klein, R. M.: Polyarteritis nodosa as a cause of perirenal and retroperitoneal hemorrhage. Radiology 94:143, 1970.

Carter, R., Vannix, R., Hinshaw, D. B., et al.: Acute inferior mesenteric vascular occlusion, a surgical syndrome. Amer. J. Surg. 98:271, 1959.

Chisolm, A. J., and Sprayregen, S.: Angiographic manifestations of ruptured abdominal aortic aneurysms. Amer. J. Roentgenol. 127:769, 1976.

Citron, B. P., Halpern, M., McCarron, M., et al.: Necrotizing angiitis associated with drug abuse. New Eng. J. Med. 283:1003, 1970.

Clark, R. A., and Rösch, J.: Arteriography in the diagnosis of large bowel bleeding. Radiology 94:83, 1970.

Crummy, A. B., Whittaker, W. B., Morrissey, J. F., et al.: Intestinal infarction secondary to retroperitoneal fibrosis. New Eng. J. Med. 285:28, 1971.

Danaraj, T. J., Wong, H. O., and Thomas, M. A.: Primary arteritis of aorta causing renal artery stenosis and hypertension. Brit. Heart J. 25:153, 1963.

D'Cruz, I. A., Kulkarni, T. P., Gandhi, M. J., et al.: Aortitis of unknown etiology. Angiology 21:49, 1970.

Demos, N. J., Bahuth, J., and Urnes, P. D.: Comparative study of arteriosclerosis in the inferior and superior mesenteric arteries. Ann. Surg. 155:599, 1961.

Derrick, J. R., and Logan, W. D.: Mesenteric arterial insufficiency. Surgery 44:823, 1958.

Deutch, V., Wexler, L., and Deutch, H.: Takayasu's arteritis: An angiographic study with remarks on ethnic distribution in Israel. Amer. J. Roentgenol. 122:13, 1974.

Deykin, D.: The clinical challenge of disseminated intravascular coagulation. New Eng. J. Med. 283:636, 1970.

Dinsmore, R. E., Willerson, J. T., and Buckley, M. J.: Dissecting aneurysm of the aorta: Angiographic features affecting prognosis. Radiology 105:567, 1972.

Doppman, J., Shapiro, R., and Conte, M.: Aneurysm of the hepatic artery: The importance of angiographic visualization. Amer. J. Roentgenol. 90:578, 1963.

Dotter, C. T.: Arteriosclerosis. Seminars Roentgenol. 5:228, 1970.

Dunbar, J. D., Molner, W., Beman, F., et al.: Compression of the celiac trunk and abdominal angina. Amer. J. Roentgenol. 95:731, 1965.

Dvorak, A., and Gazzaniga, A.: Dissecting aneurysm of the gastroduodenal artery. Ann. Surg. 169:425, 1969.

Ende, N.: Infarction of the bowel in cardiac failure. New Eng. J. Med. *258*:879, 1958.

Farrell, W. J., Nolan, J. J., and Tessitore, A.: Unilateral leg edema, migraine and methysergide. J.A.M.A. *207*:1909, 1969.

Ferris, E. J., Vittimberga, F. J., Byrne, J. J., et al.: The inferior vena cava after ligation and plication. Radiology *89*:1, 1967.

Glenn, F., Keefer, E. B. C., Speer, D. S., et al.: Coarctation of the lower thoracic and abdominal aorta immediately proximal to celiac axis. Surg. Gynec. Obstet. *94*:561, 1952.

Goldman, R. L.: Submucosal arterial malformation (aneurysm) of the stomach with fatal hemorrhage. Gastroenterology *46*:589, 1964.

Goldstone, J., Moore, W. S., and Hall, A. D.: Chronic occlusion of the superior and inferior mesenteric veins: Report of a case. Amer. Surg. *36*:235, 1970.

Gotsman, M. S., Beck, W., and Schrire, V.: Selective angiography in arteritis of the aorta and its major branches. Radiology *88*:232, 1967.

Graham, J. R., Suby, H. I., LeCompte, P. R., et al.: Fibrotic disorders associated with methysergide therapy for headache. New Eng. J. Med. *274*:359, 1966.

Grollman, J. H., Lecky, J. W., and Rosch, J.: Miscellaneous disease of arteries or, all arterial lesions aren't fatty. Seminars Roentgenol. *5*:306, 1970.

Gupta, S., and Cope, V.: Hepatic artery aneurysms as a cause of gastrointestinal blood loss. Brit. J. Radiol. *45*:726, 1972.

Hachiya, J.: Current concepts of Takayasu's arteritis. Seminars Roentgenol. *5*:245, 1970.

Harris, R. D., Anderson, J. E., and Coel, M. N.: Aneurysms of the small pancreatic arteries: A cause of upper abdominal pain and intestinal bleeding. Radiology *115*:17, 1975.

Hassani, S., and Bard, R.: Ultrasonic diagnosis of abdominal aortic aneurysms. J. Nat'l. Med. Assn. *66*:298, 1974.

Hedberg, C. A., and Kirsner, J. B.: Editorials: Mesenteric vascular insufficiency. Ann. Intern. Med. *63*:535, 1965.

Hoehn, J. G., Bartholomew, L. G., Osmundson, P. J., et al.: Aneurysms of the mesenteric artery. Amer. J. Surg. *115*:832, 1968.

Holstein, J., and Stecken, A.: Uber die Beziehungen zwischen Altersulkus und Verkalkung der Arteria gastrica sin im Röntgenbild. Fortschr. Rontgenstr. *92*:644, 1960.

Howieson, J. L.: Hepatic artery aneurysm. Radiology *81*:598, 1963.

Hynes, D. M., and Grainger, R. G.: The angiographic demonstration of coarctation of aorta and similar anomalies. Clin. Radiol. *19*:438, 1968.

Itzchak, Y., and Glickman, M. G.: Splenic vein thrombosis in patients with a normal size spleen. Invest. Radiol. *12*:158, 1977.

James, A. E. Jr., Eaton, S. B., Blazek, J. V., et al.: Roentgen findings in pseudoxanthoma elasticum (PXE). Amer. J. Roentgenol. *106*:642, 1969.

Johnsson, K.-Å.: Angiography in two cases of ergotism. Acta Radiol. *57*:280, 1962.

Jordon, P. H. Jr., Boulafendis, D., and Guinn, G. A.: Factors other than major vascular occlusion that contribute to intestinal infarction. Ann. Surg. *171*:189, 1970.

Kanter, I. E., Schwartz, A. J., and Fleming, R. J.: Localization of bleeding point in chronic and acute gastrointestinal hemorrhage by means of selective visceral arteriography. Amer. J. Roentgenol. *103*:386, 1968.

Kater, R. M. H.: Takayasu's disease with gastrointestinal symptoms. Aust. Ann. Med. *16*:80, 1967.

Kendall, B.: Collateral flow to the portal system in obstruction of the iliac veins and inferior vena cava. Brit. J. Radiol. *38*:798, 1965.

Kittredge, R. D., and Anderson, J. W.: Coarctation of the lower thoracic and abdominal aorta. Radiology *79*:799, 1962.

Klatte, E. C., Brooks, A. L., and Rhamy, R. K.: Toxicity of intra-arterial barbiturates and tranquilizing drugs. Radiology *92*:700, 1969.

Kreel, L.: Recognition and incidence of splenic artery aneurysms: A historical review. Aust. Radiol. *16*:126, 1972.

Kuniaki, H., Meaney, T. F., Zelch, J. V., et al.: Aortographic analysis of aortic dissection. Amer. J. Roentgenol. *112*:769, 1974.

Lande, A.: Takayasu's arteritis and congenital coarctation of the descending thoracic and abdominal aorta. Amer. J. Roentgenol. *127*:227, 1976.

Lande, A., and Rossi, P.: The value of total aortography in the diagnosis of Takayasu's arteritis. Radiology *114*:287, 1975.

Leopold, G. R., Goldberger, L. E., and Bernstein, E. F.: Ultrasonic detection and evaluation of abdominal aortic aneurysms. Surgery *72*:939, 1972.

Matz, E. M., and Kahn, P. C.: Occlusion of the celiac, superior mesenteric and inferior mesenteric arteries. Vasc. Dis. *5*:130, 1968.

McClelland, R. N., and Duke, J. H.: Successful resection of an idiopathic aneurysm of the superior mesenteric artery. Ann. Surg. *164*:167, 1966.

Meaney, T. F., and Kistner, R. L.: Evaluation of intraabdominal disease of an obscure cause. Arch. Surg. *94*:811, 1967.

Mikkelsen, W. P., and Zaro, J. A. Jr.: Intestinal angina. New Eng. J. Med. *260*:912, 1959.

Ming, S., and Levitan, R.: Acute hemorrhagic necrosis of the gastrointestinal tract. New Eng. J. Med. *263*:59, 1960.

Mojab, K., Lim, L., Esfahani, F., et al.: Mycotic aneurysm of the hepatic artery causing obstructive jaundice. Amer. J. Roentgenol. *128*:143, 1977.

Morris, G. C., Jr., and DeBakey, M. E.: Abdominal angina—Diagnosis and surgical treatment. J.A.M.A. *176*:89, 1961.

Morris, G. C., Jr., DeBakey, M. E., and Bernhard, V.: Abdominal angina. Surg. Clin. N. Amer. *46*:919, 1966.

Naiken, V., Shapiro, J. H., and Tellem, M.: Celiac axis aneurysm. Angiology *13*:138, 1962.

Nebesar, R. A., Kornblith, P. L., Pollard, J. J., et al.: Celiac and Superior Mesenteric Arteries. Boston, Massachusetts, Little, Brown and Company, 1969.

Nordentoft, E. L., and Larsen, E. A.: Rupture of a jejunal intramural aneurysm causing massive intestinal bleeding. Acta Chir. Scand. *133*:256, 1967.

Olin, T. B., and Reuter, S. R.: Splenic infarction secondary to a splenic artery aneurysm. Vasc. Dis. *3*:269, 1966.

Owens, J. C., and Coffey, R. J.: Aneurysm of the splenic artery, including a report of 6 additional cases. Surg. Gynec. Obstet. Int. Abstr. Surg. *97*:313, 1953.

Palubinskas, A. J., and Ripley, H. R.: Fibromuscular

hyperplasia in extrarenal arteries. Radiology 82:451, 1964.

Phillips, J. C., and Howland, W. J.: Mesenteric arteritis in systemic lupus erythematosus. J.A.M.A. 206:1569, 1968.

Pollard, J. J., and Nebesar, R. A.: Abdominal angiography. New Eng. J. Med. 279:1148, 1968.

Pugh, J. I., and Stringer, P.: Abdominal periarteritis nodosa. Brit. J. Surg. 44:302, 1956.

Pugeda, F., and Hinshaw, J. R.: Preoperative diagnosis and treatment of a splenic artery aneurysm ruptured into the stomach. Amer. Surg. 36:473, 1970.

Ranniger, K., Menguy, R., Kittle, C. F., et al.: Angiographic diagnosis of an intrahepatic aneurysm as a cause of unexplained bleeding. Radiology 90:507, 1968.

Ratner, I. A., and Swenson, O.: Mesenteric vascular occlusion in infancy and childhood. New Eng. J. Med. 263:1122, 1960.

Reiner, L., Jiminez, A., and Rodriguez, F. L.: Atherosclerosis in the mesenteric circulation. Observations and correlations with aortic and coronary atherosclerosis. Amer. Heart J. 66:200, 1963.

Reiner, L., Platt, R., Rodriguez, F. L., et al.: Injection studies on the mesenteric arterial circulation. II. Intestinal infarction. Gastroenterology 39:747, 1960.

Reuter, S. R.: Accentuation of celiac compression by the median arcuate ligament of the diaphragm during deep expiration. Radiology 98:561, 1971.

Reuter, S. R.: Development of collateral vessels in an acute occlusion of the common hepatic artery. Amer. J. Roentgenol. 97:473, 1966.

Reuter, S. R., and Bookstein, J. J.: Angiographic localization of gastrointestinal bleeding. Gastroenterology 54:876, 1968.

Reuter, S. R., Fry, W. J., and Bookstein, J. J.: Mesenteric artery branch aneurysms. Arch. Surg. 97:497, 1968.

Reuter, S. R., Kanter, I. E., and Redman, H. C.: Angiography in reversible colonic ischemia. Radiology 97:371, 1970.

Reuter, S. R., and Redman, H. C.: Intrasplenic arterial aneurysms. J. Canad. Ass. Radiol. 19:200, 1968.

Robins, J. M., and Bookstein, J. J.: Regressing aneurysms in periarteritis nodosa. Radiology 104:39, 1972.

Rosenburger, A., Munk, J., Schramek, A., et al.: The angiographic appearance of thromboangiitis obliterans (Buerger's disease) in the abdominal visceral vessels. Brit. J. Radiol. 46:337, 1973.

Sacks, R. P., Sheft, D. J., and Freeman, J. H.: The demonstration of the mesenteric collateral circulation in young patients. Amer. J. Roentgenol. 102:401, 1968.

Saw, E. C., Arbegast, N. R., Schmalhorst, W. R., et al.: Splenic artery aneurysms. Arch. Surg. 106:660, 1973.

Schwartz, S., Boley, S., Lash, J., et al.: Occlusion of the colon and its relationship to ulcerative colitis. Radiology 80:625, 1963.

Shaw, R. S., and Maynard, E. P., III: Acute and chronic thrombosis of the mesenteric arteries associated with malabsorption. New Eng. J. Med. 258:874, 1958.

Siegelman, S. S., Sprayregen, S., Strasberg, Z., et al.: Aortic dissection and the left renal artery. Radiology 95:73, 1970.

Siegelman, S. S., Sprayregen, S., and Boley, S. J.: Angiographic diagnosis of mesenteric arterial vasoconstriction. Radiology 112:533, 1974.

Smith, S. L., Sutton, R. H., and Ochsner, S. F.: Roentgenographic aspects of intestinal ischemia. Amer. J. Roentgenol. 116:249, 1972.

Stachenfeld, R. A., Gordimer, H., Friedenberg, R. M., et al.: Aneurysm of the left gastric artery: Preoperative angiographic diagnosis. Radiology 83:1026, 1964.

Stanley, J. C., Thompson, N. W., and Fry, W. J.: Splanchnic artery aneurysms. Arch. Surg. 101:689, 1970.

Steelquist, J. H.: Aneurysm of the hepatic artery. Amer. J. Surg. 89:1241, 1955.

Stein, H. L., and Steinberg, I.: Selective aortography, the definitive technique for diagnosis of dissecting aneurysm of the aorta. Amer. J. Roentgenol. 102:333, 1968.

Steinberg, I.: Diagnosis of aneurysms of the hepatic and splenic arteries by intravenous abdominal aortography. New Eng. J. Med. 263:341, 1960.

Sutton, D., and Lawton, G.: Angiographic diagnosis of aneurysms involving the hepatic artery. Clin. Radiol. 24:43, 1973.

Sutton, D., and Lawton, G.: Celiac stenosis or occlusion with aneurysm of the collateral supply. Clin. Radiol. 24:49, 1973.

Thomas, J. R.: Osler's disease with a dissecting aneurysm of the aorta. Arch. Intern. Med. 116:448, 1965.

Thompson, J. F., Mazella, S. F., and Thistlethwaite, J. R.: Aneurysm of the celiac artery. Ann. Surg. 161:83, 1965.

Touloukian, R. J., Zikria, B. A., and Ferrer, J. M.: Segmental small bowel infarction associated with abdominal angina. Amer. J. Gastroent. 46:347, 1966.

Weaver, D. H., Fleming, R. J., and Barnes, W. A.: Aneurysm of the hepatic artery: The value of arteriography in surgical management. Surgery 64:891, 1968.

Weidner, W., Fox, P., Brooks, J. W., et al.: The roentgenographic diagnosis of aneurysms of the superior mesenteric artery. Amer. J. Roentgenol. 109:138, 1970.

Weintraub, R. A., and Abrams, H. L.: Mycotic aneurysms. Amer. J. Roentgenol. 102:354, 1968.

West, J. E., Bernhardt, H., and Bowers, R. F.: Aneurysms of the pancreaticoduodenal artery. Amer. J. Surg. 115:835, 1968.

Westcott, J. L., and Ziter, F. M. H.: Aneurysms of the splenic artery. Surg. Gynecol. Obstet. 136:541, 1973.

Wholey, M. H., Bron, K. M., and Haller, J. D.: Selective angiography of the colon. Surg. Clin. N. Amer. 45:1283, 1965.

Wirtanen, G. W., and Kaude, J. V.: Inferior phrenic artery collateralization in hepatic artery occlusion. Amer. J. Roentgenol. 117:615, 1973.

Wyatt, G. M., Rauchway, M. I., and Spitz, H. B.: Roentgen findings in aorto-enteric fistulae. Amer. J. Roentgenol. 126:714, 1976.

Chapter 4

TUMORS

NEOPLASMS

The angiographic appearance of some gastrointestinal neoplasms was known before the development of percutaneous transfemoral arterial catheterization; however, angiography was seldom used to evaluate patients with tumors because of the morbidity associated with cut-down tech-niques and the toxicity of the available contrast media. Since the development of percutaneous catheterization techniques, numerous reports have described the angiographic manifestations of individual neoplasms in the gastrointestinal tract. It has become apparent that most gastrointestinal tumors have a spectrum of angiographic abnormalities; this is well recognized for most lesions examined.

106

General Angiographic Characteristics of Gastrointestinal Neoplasms

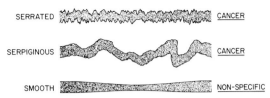

Figure 4–1. Types of arterial encasement by tumor. Serrated encasement is specific for infiltration by a tumor and is not seen in other types of disease. Serpiginous encasement is also reasonably specific for carcinoma but is occasionally caused by severe fibrosis, such as occurs in longstanding, relapsing pancreatitis or following extensive radiation therapy. Smooth encasement is frequently caused by a tumor but is also frequently seen in other types of diseases, particularly in inflammatory diseases. It is therefore nonspecific and should not be used as a criterion for the diagnosis of cancer.

Angiographic abnormalities caused by gastrointestinal neoplasms vary with the histology of the lesions and are limited, since the number of responses available to blood vessels are few. These abnormalities are the same as those caused by any neoplasm and are as follows:

1. Invasion of normal arteries and veins by the tumor (encasement).
2. Displacement of arteries and veins by the tumor (displacement).
3. Vascular neoformation within the tumor (tumor vessels).
4. Filling of necrotic areas in the tumor with contrast medium (pools, lakes or puddles of contrast medium).
5. Prolonged capillary perfusion or increased capillary permeability (tumor blush or stain, increased contrast accumulation).
6. Arteriovenous shunting.

Invasion of Arteries and Veins

Most adenocarcinomas of the stomach, small bowel, colon, pancreas and liver are invasive, infiltrative lesions. Histologically, they vary from anaplastic to well differentiated. The more anaplastic and scirrhous a lesion is, the more invasive it becomes. Therefore, the demonstration of arterial or venous encasement is a particularly important part of the evaluation of gastrointestinal tumors. The exact histologic nature of vascular invasion by infiltrating carcinoma has never been established, though the angiographic appearance is well recognized.

The pathognomonic appearance of neoplastic invasion of an artery is called "serrated" or "serpiginous" encasement (Fig. 4–1). The term "serrated" describes the irregular, saw-toothed appearance seen in the walls of arteries encased by tumors (Fig. 4–2), while "serpiginous" describes the manner in which arterial pathways are abruptly angulated by tumors (Fig. 4–3). In fact, the changes caused by tumors range from serration and abrupt angulation to smooth encasement (Fig. 4–4). Carcinoma can be diagnosed only when the character-

istic serrated or serpiginous abnormalities are present. Smooth narrowing of arteries is a nonspecific finding and is more frequently seen in benign diseases, such as atherosclerosis or inflammation. In general, serrated encasement is seen in larger arteries, such as the hepatic, splenic, left gastric, superior mesenteric and gastroduodenal arteries, while serpiginous encasement is more common in smaller branches (Fig. 4–5). Smaller arteries tend to become completely distorted by the tumor, resulting in abrupt angulation and frequent variations in caliber.

The same arterial changes are caused by tumors whether the arteries are several microns or several millimeters in diameter. In general, the larger the vessel involved, the more certain the examiner can be of the diagnosis. This is partly true because larger arteries have more familiar, predictable courses, and any deviation from the normal pattern is readily discerned as an abnormality. Third and fourth order branches of the major vessels, however, have unpredictable courses through an organ, and normal changes in the direction of the vessel may simulate angulation. For this reason, two projections, anteroposterior and oblique, are usually obtained so that the course of arteries can be determined in three dimensions. Magnification angiography can also be used to enlarge the abnormalities in the course and caliber of arteries, and superselective injections can be used to assure that

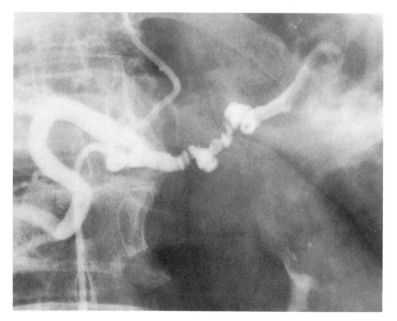

Figure 4–2. Serrated encasement of a major artery by carcinoma. Arterial phase of a celiac angiogram in a 61 year old man with carcinoma of the body and tail of the pancreas. The splenic artery is encased by the tumor and has a sawtoothed or serrated appearance. This type of encasement is characteristic for carcinoma and is not caused by benign diseases.

the second, third and fourth order branches are completely filled with contrast medium. These techniques extend the range of diagnostic certainty to smaller arteries.

In addition to being encased, arteries can be completely occluded by tumors. Arterial occlusion, like smooth narrowing, is not as specific a finding for the diagnosis of carcinoma as is serrated or serpiginous encasement, since other diseases, particularly atherosclerosis, can occlude arteries.

Veins may also be invaded or compressed by neoplasms (Fig. 4–6). Such compression or occlusion is frequently demonstrated only by the presence of a venous collateral circulation. Because of the decreased concentration of contrast medium in the veins, these vessels are difficult to evaluate. A careful search for venous abnormalities should be made in each angiogram performed for tumor. Occasionally, the presence of a venous abnormality lends support to the angiographic diagnosis of neoplasm. The serrated changes that

Figure 4–3. Serpiginous encasement by carcinoma. Splenic angiogram in a 67 year old woman with carcinoma of the body and tail of the pancreas. Subtraction technique. The proximal and midportions of the splenic artery are narrowed (➡), as is the proximal portion of the superior polar artery (▶). The abrupt angulations and changes in the caliber of the artery are typical for serpiginous encasement. In addition, the left gastric artery (➡) is also encased by the tumor.

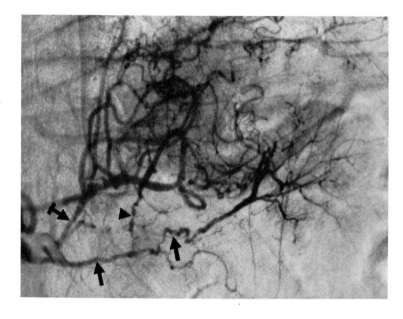

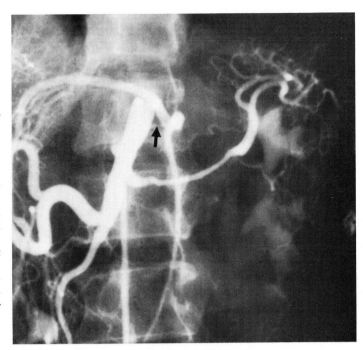

Figure 4-4. Smooth encasement of a major artery by carcinoma. Arterial phase of a celiac angiogram in a 65 year old woman with carcinoma of the tail of the pancreas. The splenic artery is narrowed for a length of 5 cm. On either side of the narrowing the vessel appears normal. In addition, the left gastric artery is occluded (➡), and a left hepatic artery arising from it receives blood flow over the right gastric–left gastric arcade. Thus, although the lumen in the narrowed segment is relatively smooth and does not exhibit the serrations seen in Figure 4–1, the occluded left gastric artery allows a definitive diagnosis. (From Reuter, S. R.: Angiography in the diagnosis of gastrointestinal cancer. Proc. Cancer Conf., p. 447, 1968.)

occur in arteries are not seen in veins. Perhaps the invasion which causes serrated change in an artery occludes the more flexible vein. Intraluminal tumor is occasionally seen in the portal or other large veins (Fig. 4–7).

Vascular Displacement

Both benign and well differentiated malignant neoplasms may displace rather than invade the surrounding arteries as they expand (Fig. 4–8). Even invasive neoplasms

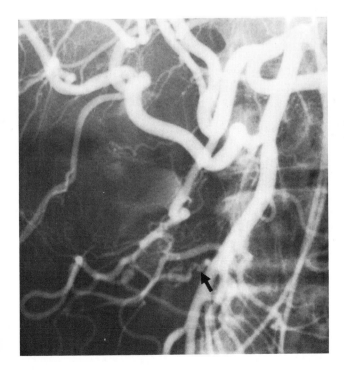

Figure 4-5. Serpiginous encasement of a small pancreatic artery by carcinoma. Arterial phase of a combined celiac–superior mesenteric angiogram in a 73 year old woman with carcinoma of the head of the pancreas. There are abrupt angulations and changes in caliber of the inferior pancreaticoduodenal artery over a 1 cm segment (➡). Although these changes involve only a short segment of a small pancreatic artery, they are characteristic enough of carcinoma to allow a firm diagnosis.

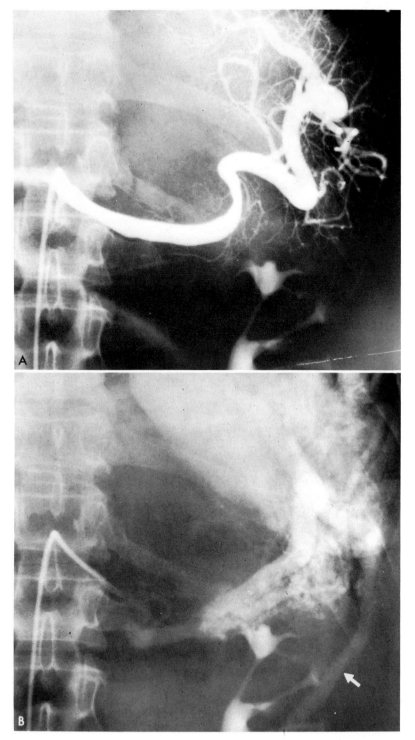

Figure 4–6. Occlusion of a major vein by sarcoma. Splenic angiogram in a 67 year old man with gastric lymphosarcoma.

A. Arterial phase. The splenic artery is stretched downward and narrowed by the gastric mass. The intrasplenic arteries have a normal appearance.

B. Venous phase. The splenic vein narrows and ends abruptly in its midportion. In the lower right-hand corner of the film, a collateral epiploic vein (⟹) bypasses the occlusion, delivering splenic blood flow to the portal vein.

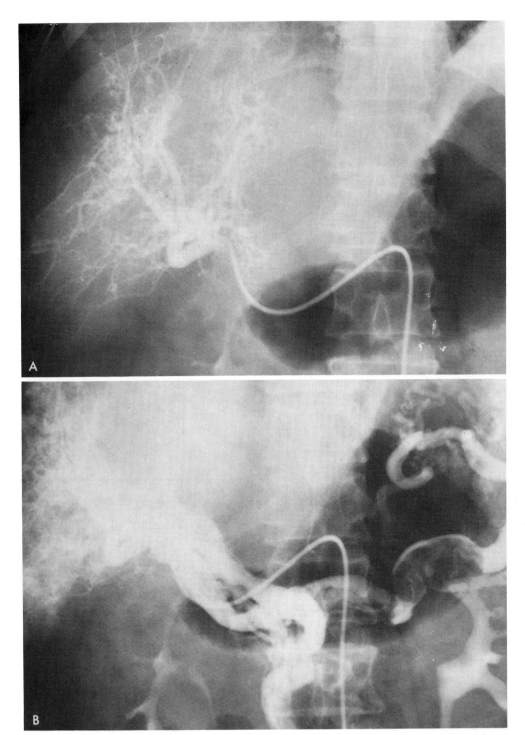

Figure 4-7. Growth of hepatoma into the portal vein. Hepatic angiogram in a 60 year old man with obstructive jaundice.

A. Arterial phase. The hepatic artery and its branches are dilated, and numerous tumor vessels are seen throughout the right lobe of the liver.

B. Venous phase. Arteriovenous shunting has occurred through the tumor, and there is dense opacification of the portal, splenic and superior mesenteric veins. Frondlike strands of tumor extend down the portal vein, and tumor thrombus can be seen in the midsplenic vein. These findings were confirmed at autopsy.

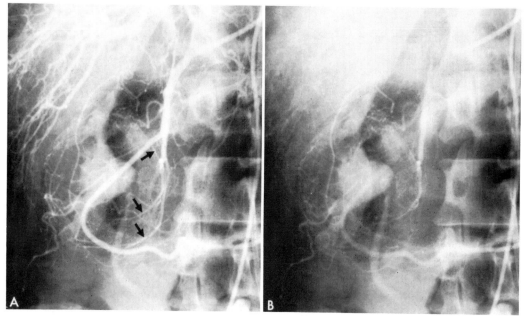

Figure 4–8. Displacement of arteries by tumor. Gastroduodenal angiogram in a 28 year old man with a duodenal leiomyosarcoma.

    A. Early arterial phase. Duodenal branches of the gastroduodenal artery (➡) are stretched around the tumor mass.

    B. Late arterial phase. A few tumor vessels are present, and contrast accumulation in the lesion is minimally increased. The distortion of the duodenal sweep can be appreciated by the appearance of the air in the duodenum. This tumor is at the poorly vascularized end of the spectrum for leiomyosarcoma.

generally cause some vascular displacement. Displacement of vessels, however, is not diagnostic of neoplasm, since it is frequently the primary angiographic abnormality caused by cysts, abscesses and other benign masses. When arteries or veins are displaced by a mass and show other angiographic evidence of neoplasm, however, the displacement becomes an additional positive diagnostic sign.

Vascular Neoformation

As a tumor grows, it develops its own blood supply. The nutrient vessels within the tumor are not normal arteries since they do not have an endothelium or a muscular layer. They are, however, vascular channels and often fill with contrast medium during the angiogram. They generally are short, serpiginous, abruptly angulated and of variable diameter. Origins and terminations often cannot be defined (Fig. 4–9). Although superselective injections

and magnification angiography improve their demonstration, these vessels are frequently below the limits of resolution of current angiographic systems. It is often difficult to define a single vascular tumor neoformation. Rather, a number of these small channels seem to fuse, giving the appearance of increased vascularity. Vascular neoformation is often referred to as "tumor vessels" or "tumor neovascularity" and is usually diagnostic of a neoplasm. Abnormal channels may develop around hemorrhage or in inflammatory disease, particularly when granulation tissue is present, and these channels can simulate tumor vessels. In general, however, neovascularity indicates a neoplasm.

Filling of Necrotic Areas with Contrast Medium

On occasion, areas of necrosis within tumors communicate with the tumor vessels or with blood vessels that the tumor

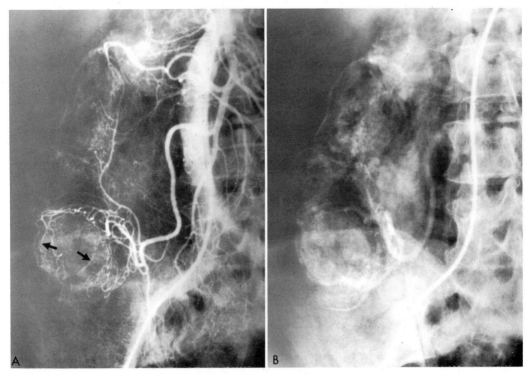

Figure 4-9. Tumor vessels in a colon carcinoma. Superior mesenteric angiogram in a 70 year old woman with carcinoma of the ascending colon.

A. Arterial phase. Vasa recta in the proximal ascending colon are stretched around the tumor and are invaded (➡). Numerous small serpiginous tumor vessels are seen through the tumor.

B. Venous phase. The increase in contrast accumulation in the tumor is only moderate. Venous drainage is dense.

has invaded. This leads to filling of these spaces with contrast medium at angiography and the appearance of "pools" or "lakes" of contrast medium (Fig. 4–10). Probably more often, necrotic areas within tumors are not filled with contrast medium, and the appearance is one of hypovascularity. This perhaps occurs most frequently in necrotic hypernephromas. When the necrotic areas within tumors do fill with contrast medium, the margins of the area are irregular and poorly defined. This is in contrast to the well defined, dilated vascular spaces seen in cavernous hemangiomas.

Increased Accumulation of Contrast Medium

The mechanisms of "increased contrast accumulation," "tumor blush" or "tumor stain" are not well understood. This entity is seen as an area of diffuse, increased den-

sity of contrast medium compared with the accumulation seen in the surrounding normal tissues (Fig. 4–11). The contrast medium which causes this "blush" may be in the interstitial spaces of the tumor or within many small vascular channels or both. It is generally seen in tumors that are histologically vascular and is rarely present in scirrhous, invasive lesions. When contrast accumulation is increased, it is an excellent indicator of tumor size. Contrast accumulation throughout a tumor may be homogeneous or mottled. This change is not specific for tumor and is more often a finding in inflammatory disease.

Arteriovenous Shunting

Arteriovenous shunts are present in some of the more vascular tumors. The increased blood flow through the tumor is seen as early opacification of the veins or as opaci-

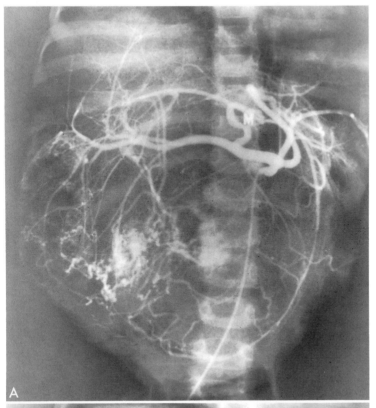

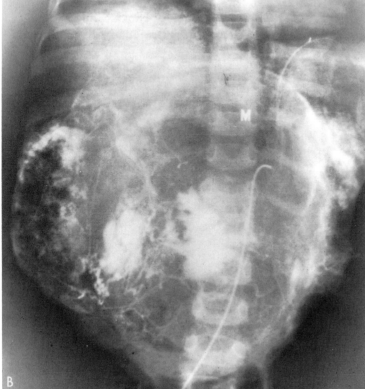

Figure 4–10. Vascular lakes. Celiac angiogram in a 22 month old girl with hemangiosarcoma.

A. Arterial phase. Hepatic artery branches are stretched and invaded. Several large, irregular vascular spaces in the right lobe of the liver fill with contrast medium.

B. Venous phase. The abnormal spaces remain filled. The smaller spaces probably represent the endothelial-lined cavities seen in a cavernous hemangioma, but the larger spaces appear to represent necrotic areas. (Courtesy of Dr. A. J. Palubinskas. From Moss, A. A., Clark, R. E., Palubinskas, A. J., and de Lorimier, A. A.: Angiographic appearance of benign and malignant tumors in infants and children. Amer. J. Roentgenol. *113*:64, 1971.)

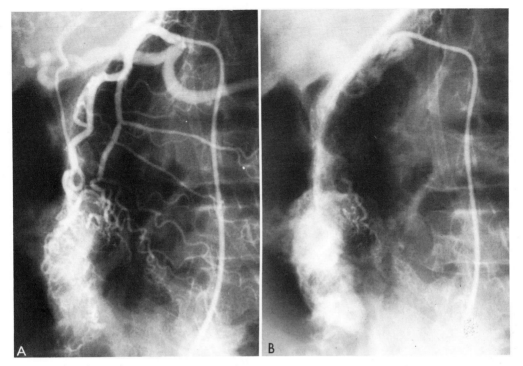

Figure 4–11. Increased contrast accumulation in a gastric carcinoma. Left gastric angiogram in a 66 year old woman with carcinoma of the antrum of the stomach.

A. Arterial phase. A dilated left gastric artery supplies several dilated branches to the antrum of the stomach. Some of these branches are invaded by carcinoma.

B. Venous phase. There is delayed emptying of infiltrated arteries. The tumor is unusually hypervascular for a gastric carcinoma, and a great deal of increased contrast accumulation is seen throughout the tumor. The increased contrast accumulation stands out against the air in the remainder of the stomach.

fication of veins not usually seen (Fig. 4–12). This is always accompanied by increased density of the contrast medium in the veins. While early venous drainage and dense venous drainage go hand in hand, the converse is not always true; venous drainage from a tumor can be dense without being early. The normal appearance time of contrast medium in veins varies from patient to patient. Therefore, a definitive diagnosis of early venous drainage should be made when veins opacify while the arteries to the area are still filled with contrast medium or when veins in one area fill several seconds earlier than veins from the remaining tissue. The latter finding is not as definitive in the venous system of the bowel since a food bolus causes a relatively early filling of veins. Also, these criteria apply only to injection times of 3 to 4 seconds or less, since these findings can be simulated by long injections of contrast me-

dium. Arteriovenous shunting is not common in most gastrointestinal tumors, and this finding is more indicative of a benign process such as inflammation or an arteriovenous malformation.

Several of these angiographic abnormalities are usually present in a gastrointestinal neoplasm; the greater the number present, the greater the certainty of diagnosis. In general, infiltrative, scirrhous lesions cause arterial invasion and tumor vessel formation. Well differentiated and benign lesions cause tumor vessel formation, vascular displacement, increased contrast accumulation and, perhaps, arteriovenous shunting.

The statement has been made that differentiation between malignant and benign neoplasms is possible on the basis of the angiographic findings. This is only partially true. Within any given organ, malignant tumors can generally be differentiated from

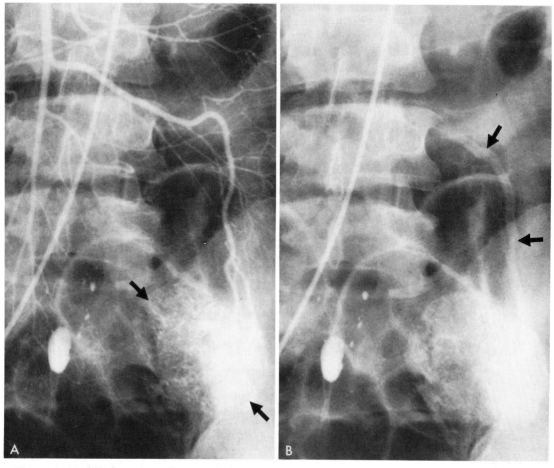

Figure 4–12. Early venous drainage. Superior mesenteric angiogram in a 54 year old man with an ileal leiomyoma.

A. Arterial phase. An ileal branch of the superior mesenteric artery is dilated and supplies many tumor vessels through a hypervascular mass in the midileum. The tumor is well circumscribed (➡).

B. Parenchymal phase. The contrast accumulation through the tumor is relatively homogeneous. Contrast medium draining from the tumor fills a dilated ileal vein before any of the other veins draining the bowel have opacified (➡).

those which are usually benign. For example, the differentiation between an islet cell adenoma and an adenocarcinoma of the pancreas is not difficult. Likewise, a hepatic angioma and a cholangiocarcinoma can be differentiated; however, such differentiation is impossible in any neoplasm that has both a benign and a malignant phase. Thus, leiomyoma cannot be differentiated from leiomyosarcoma, lymphoma from lymphosarcoma or benign islet cell adenoma from malignant islet cell adenoma. Both phases of these tumors have the same angiographic abnormalities, and the malignant form can only be identified

by local invasion or the presence of liver metastases.

Localization of a tumor to a given part of the gastrointestinal tract and visualization of its extent are important parameters in the angiographic evaluation of gastrointestinal neoplasms. Generally, the organ of origin can be identified by determining which arteries provide the major blood supply to the tumor. This evaluation requires a thorough knowledge of visceral arterial anatomy and its many variations. Even when a tumor has infiltrated widely, it usually maintains a predominant blood supply from the organ of origin. This blood supply is most easily identified in vascular tumors. The extent of tumor growth is also more easily demonstrated in vascular tumors and can be defined by the extent of tumor vessels, extent of arterial invasion and extent of contrast accumulation within the lesion. In the less vascular, more infiltrative lesions, an exact definition of the tumor size is often difficult and depends on the demonstration of the extent of vascular invasion, including venous invasion. Inflammatory response around a neoplasm can make it appear larger than it is. In spite of this, the correlation of tumor size seen at angiography and at operation or autopsy has generally been good.

Indications for the Use of Angiography in the Evaluation of Gastrointestinal Neoplasms

Angiography should be used in the evaluation of suspected gastrointestinal neoplasms when the more routine studies, including plain films, barium examinations, ultrasound and isotopic examinations, have not been definitive. In most of the alimentary tract, barium examinations are accurate in diagnosing tumors. This is particularly true in the esophagus, stomach and colon. In the esophagus, the accuracy is so good and the arterial supply so diffuse that the usefulness of angiography has not even been evaluated. The angiographic abnormalities that occur with gastric tumors have been described, but angiography has little role in the evaluation of these lesions. The same is true in the colon. The only part of the alimentary canal in which angiography has proved to be of diagnostic value is the small bowel. Small tumors may be missed by even a careful small bowel series, or the changes in the barium column may not be sufficiently characteristic to allow a definite preoperative diagnosis. Therefore, angiography is useful in the evaluation of small bowel tumors.

Angiography is most useful in evaluating tumors of the liver and pancreas. The accuracy of plain films and barium studies in the examination of these organs is poor. Ultrasound can differentiate solid and cystic masses in the pancreas and diagnose fluid-filled masses in the liver but has not been particularly helpful in demonstrating solid hepatic tumors. Computerized tomography may be an accurate procedure for the diagnosis of abdominal tumors. Isotopic examinations are good screening procedures for diagnosing hepatic lesions but have had little value in diagnosing pancreatic tumors.

Although angiography is still widely used for the diagnosis of pancreatic and hepatic masses, it has become even more important in assessing the resectability and curability of tumors diagnosed by other methods. Resectability is evaluated by observing the extent of the tumor and the arteries, veins and organs that it involves. Potential curability is determined by assessing the extent of the lesion, the presence of venous invasion (particularly mesenteric and portal venous invasion) and the presence of hepatic metastases. Both angiographic and isotopic examinations are useful in the evaluation of suspected hepatic metastases, and the methods are complementary (Rossi and Gould, 1970; Lerona et al., 1974). Isotopes tend to be more accurate in the evaluation of hypovascular metastases, while angiography is more accurate in the evaluation of hypervascular metastases. Computerized tomography will also have a role in the evaluation of hepatic metastases.

Finally, angiography has been useful in the demonstration of variant blood supply to the viscera. A preoperative knowledge of visceral vascular variations forewarns the surgeon of crucial arteries that may be sacrificed during radical tumor surgery. In practice, the usefulness of this procedure depends on the surgeon; some prefer to have an accurate preoperative "road map" of the vascular variations that will be encountered, while others feel this is not important.

Angiographic Abnormalities in Neoplasms of the Alimentary Tract

In general, tumors with a similar histology have a similar angiographic appearance, regardless of their source of origin in the alimentary canal. Therefore, the following summary of alimentary canal tumors describes the abnormalities for each histologic type, pointing out regional differences as they occur.

Benign Neoplasms and Their Malignant Counterparts

The benign neoplasms that occur in the stomach, small bowel and colon are adenomas or adenomatous polyps, myomas or leiomyomas, neurofibromas, lipomas, carcinoid tumors and angiomas. Most of these tumors may be premalignant and have malignant counterparts. As mentioned earlier, however, when a benign tumor crosses the line and becomes malignant, identification of this change by the presence of characteristic angiographic abnormalities is impossible. Malignancy can be determined only by the identification of the local extension of the tumor or the presence of metastases to the liver or elsewhere.

ADENOMA. The angiographic abnormalities of adenomatous polyps have not been described to date. The authors have seen one patient in whom an adenomatous polyp was discovered incidentally during angiography for other purposes. The lesion had a few tumor vessels and appeared somewhat hypervascular compared with the remaining bowel (Fig. 4–13). No early venous drainage was present, nor was the venous drainage intense. The very absence of reports describing adenomatous polyps indicates that the findings are minimal. Twelve per cent of patients coming to autopsy have such lesions. Therefore, by now a large number of polyps detected incidentally at angiography should have been reported if abnormal findings are common. At the same time, one may conjecture that angiographic abnormalities similar to those seen in adenocarcinomas of the intestinal tract might be seen in larger adenomatous polyps.

Villous adenomas of the colon have moderate tumor neovascularity accompanied by a moderate contrast accumulation in the parenchymal phase of angiography and early, dense venous drainage (Fig. 4–14). Both the feeding arteries and the draining veins may dilate if the tumor is large (Riba and Lunderquist, 1973). Malignant change

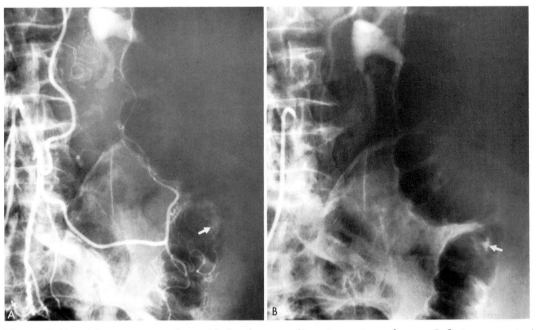

Figure 4–13. Adenomatous polyp with focal areas of carcinomatous change. Inferior mesenteric angiogram in a 76 year old man with chronic lower gastrointestinal bleeding and anemia.
A. Arterial phase. Vasa recta in the distal descending colon supply a few abnormal vessels (⟹) along the antimesenteric border of the bowel.
B. Venous phase. Contrast accumulation in the polyp is irregularly increased (⟹).

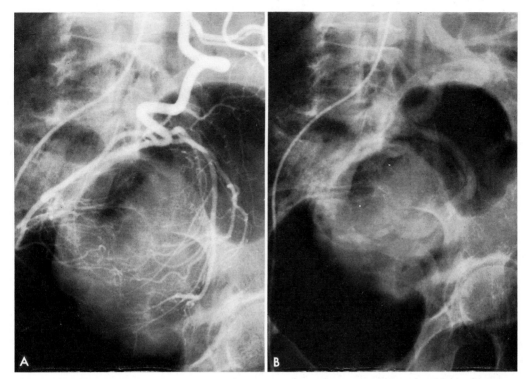

Figure 4-14. Villous adenoma. Inferior mesenteric angiogram in a 69 year old man with watery diarrhea.

A. Arterial phase. The inferior mesenteric artery is dilated and the superior hemorrhoidal branches supply numerous dilated vasa recta throughout a large villous adenoma at the rectosigmoid. A moderate number of tumor vessels are seen through the lesion.

B. Venous phase. Contrast accumulation is moderately increased, and dilated hemorrhoidal and inferior mesenteric veins drain the lesion. The tumor mass stands out against the air in the rectum and sigmoid colon.

can be detected only by the presence of distant metastases. Since these tumors are usually demonstrated at barium enema and since a typical syndrome is often present, angiography has little use in their diagnosis.

LEIOMYOMA AND NEUROGENIC TUMORS. Leiomyomas of the small bowel are generally hypervascular (Kaude et al., 1972), while those arising in the stomach may be either hypervascular or poorly vascularized. There is no histologic basis for this difference in appearance. The angiographic abnormalities in small bowel leiomyomas include a moderate number of tumor vessels, dilated vascular channels or venous lakes, displacement of normal arteries around the tumor, invasion of arteries within the tumor and early and dense venous drainage (Figs. 4–8 and 4–15). Thus,

most of the criteria for an angiographic diagnosis of tumor are present, and these lesions usually stand out from the normal surrounding bowel. In general, leiomyomas appear well encapsulated. When the encapsulated appearance is not present and the tumor is large, malignant degeneration of the leiomyoma can be postulated.

Gastric leiomyomas (Fig. 4–16) may become large before being discovered and present as an abdominal mass rather than as a gastric lesion. They frequently arise from the greater curvature of the stomach. It is, therefore, important to identify the course of the right gastroepiploic artery and look carefully for invasion of its branches or tumor vessels in its distribution.

Tumors of neurogenic origin which occur in the alimentary tract tend also to be hypervascular (Capdeville et al., 1970), and

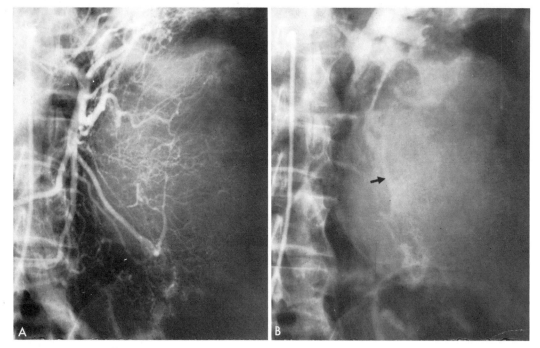

Figure 4–15. Small bowel leiomyoma. Superior mesenteric angiogram in a 58 year old man with an abdominal mass.

A. Arterial phase. Dilated distal jejunal and proximal ileal branches of the superior mesenteric artery supply many tumor vessels throughout a large mass in the left midabdomen.

B. Venous phase. There is a moderately homogeneous increase in contrast accumulation throughout the tumor, and a dilated vein (➡) is present. Most of this leiomyoma is in the mesentery.

the angiographic findings in these unusual tumors are similar to those described for leiomyomas.

CARCINOID TUMORS. Most carcinoid tumors are found near the terminal ileum and are fairly large. The tumors that have been described have invaded the mesentery, and the angiographic manifestations are related primarily to how this invasion occurs (Reuter and Boijsen, 1966; Boijsen et al., 1974). As the lesion infiltrates, it thickens and foreshortens the mesentery, leading to a typical "kinking" of the small bowel loops which is the hallmark of the carcinoid tumor on a small bowel series (Fig. 4–17). The foreshortening makes the mesenteric arteries very tortuous and frequently narrowed and draws them into a stellate pattern. The area appears hypervascular (Fig. 4–18), but in reality the number of arteries is not increased; instead, the vessels are contracted into a smaller area. Another arterial change of carcinoid

tumor is smooth narrowing of the mesenteric arteries distant from the tumor itself. In the capillary phase, there is frequently little or no increased accumulation of contrast medium, and generally no "tumor blush" is present. Similarly, no early or dense venous drainage is present. Any process that thickens and contracts the mesentery can cause a similar angiographic appearance. For example, chronic sclerosing fibrinous peritonitis (retractile mesenteritis), a rare entity, or carcinoma of the pancreas invading the mesentery may result in these findings.

ANGIOMA. Angiomas occur throughout the alimentary tract. They are generally single but may be multiple in syndromes such as hereditary hemorrhagic telangiectasia. These lesions are usually a centimeter or less in diameter. Venous drainage is often early and dense (Fig. 4–19). Gastrointestinal angiomas may remain asymptomatic for life and are generally detected only

Text continued on page 125.

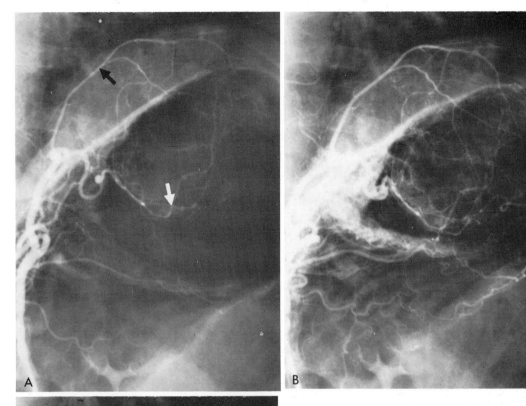

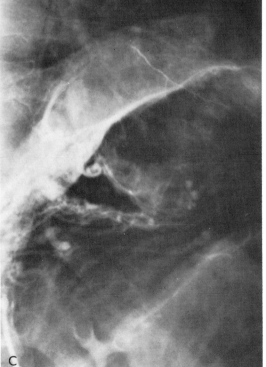

Figure 4–16. Gastric leiomyoma. Left gastric angiogram in a 48 year old woman with a mass in the fundus of the stomach on an upper gastrointestinal series.

A. Early arterial phase. The branches of the left gastric artery to the fundus are displaced around a mass (⇒). About half of the mass lies outside the air-filled stomach, while the other half is intraluminal.

B. Late arterial phase. Several tumor vessels are seen throughout the tumor, but it is not markedly hypervascular.

C. Venous phase. There is minimal, irregular accumulation of contrast medium through the tumor. Venous drainage from the tumor is neither early nor dense.

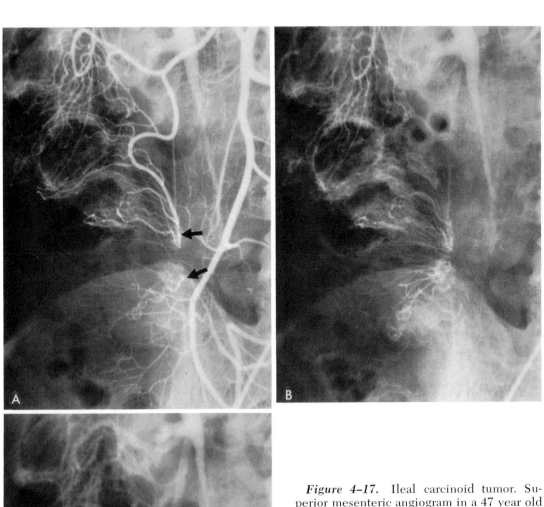

Figure 4–17. Ileal carcinoid tumor. Superior mesenteric angiogram in a 47 year old man with a right lower quadrant mass.

A. Early arterial phase. The anastomosis between the right colic and ileocolic arteries is discontinuous, and serpiginous encasement of arteries can be seen (➡).

B. Late arterial phase. Tumor vessels and serpiginous encasement of arteries are seen in the terminal ileum. The vasa recta of the terminal ileum appear to radiate from the primary area of arterial invasion, giving a stellate appearance.

C. Venous phase. There is minimal, homogeneously increased contrast accumulation through the tumor. Venous drainage is neither early nor dense.

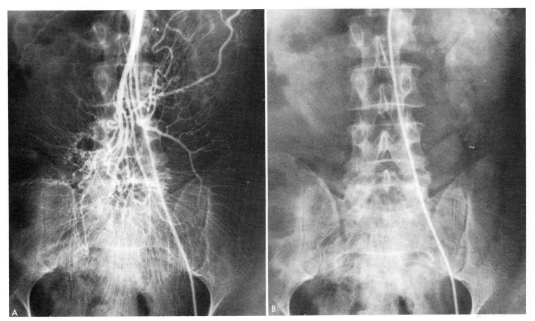

Figure 4–18. Ileal carcinoid tumor. Superior mesenteric angiogram in a 54 year old man with severe diarrhea.

A. Arterial phase. The superior mesenteric artery is not dilated, but several of the branches of the ileocolic artery and terminal superior mesenteric artery are retracted and drawn into a stellate pattern with the vasa recta radiating from the mesenteric mass.

B. Capillary phase. There is no increase in contrast accumulation in the region of the tumor. No veins are seen draining the area. These findings are characteristic of carcinoid tumor which has invaded the mesentery.

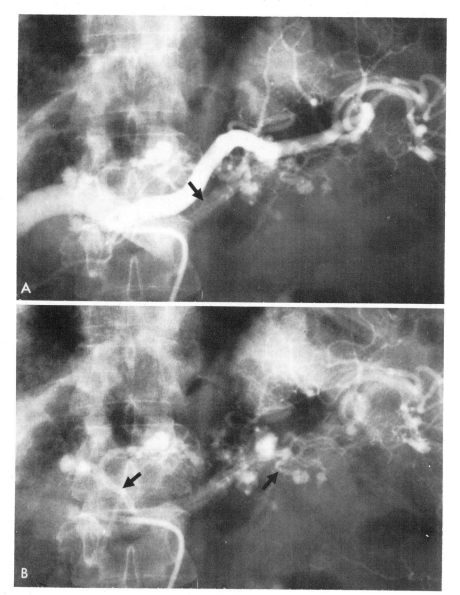

Figure 4–19. Multiple small angiomas. Celiac angiogram in a 66 year old patient with hereditary telangiectasia.

A. Early arterial phase. Several small angiomas in the pancreas are supplied by splenic artery branches. Arteriovenous shunting through the angiomas leads to early splenic vein opacification (➡).

B. Venous phase. The veins draining the angiomas are well demonstrated (➡).

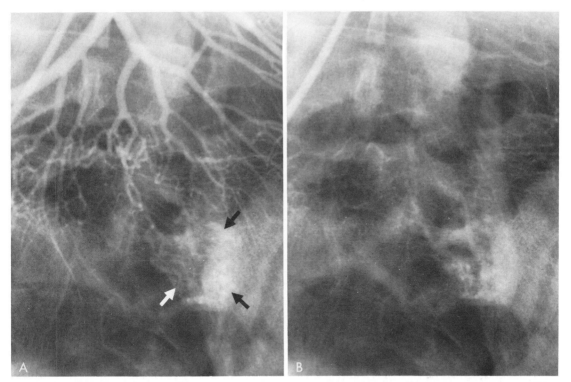

Figure 4–20. Ileal hemangioma. Superior mesenteric angiogram in a 17 year old man with recurrent gastrointestinal bleeding.

A. Arterial phase. The ileal branch of the superior mesenteric artery supplying the hemangioma is not dilated. Several irregular vascular spaces are seen (⇉).

B. Venous phase. The vascular spaces retain the contrast medium long into the venous phase. No dense or early venous drainage is apparent. The appearance of the tumor is identical to that of an hepatic hemangioma.

if they bleed. Such angiomas are the most common abnormal finding on angiograms performed because of chronic, recurrent bleeding (see Chapter 6).

Cavernous hemangiomas also occur in the gastrointestinal tract. Grieco and Bartoni (1967) described phleboliths in such a patient. The angiographic findings in cavernous hemangiomas of the gastrointestinal tract are the same as the findings in hemangiomas in other parts of the body (Fig. 4–20).

Adenocarcinoma

Adenocarcinomas of the alimentary tract have a wide spectrum of angiographic abnormalities. This variation is due to several factors. One is the degree of differentiation of each carcinoma. Other factors include the amount of inflammatory reaction that is caused in adjacent tissues by the tumor and the degree of bowel obstruction which the tumor causes (Miller et al., 1969). Both inflammation and increased intraluminal pressure can lead to hypervascularity and dense, early venous drainage.

Most gastrointestinal adenocarcinomas are infiltrating and scirrhous. The primary angiographic abnormality, therefore, is infiltration of existing arteries, either in the wall of the stomach or in the intestine. Some degree of arterial infiltration is present in almost all gastrointestinal carcinomas (Fig. 4–21). The number of tumor vessels may vary from none to many. In general, the degree of contrast accumulation within these tumors is proportional to the number of tumor vessels, and "tumor blush" may be absent or relatively dense. Similarly, tumors with a relatively large number of tumor vessels and increased contrast accumulation tend to have dense venous drainage (Fig. 4–22), whereas more poorly vascularized lesions do not have early venous drainage or increased density

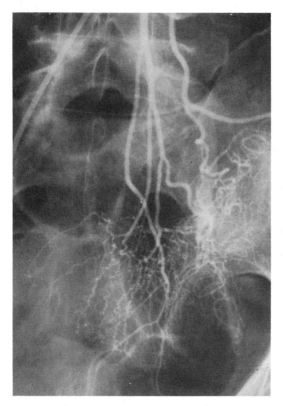

Figure 4-21. Encasement of vasa recta by a sigmoid colon carcinoma. Arterial phase of an inferior mesenteric angiogram in a 63 year old man. The vasa recta are invaded and distorted by the tumor, and several tumor vessels are present in the region. In addition, the mesenteric branches along the mesenteric side of the bowel are angulated, indicating growth of the tumor through the bowel wall into the mesentery.

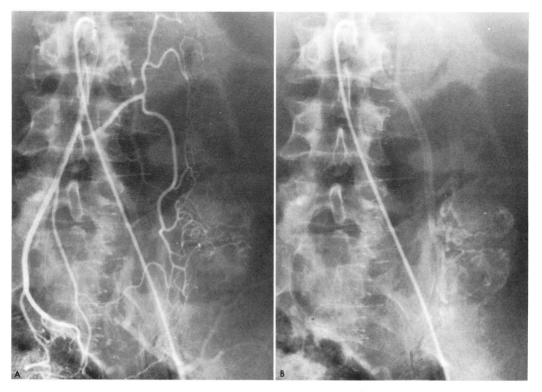

Figure 4-22. *See opposite page for legend.*

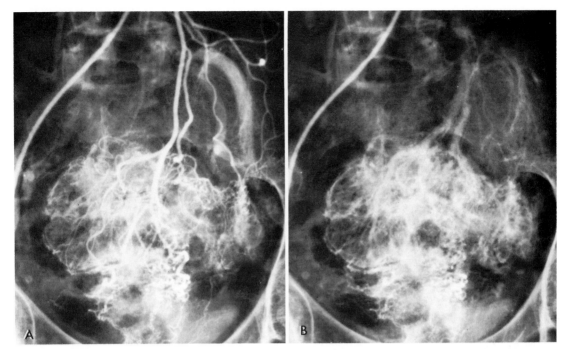

Figure 4-23. Inflammatory reaction surrounding a colon carcinoma. Inferior mesenteric angiogram in a 79 year old woman with a rectal mass.

A. Arterial phase. Extensive hypervascular changes are present throughout the rectum and sigmoid colon. Tumor vessels, however, are only present in the walls of the rectum.

B. Venous phase. Dense venous drainage is seen from the entire sigmoid colon and rectum, and a great deal of contrast accumulation is noted in the mucosa of the bowel. These findings are typical of inflammatory bowel disease. Carcinoma of the colon is rarely this hypervascular. At operation, the carcinoma was confined to the rectum.

of contrast medium in the veins. Any inflammation adjacent to the tumor accentuates the concentration of contrast medium in the veins (Fig. 4-23).

The normal arrangement of the gastric artery branches and vasa recta is regular. In the distended stomach, the branches of the gastric and gastroepiploic arteries cross it in an undulating but parallel manner (see Fig. 2-3). The same is true of the vasa recta across the wall of the distended bowel.

Most alimentary tract carcinomas disrupt this regular arrangement of vessels; bowel tumors, particularly, tend to spread adjoining vasa recta around the tumor in a "parenthesis" configuration. Gaseous distention of the stomach or the colon is helpful because it straightens the normal vasa recta, accentuating their distortion by tumor.

An assessment of the degree of infiltration of alimentary tract carcinomas is im-

Figure 4-22. Increased concentration of contrast medium in veins draining a descending colon carcinoma. Inferior mesenteric angiogram in a 50 year old man.

A. Arterial phase. Vasa recta in the mid-descending colon are displaced around a mass which has several fine tumor vessels.

B. Venous phase. The veins in the bowel around the tumor are dilated and tortuous, and the contrast medium in them is denser than in veins in the surrounding bowel. The central flow defect in the inferior mesenteric vein is caused by blood from the surrounding bowel mixing with the contrast medium from the tumor.

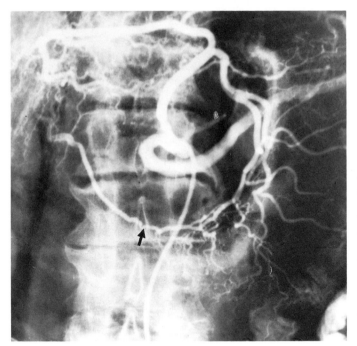

Figure 4–24. Invasion of the right gastric artery by a carcinoma of the body and antrum of the stomach. Arterial phase of a left gastric angiogram in a 71 year old man. The contrast medium has refluxed through the left gastric artery to the right gastric artery. A left hepatic artery arises from the left gastric artery. There are abrupt angulations and changes in caliber of a 1 cm segment of the right gastric artery (➡), indicating extension of the tumor through the wall of the stomach. In addition, several tumor vessels and infiltrated gastric artery branches are seen in the body of the stomach. (From Reuter, S. R., Redman, H. C., Miller, W. J., and Hoskins, P. A.: Gastric angiography. Radiology *94:* 272, 1970.)

portant. As long as the infiltrated arteries are within the gastric wall or are vasa recta on the surface of the bowel, the tumor has not invaded beyond the wall. However, when the marginal artery of Drummond, mesenteric artery branches, left or right gastroepiploic artery or the right gastric–left gastric arcade is invaded, the lesion has extended beyond the wall of the viscus (Fig. 4–24). A positive angiographic finding is more reliable in this assessment than a negative finding.

Lymphoma

Very few angiograms have been performed in patients with alimentary tract lymphomas. In general, lymphoma is a poorly vascularized lesion at angiography (Figs. 4–6 and 4–25). The primary findings have been displacement and distortion of vascular anatomy with some infiltration of arteries in the bowel wall or stomach but with few tumor vessels and minimal increased contrast accumulation. Early venous drainage is unusual. Angiographic differentiation of lymphoma from lymphosarcoma is not possible.

Metastases to the Alimentary Canal

Most metastases to the stomach and bowel occur by direct extension of an adjacent carcinoma or by peritoneal seeding. Thus, carcinoma of the pancreas can infiltrate gastric as well as pancreatic arteries (see Fig. 4–3). Since both gastric and pancreatic carcinomas are infiltrating, scirrhous lesions, it is occasionally impossible to determine the origin of the tumor by angiography. Similarly, biliary carcinomas may invade the duodenum or common duct, and pancreatic carcinomas may infiltrate the duodenum or jejunum (Fig. 4–26). Other tumors that metastasize to small bowel are ovarian tumors, melanomas and choriocarcinomas. Ovarian tumors and melanomas are usually poorly vascularized and primarily distort existing intestinal arteries. A choriocarcinoma, however, is extremely vascular wherever it metastasizes, and contrast accumulation in the capillary phase is prominent (Fig. 4–27). The presence of the primary tumor is generally known prior to angiography.

Occasionally tumors metastasize to the

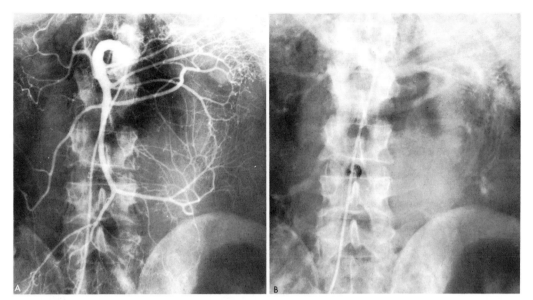

Figure 4-25. Small bowel lymphoma. Superior mesenteric angiogram in a 50 year old man.

A. Arterial phase. A poorly vascularized tumor mass displaces the superior mesenteric artery and its jejunal and ileal branches in a curvilinear manner.

B. Venous phase. Contrast accumulation is only minimally increased in the tumor, and no early or dense venous drainage is apparent. Jejunal veins are elevated by the mass. (Courtesy of Dr. Lawrence Campbell.)

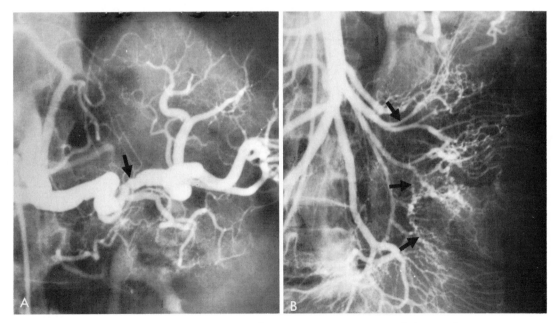

Figure 4-26. Infiltration of the mesentery by pancreatic carcinoma. Celiac and mesenteric angiograms in a 60 year old man.

A. Arterial phase of a celiac angiogram. The splenic artery is encased by the tumor (➡) and has a serrated appearance. Several tumor vessels are seen in the tumor.

B. Arterial phase of a superior mesenteric angiogram. The jejunal branches are invaded by the tumor (➡).

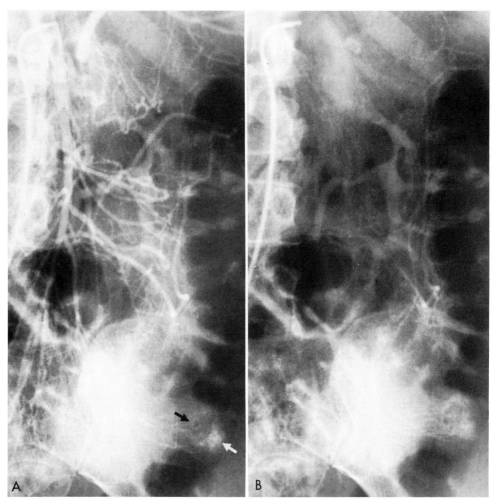

Figure 4–27. Ileal metastasis from choriocarcinoma. Superior mesenteric angiogram in a 23 year old woman with disseminated choriocarcinoma.

A. Arterial phase. An ileal branch of the superior mesenteric artery supplies several tumor vessels in a hypervascular lesion in the proximal ileum (⇉).

B. Venous phase. The accumulation of contrast in the metastasis is increased. The center of the metastasis is hypovascular, probably indicating central necrosis.

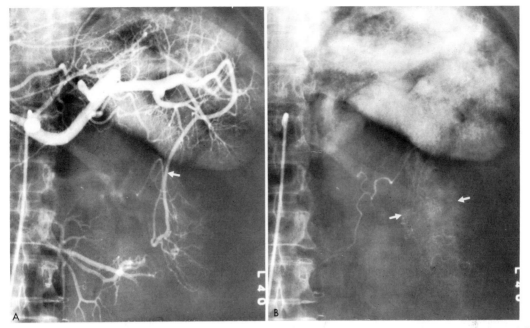

Figure 4–28. Omental metastasis. Celiac angiogram in a 61 year old woman with carcinoma of the ovary metastatic throughout the abdomen.

A. Arterial phase. An epiploic branch of the splenic artery (⟹) is dilated and supplies numerous infiltrated, dilated branches throughout the metastasis. A proximal jejunal branch supplies the lower portion of the tumor.

B. Capillary phase. Contrast accumulation is increased throughout the metastasis (⟹).

mesentery and greater omentum. When this occurs, the arteries in the mesentery and omentum become distorted. Deutch et al. (1971) have observed dilatation of epiploic branches in patients with metastatic involvement of the omentum (Fig. 4–28). However, one must be cautious in the interpretation of this finding, since the omentum frequently participates in the walling off of intraabdominal abscesses, which may result in a similar appearance.

Problems in the Differential Diagnosis of Alimentary Tract Tumors

Although few diseases cause angiographic changes similar to carcinoma of the alimentary tract, it is occasionally difficult to establish whether minor arterial changes are significant or lie within the range of normal variation. Generally, small vessel atherosclerosis can be identified by the wide extent of vascular abnormalities.

Probably the most troublesome diagnostic problem is differentiating between carcinoma and inflammatory disease. However, inflammatory disease of the intestines usually involves much longer segments of bowel than are involved by tumor and does not disturb the anatomic arrangement of arteries and veins in the bowel wall as much. One of the hallmarks of active inflammatory disease in the bowel is dense venous drainage from the entire affected segment of bowel. This is unusual in bowel tumors. Abscesses and granulation tissue may have disturbing neovascularity as well as demonstrate a mass effect. Inflammatory disease is described in Chapter 7.

Carcinoma must be diagnosed with caution when there has been previous surgery in the area being examined. The intraoperative ligation of blood vessels with the subsequent development of collateral vessels and fibrosis may simulate neoplasm.

Hepatic Neoplasms

Angiography, isotopic scanning, ultrasound and computerized tomography are the primary diagnostic methods in the evaluation of hepatic masses. Of these, only angiography can yield specific information about their nature and about the hepatic segments and arteries involved. These factors are important to the surgeon in planning a hepatic resection for tumor, and angiography should precede any liver resection.

Benign Hepatic Tumors

Benign tumors of the liver rarely cause symptoms and are generally discovered incidentally during angiography performed for other reasons. The most common benign tumor is the angioma. Adenomas and focal nodular hyperplasias are uncommon. All other benign hepatic tumors are rare.

ANGIOMA. Hepatic angiomas occur either as cavernous hemangiomas or as hemangioendotheliomas.

The cavernous type of hemangioma is seen primarily in women. Although irregular amorphous calcifications in cavernous hemangiomas are sometimes seen on plain films, the typical phlebolith does not occur in hepatic hemangiomas. The angiographic appearance is the same as elsewhere in the body. The hepatic artery and its major branches are not dilated. In the late arterial phase, small groups of dilated vascular spaces fill with contrast medium (Figs. 4–29 and 4–30). These spaces are coarse and have irregular walls but are well marginated. Contrast medium of arterial concentration is retained in the spaces long into the venous phase, since blood flow is extremely slow. On occasion, a large portion of the liver may be involved with such hemangiomas (Fig. 4–31), which may cause hemobilia.

Cavernous hemangiomas can usually be differentiated from hepatomas because the vascular spaces in hepatomas do not retain the contrast medium nearly as long as those of the angioma. The major branches of hepatic arteries supplying cavernous hemangiomas generally do not dilate, while those to a hepatoma usually do. No vascular infiltration or tumor vessels are present in hemangiomas. Draining veins are sometimes seen with hepatomas but are rare in hemangiomas, except in infants with giant cavernous hemangiomas. Occa-

sionally an angioma may be misdiagnosed as a hypervascular liver metastasis in patients with endocrine or renal carcinomas.

The hemangioendothelioma type of angioma has been reported in patients who had received Thorotrast (Curry et al., 1975). However, almost all hemangioendotheliomas occur in children. Because of the very cellular nature of these angiomas, their appearance is somewhat different from the cavernous hemangiomas. Although the amorphous spaces which retain contrast medium into the venous phase occur, these tumors also cause arteriovenous shunting, and early venous drainage to the hepatic vein is characteristic. Hemangioendotheliomas of childhood become malignant, resulting in hemangioendothelial sarcomas. Although hemangioendothelial sarcomas retain the angiographic characteristics of the hemangioendothelioma, they may be larger, and the mass of the tumor causes more displacement and distortion of the hepatic artery branches (see Fig. 4–10). Fredens (1969) reported an endothelial sarcoma in a child. The lesion appeared avascular and cystic at angiography. Moss et al. (1971) reported a hemangiosarcoma that was hypervascular.

The giant hepatic hemangioma of infancy must be diagnosed early because the arteriovenous shunting leads to congestive heart failure. The typical angiographic appearance is a markedly dilated hepatic artery supplying multiple dilated vascular channels throughout the tumor (Fig. 4–32). The arteriovenous shunting causes dense filling of hepatic veins (Fig. 4–33). In addition to establishing the diagnosis, angiography can demonstrate the extent of the lesion, since giant hemangiomas involving only a single lobe of the liver can be resected. Alternatively, the hepatic artery can be ligated (de Lorimier et al., 1967) or embolized. If congestive heart failure can be avoided, these lesions generally involute within the first year of life.

ADENOMA. Hepatic adenomas are uncommon benign tumors occurring in women primarily of childbearing age. During the past 5 years, however, the reported incidence of these tumors has increased markedly, and an association between adenomas and oral contraceptives has been postulated (Baum et al., 1973). The exact

Text continued on page 136.

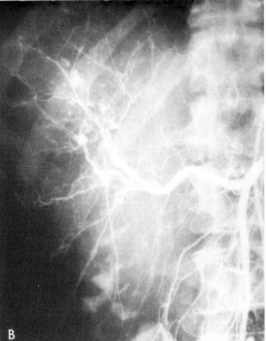

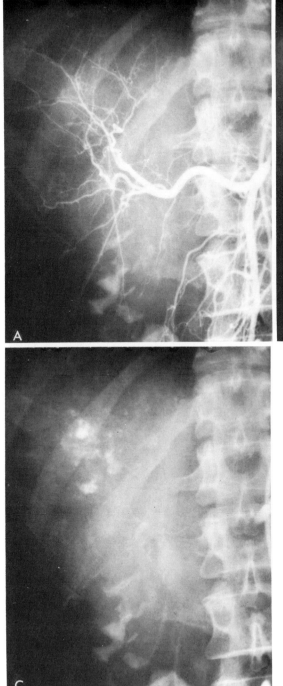

Figure 4-29. Hepatic hemangioma. Superior mesenteric angiogram in a 43 year old woman.

A. Early arterial phase. The right hepatic artery is replaced to the superior mesenteric artery. The hepatic artery branches appear normal.

B. Midarterial phase. Amorphous but sharply defined vascular spaces begin to fill with contrast medium of arterial density.

C. Late venous phase. The vascular spaces retain the contrast medium long after the veins have cleared.

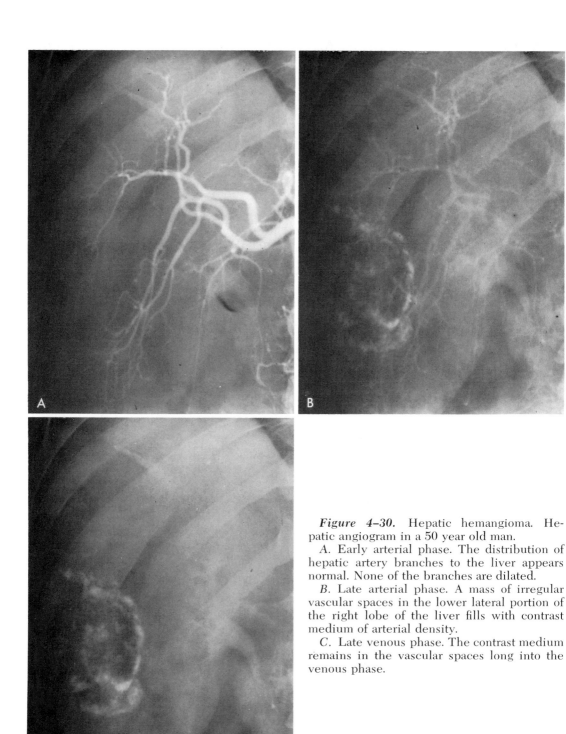

Figure 4-30. Hepatic hemangioma. Hepatic angiogram in a 50 year old man.

A. Early arterial phase. The distribution of hepatic artery branches to the liver appears normal. None of the branches are dilated.

B. Late arterial phase. A mass of irregular vascular spaces in the lower lateral portion of the right lobe of the liver fills with contrast medium of arterial density.

C. Late venous phase. The contrast medium remains in the vascular spaces long into the venous phase.

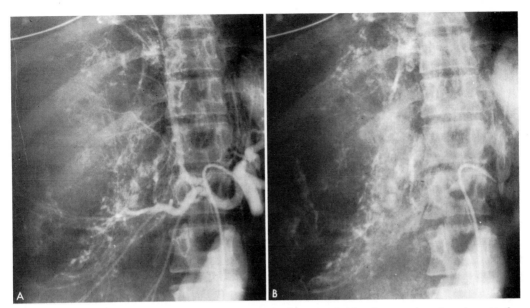

Figure 4–31. Large cavernous hemangioma of the liver with bleeding and an intrahepatic hematoma. Celiac angiogram in a 29 year old woman.

A. Arterial phase. The hepatic artery branches are not dilated but are stretched around the hematoma in the right lobe of the liver. The vascular spaces of the hemangioma have begun to fill.

B. Late venous phase. The defect in the hepatogram from the hematoma is apparent. The dilated vascular spaces in the hemangioma retain contrast medium of arterial density.

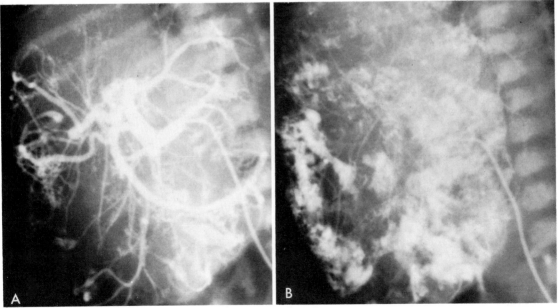

Figure 4–32. Giant hemangioma of infancy. Hepatic angiogram in an 8 day old boy with a hepatic mass.

A. Early arterial phase. The hepatic artery branches are markedly dilated, and there is early filling of abnormal vascular spaces.

B. Late arterial phase. The tumor has replaced most of the right lobe of the liver. The contrast medium remains in the abnormal vascular spaces into the venous phase. Arteriovenous shunting is not a prominent part of this infant's tumor.

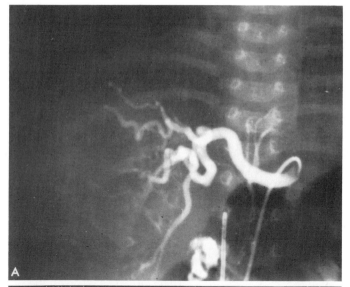
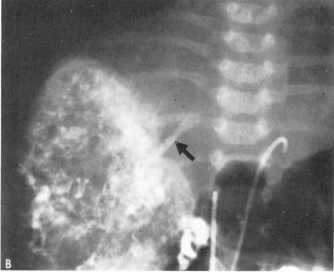

Figure 4–33. Giant hemangioma of infancy. Hepatic angiogram in a 7 week old boy with an enlarging abdominal mass and congestive failure.

A. Arterial phase. The hepatic artery and its branches are markedly dilated and tortuous.

B. Venous phase. The vascular spaces in the hemangioma retain contrast medium of arterial density. In addition, there is dense filling of the hepatic vein (➡) indicating the arteriovenous shunting in the tumor. (Courtesy of Dr. A. J. Palubinskas. From Moss, A. A., Clark, R. E., Palubinskas, A. J., and de Lorimier, A. A.: Angiographic appearance of benign and malignant tumors in infants and children. Amer. J. Roentgenol. *113*:65, 1971.)

incidence of these lesions is unknown because they are asymptomatic until discovered incidentally at operation or angiography or when they bleed. There is no evidence that adenomas are premalignant (Ishak and Rabin, 1975), but they should be resected because of their tendency to bleed. The diagnosis should be considered in any young woman with spontaneous intraabdominal hemorrhage.

Angiography is the most useful diagnostic examination in patients with suspected adenomas. Even small adenomas are readily detectable (Ameriks et al., 1975). Although the angiographic abnormalities found in a number of patients with hepatic adenomas have been reported, experience is yet too limited to determine the range of angiographic findings occurring in these lesions. In general, however, hepatic adenomas appear as rounded hypervascular masses which displace the hepatic arteries as they grow and which are fed by numerous vascular branches perforating from the periphery (Figs. 4–34 and 4–35). Although there is a rich and fairly coarse neovascularity throughout the tumors, "pooling" or "laking" has not been described. Adenomas tend to displace rather than invade portal vein

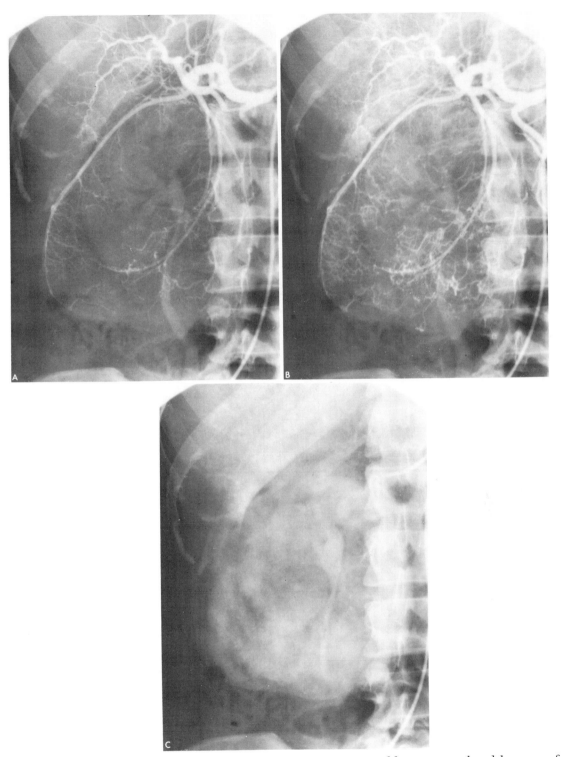

Figure 4–34. Hepatic adenoma. Hepatic angiogram in 29 year old woman explored because of a palpable right upper quadrant mass.

A. Early arterial phase. The hepatic artery branches are stretched around a mass in the lower right lobe of the liver. The smaller branches perforate toward the center of the tumor from the displaced branches.

B. Midarterial phase. Several tumor vessels are visualized throughout the lesion.

C. Parenchymal phase. There is increased accumulation of contrast medium throughout the tumor, which has a nonhomogeneous, "lumpy" appearance. (Courtesy of Dr. Joseph J. Bookstein.)

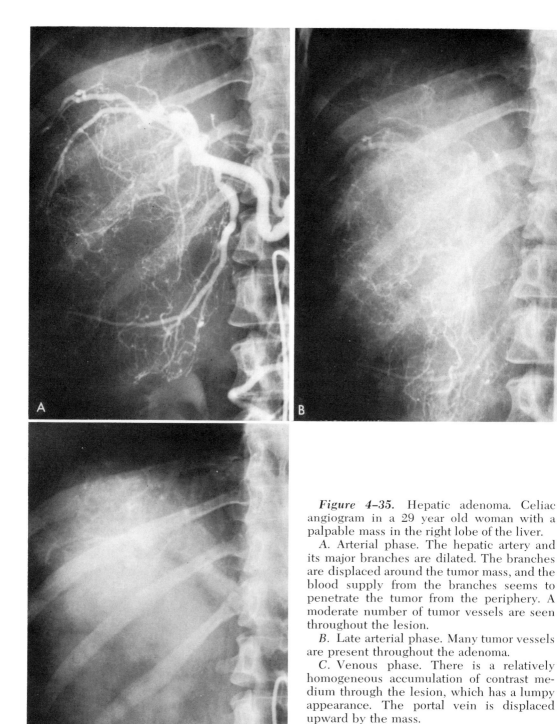

Figure 4–35. Hepatic adenoma. Celiac angiogram in a 29 year old woman with a palpable mass in the right lobe of the liver.

A. Arterial phase. The hepatic artery and its major branches are dilated. The branches are displaced around the tumor mass, and the blood supply from the branches seems to penetrate the tumor from the periphery. A moderate number of tumor vessels are seen throughout the lesion.

B. Late arterial phase. Many tumor vessels are present throughout the adenoma.

C. Venous phase. There is a relatively homogeneous accumulation of contrast medium through the lesion, which has a lumpy appearance. The portal vein is displaced upward by the mass.

radicles. The primary diagnostic problem is in differentiating hepatoma and focal nodular hyperplasia from adenoma. The angiographic characteristics of hepatomas are described later. Generally, hepatomas occur in an older age group and are more common in men. However, when a well differentiated hepatoma occurs in a young woman, the angiographic differentiation from adenoma may be very difficult (Fig. 4–36). Since the treatment for both hepatoma and adenoma is surgical excision, the differentiation is not critical, and assessment of resectability becomes an important part of the angiogram. Differentiation of an adenoma from focal nodular hyperplasia may be more difficult.

FOCAL NODULAR HYPERPLASIA. This uncommon entity, also called hamartoma, is an hepatic tumor which forms around central areas of scar tissue. Multiple fine septa subdivide the nodule into smaller units. Characteristically, large veins and arteries are present at the periphery of the lesion and in the scars, while smaller vessels are scattered throughout the septa (Ishak and Rabin, 1975). The etiology and pathogenesis of the lesion remain undetermined. Although probably not caused by oral contraceptives (Ishak and Rabin, 1975), focal nodular hyperplasia may grow under the influence of hormones, as has been shown for hemangiomas and adenomas. When the lesions are small, the arteries supplying them break up into many small branches which permeate the lesions, causing a reticular pattern. These branches are not dilated, but the overall impression is one of increased vascularity. Tumor vessels are not seen. In the hepatogram phase a fine homogeneous granularity is present throughout the tumor (Fig. 4–37), and sometimes there is a lucent ring around the periphery (Fig. 4–38). In larger tumors, a dilated hepatic artery branch frequently perforates toward the center of the lesion and then breaks into a radiating group of branches (Fig. 4–38). However, this configuration may not be seen, and the tumors may appear similar to adenomas. In the hepatogram phase the contrast accumulation through the lesion appears homogeneously granular or nodular.

When the typical angiographic findings of either adenoma or focal nodular hyperplasia occur, the differential diagnosis can be suggested. However, the two tumors may have similar appearances, and the angiographic differentiation may not be as easy as the literature implies. Moreover, there is an even greater similarity in the histologic appearances of the two lesions, and until the pathologists develop a standard nomenclature and consistent diagnostic criteria, it will be difficult for the radiologist to establish the angiographic criteria (Fig. 4–39).

Other benign hepatic tumors are extremely rare. These include bile duct adenomas and cystadenomas, leiomyomas, parenchymal hamartomas and myomas. To our knowledge the angiographic abnormalities occurring in these lesions have not been reported.

REGENERATING NODULES. The human liver has remarkable regenerative power. Whenever large areas of hepatic parenchyma are destroyed by resection or disease, particularly cirrhosis, the remaining liver cells proliferate. As this occurs, regenerating nodules, which may become large, are formed (Fig. 4–40). The arteries supplying the nodule penetrate toward the center and are stretched (Fig. 4–41) and sometimes distorted (Rabinowitz et al., 1974). The nodule has fewer arteries than the surrounding liver. In the hepatogram phase, the contrast accumulation through the nodule is generally homogeneous and resembles that of the remaining liver. In many instances the venous phase demonstrates a stretched and elongated prominent branch of the portal vein extending through the regenerating mass. The primary diagnostic problem is in differentiating hepatoma from a regenerating nodule, since both masses are common in patients with alcoholic cirrhosis. In general, most hepatomas are much more vascular than regenerating nodules, have areas of arterial invasion and have extensive neovascularity. Therefore, only the rare, poorly vascularized hepatoma is difficult to diagnose. The usefulness of gold or technetium scanning in the differentiation is not certain. Authors agree that there is no uptake of the colloidal nuclide by hepatomas. However, uptake by regenerating nodules has been reported to be increased (Viamonte et al., 1970) or irregularly diminished to absent (Rabinowitz et al., 1974).

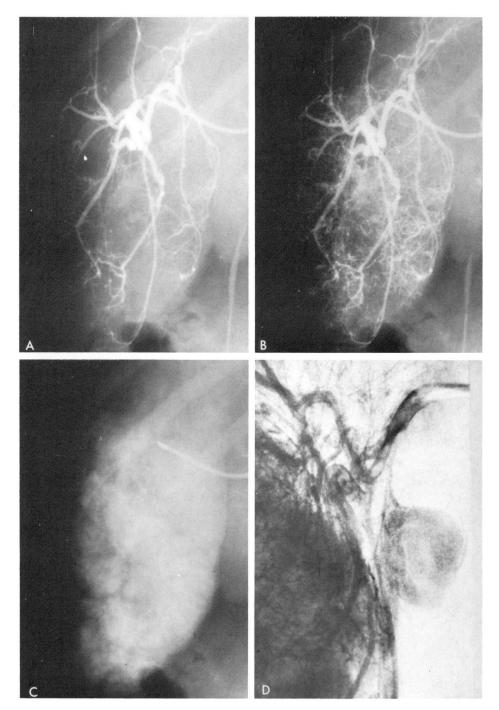

Figure 4–36. Hepatoma, clinically felt to be an adenoma. Hepatic and superior mesenteric angiograms in a 21 year old woman taking oral contraceptives.

A. Early arterial phase. Hepatic artery branches around the tumor are slightly dilated and displaced.

B. Midarterial phase. Many tumor vessels and a few abnormal vascular spaces are seen throughout the tumor. Although the hepatic artery branches are not draped around the tumor to the same extent as in the patient in Figure 4–35, the appearance of the tumor vascularity is similar.

C. Venous phase. The contrast accumulation through the tumor is diffusely nodular.

D. Subtraction film of a magnification hepatic angiogram. Late arterial phase. A secondary nodule is present in the hilum of the liver, which is separate from the major portion of the tumor. This was interpreted to represent metastatic nodes.

Figure continued on opposite page.

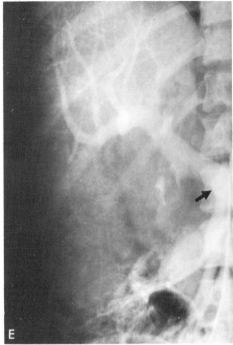

Figure 4–36. Continued. E. Venous phase of a high-dose superior mesenteric angiogram following injection of Priscoline. The impression of the secondary nodule can be seen in the proximal portion of the portal vein (➡). At operation the lesion was found to be a hepatoma with multiple metastatic nodes around the root of the mesentery.

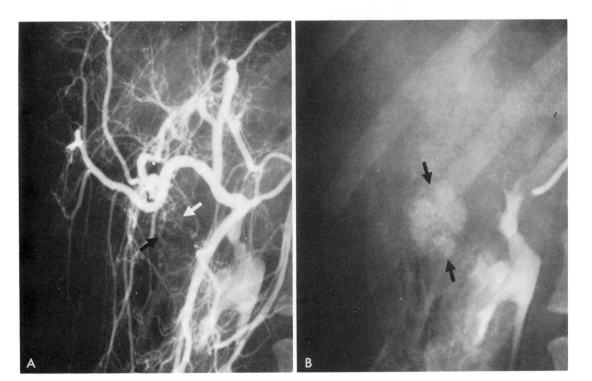

Figure 4–37. Probable focal nodular hyperplasia. Hepatic angiogram in a 30 year old woman in whom a hepatic nodule was palpated during a laparotomy for unrelated disease.

A. Arterial phase. Some slightly irregular arteries are present below the right hepatic artery in the region of the liver hilum (⇉).

B. Venous phase. A sharply marginated, hypervascular tumor is present with a fine homogeneous granularity throughout (➡).

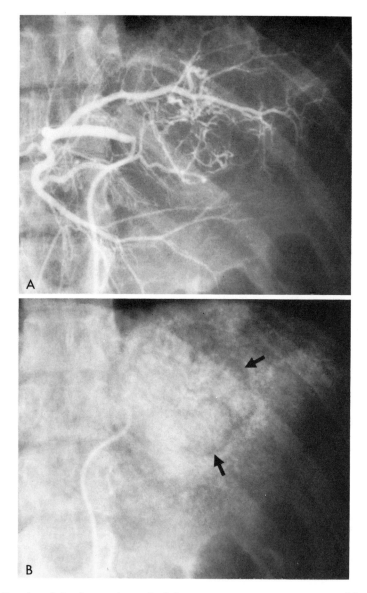

Figure 4–38.   Focal nodular hyperplasia. Left hepatic angiogram in a 34 year old woman in whom a left hepatic mass was discovered during a laparotomy for unrelated disease.

A. Arterial phase. Branches of the left hepatic artery supply a hypervascular nodule. Several of the arteries in the tumor are irregular and have a gross "spoke-wheel" pattern.

B. Venous phase. The lesion appears well marginated and has a homogenous granularity throughout. In addition, there appears to be a lucent margin to the tumor (➡).

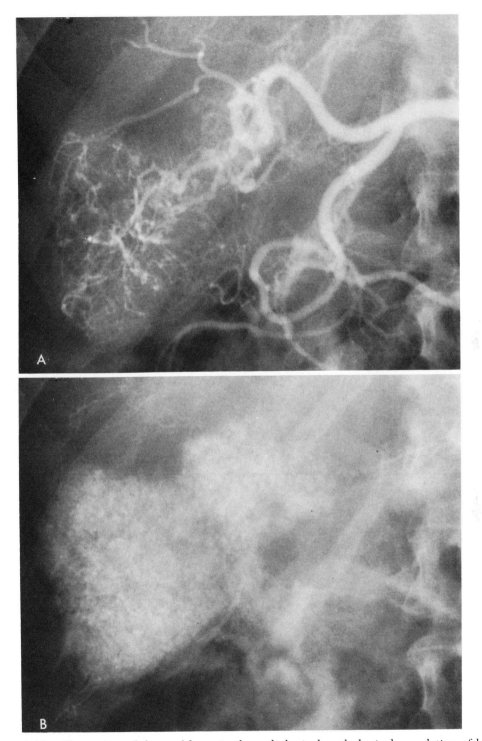

Figure 4–39. Illustration of the problems in the radiological–pathological correlation of hepatic "pill tumors." Celiac angiogram in a 42 year old woman on oral contraceptives with a large mass in the right lobe of the liver discovered incidentally during a laparotomy for unrelated disease.

A. Arterial phase. The major branch of the hepatic artery supplying the tumor penetrates toward the center of the mass and supplies several branches through the tumor and is somewhat "spoke wheel" patterned. The vessels within the tumor have an irregular distribution and have irregular walls, but tumor vessels are not seen.

B. Venous phase. The tumor mass is bilobed and has a homogeneous, coarsely granular pattern throughout.

Although this tumor has the typical angiographic appearance of focal nodular hyperplasia, the pathologists could not determine whether it was focal nodular hyperplasia or adenoma, although they favored the latter diagnosis.

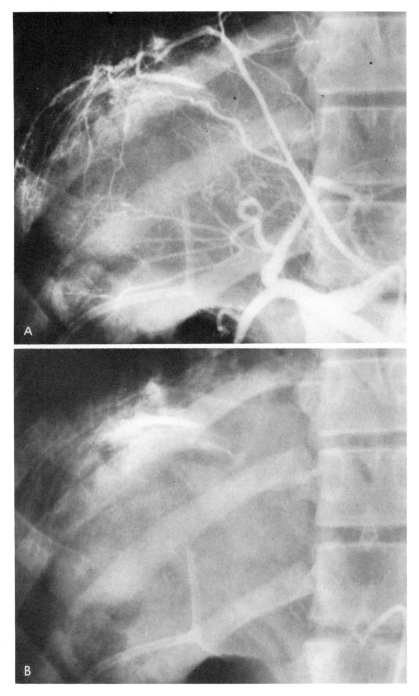

Figure 4-40. Celiac angiogram in a 17 year old man who had a right hepatic lobectomy because of hepatic trauma 3 months previously.

A. Arterial phase. Only the left and middle hepatic arteries arise from the celiac axis. The branches of the middle hepatic artery are stretched around an avascular mass. The right inferior phrenic artery is also dilated and supplies a hypervascular, inflammatory-appearing diaphragm.

B. Venous phase. The mass around which the middle hepatic artery branches are stretched has approximately the same degree of contrast accumulation as the remainder of the liver. A great deal of increased contrast accumulation is seen in the region of the diaphragm.

Because of fever and the angiographic findings, the patient was reexplored. No subphrenic abscess was seen, and a biopsy of the hepatic mass revealed regenerating liver cells.

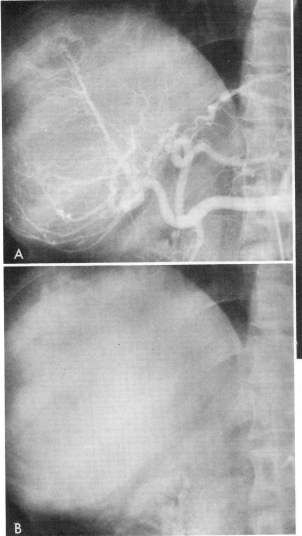
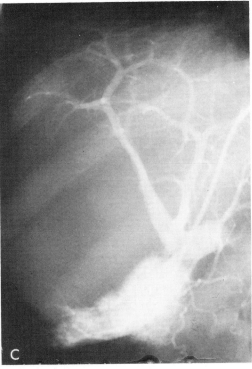

Figure 4–41. Large regenerating nodule. Celiac angiogram and wedged hepatic venogram in a 48 year old man with advanced cirrhosis.

A. Arterial phase. Several branches of the right hepatic artery are displaced around a large mass in the right lobe of the liver.

B. Venous phase. The mass has slightly greater contrast accumulation than the surrounding liver.

C. Wedged hepatic venogram. The sinusoidal filling pattern appears mildly unhomogenous, and the portal vein radicles which fill from the sinusoids are stretched around the mass.

Primary Malignant Tumors

Almost all primary malignant hepatic tumors in adults are carcinomas and arise either from the hepatic cells or from the biliary ducts. Angiography is generally performed in patients with primary hepatic carcinoma because of the presence of jaundice, ascites, severe abdominal pain or an abdominal mass. The hepatoma (or liver cell carcinoma) is more common than the biliary ductal carcinoma (or cholangiocarcinoma). Both types may be confluent, multinodular or diffuse. Fortunately, the massive confluent form is most common, since this type is easiest to diagnose by angio-graphy. A mixed form of the tumor, in which both hepatic ductal and hepatic cellular elements are present, is uncommon.

HEPATOMA. A spectrum of angiographic abnormalities occurs in hepatoma, although most hepatomas are very vascular, with a dilated hepatic arterial supply and many small, abnormal vessels throughout the tumor (Figs. 4–36 and 4–42). Abnormal vascular spaces are frequently present. Arteriovenous shunting occasionally occurs through the tumor to the portal vein, and the portal vein may be invaded (Figs. 4–7 and 4–43). When this constellation ·of angiographic findings is present, the diagnosis of hepatoma is made easily, because

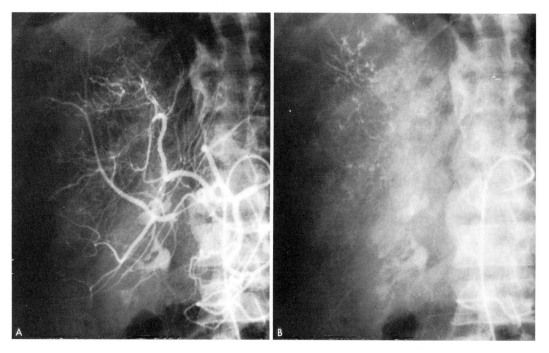

Figure 4–42. Hepatoma. Hepatic angiogram in a 63 year old man with jaundice and an enlarged liver.

A. Arterial phase. The hepatic artery branches to the right lobe are dilated and supply numerous fine tumor vessels throughout the upper portion of the lobe.

B. Venous phase. The stellate arrangement of abnormally dilated sinusoids is characteristic of hepatoma. Contrast accumulation is mottled and uneven through the right lobe of the liver. No early venous drainage is noted in this patient.

no other hepatic tumors have this appearance. Kido et al. (1971) have correlated the angiographic abnormalities in hepatomas with the histology. In general, this typical appearance was seen in well differentiated tumors. Anaplastic lesions were more poorly vascularized. When hepatomas are less vascular or multicentric, the diagnosis becomes increasingly difficult (Fig. 4–44).

An assessment of the extent of spread of the hepatoma is an important part of the angiographic evaluation, since hepatomas localized to a single lobe of the liver can be resected. This is done primarily by determining which branches of the hepatic artery participate in the tumor supply; two projections are often necessary. Equally important is excellent visualization of the portal vein and its branches. Hepatomas frequently invade the portal vein radicles in their vicinity, and splenoportography should be used as part of the preoperative evaluation of these patients. Even when the tumor appears to be localized to one lobe by the arterial abnormalities, it may

have grown along the portal vein to the other lobe, making it unresectable (Fig. 4–45). In this instance, splenoportography is preferred over high dose splenic angiography because of the greater anatomic information this study provides.

A primary diagnostic problem is differentiating hepatoma from a regenerating liver after resection, which was discussed in the preceding section. Another differential problem may be created by the very hypervascular liver metastases arising from choriocarcinoma or hypernephroma. In general, however, metastases tend to be more peripheral while the primary tumors are more central. Hemangiomas have been discussed earlier and also must be differentiated from hepatomas.

CHOLANGIOCARCINOMA. Tumors arising from the hepatic ducts are infiltrating, scirrhous adenocarcinomas and generally do not have the rich network of tumor vessels and dilated sinusoids that occur in hepatomas. The primary angiographic finding is arterial infiltration, and all such

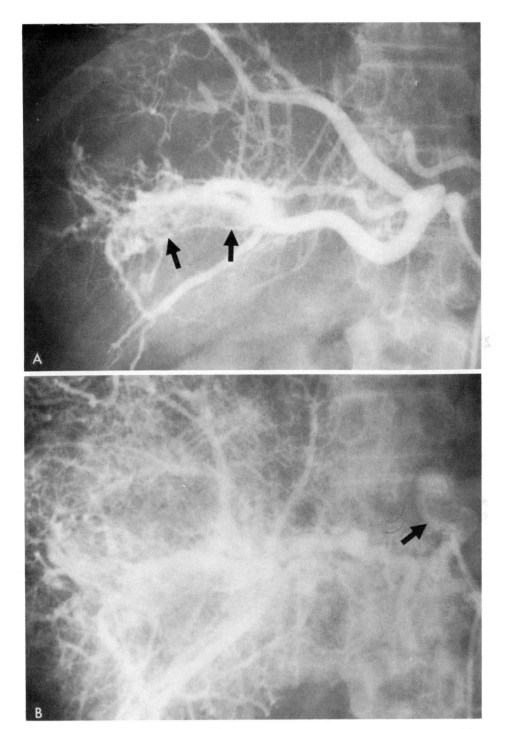

Figure 4-43. Arterio-portal shunting in hepatoma. Hepatic angiogram in a 51 year old man with chronic alcoholism.

A. Arterial phase. Several tumor vessels are seen through the right lobe of the liver, and contrast medium immediately fills the portal vein, outlining tumor in one of the major right portal vein radicles (➡).

B. Late arterial phase. Some contrast medium in the portal vein flows centrally, draining toward portal–systemic collateral veins (➡).

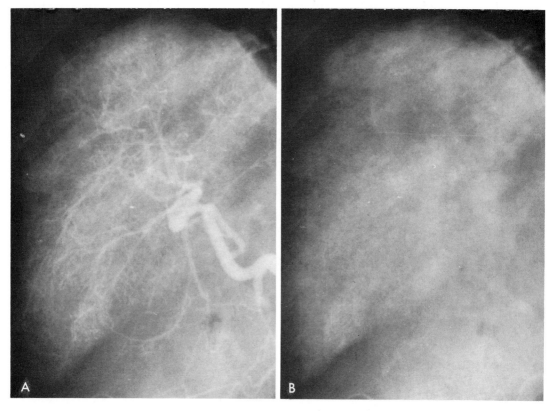

Figure 4-44. Diffuse hepatoma. Celiac angiogram in a 65 year old man with weight loss.

A. Arterial phase. Most of the hepatic arteries through the right lobe of the liver are angulated and appear to be involved by tumor. However, few tumor vessels and no abnormal vascular spaces typical of hepatoma are seen.

B. Venous phase. The hepatogram phase is irregular and nodular without arterioportal shunting. There is mild, diffuse hypervascularity. Although the hepatic angiogram is clearly abnormal and suggests tumor, the correct histologic diagnosis cannot be made from this study.

tumors large enough to be diagnosed have invaded arteries. This invasion has a typical serrated or serpiginous appearance (Fig. 4–46). The presence of other abnormal angiographic findings depends on the size of the tumor. Occasionally, cholangiocarcinomas spread through the bile ducts, and the tumor may be extensive without causing much mass effect. Large cholangiocarcinomas tend to be relatively vascular, with a moderate number of tumor vessels and increased contrast accumulation within the lesion in the capillary phase (Fig. 4–47). When the tumors are small, arterial invasion is the only abnormality. The findings may be very subtle and the diagnosis difficult (Fig. 4–48). Early or dense venous drainage from cholangiocarcinomas does not occur, and arteriovenous shunting between the hepatic artery and either the portal or hepatic veins has not been seen. Cholangiocarcinomas do not invade the portal vein or its branches as frequently as hep-

atomas. Cholangiocarcinomas can spread along the bile ducts as well as grow as local masses. Occasionally, ductal spread may predominate. In this case, mild but diffuse invasion of hepatic artery branches is seen throughout a large area of liver (Fig. 4–49).

OTHER PRIMARY MALIGNANT HEPATIC TUMORS. Although malignant hepatic tumors other than hepatomas and cholangiocarcinomas are unusual, the angiographic abnormalities in patients with hepatic angiosarcomas have been reported.

Angiosarcomas have been observed among vinyl chloride workers (Whelan et al., 1976). The few cases that have been reported showed a mild increase in vascularity around the periphery of the tumor with development of fine tumor vessels. The hepatic artery and the branches supplying the tumors were not dilated. The contrast accumulation within the lesions persisted into the venous phase, and pooling of contrast medium was observed. The

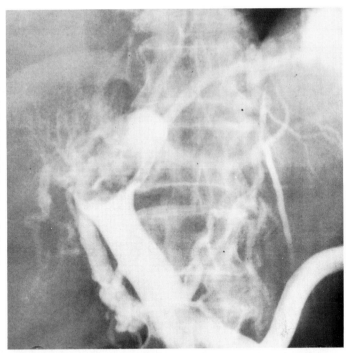

Figure 4-45. Invasion of the portal vein by hepatoma. Splenoportogram in a 66 year old man with a large hepatoma in the right lobe of the liver. The tumor grows into the confluence of the right and left portal vein radicles, occluding the right and partially occluding the left. This lesion is not resectable. Splenoportography is an important adjunct to the angiographic assessment of operability of hepatomas. (From Reuter, S. R., Redman, H. C., and Siders, D. B.: The spectrum of angiographic findings in hepatoma. Radiology *94*:90, 1970.)

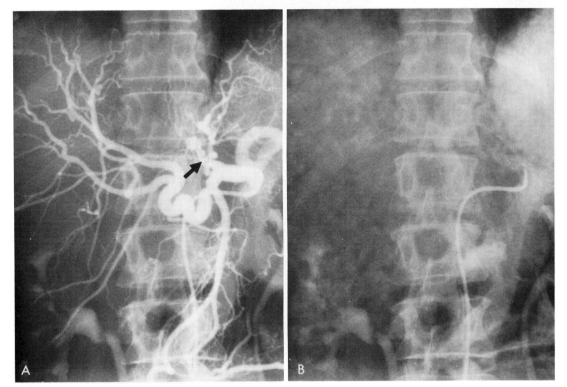

Figure 4-46. Cholangiocarcinoma. Common hepatic angiogram in a 53 year old man with a 6 month history of painless jaundice.

A. Arterial phase. The left hepatic artery is encased by tumor (➡), and its primary branches are markedly irregular. No tumor vessels are seen.

B. Parenchymal phase. There is no increased contrast accumulation through the tumor. The hepatogram phase has a mild, diffusely nodular appearance caused by obstructive jaundice.

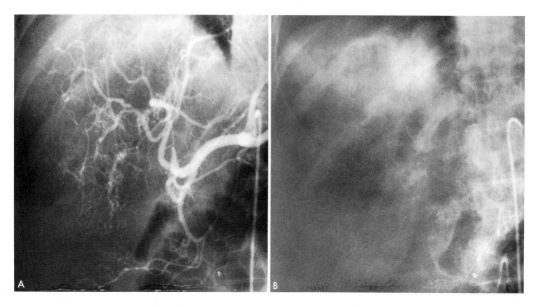

Figure 4–47. Hypervascular cholangiocarcinoma. Celiac angiogram in a 64 year old man with obstructive jaundice.

A. Arterial phase. Several branches of the right hepatic artery are invaded in the hilum and medial right lobe of the liver. Numerous tumor vessels are present throughout the lower portion of the right lobe of the liver.

B. Capillary phase. Contrast accumulation is minimally increased in the area of the tumor vessels. Large cholangiocarcinomas tend to appear hypervascular compared with the normal liver parenchyma, but still have only minimally increased contrast accumulation.

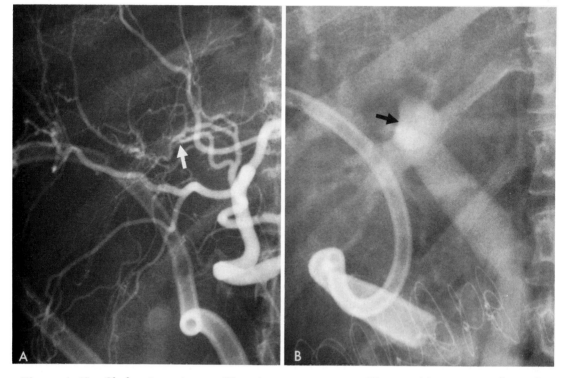

Figure 4–48. Cholangiocarcinoma. Hepatic angiogram in a 37 year old woman with painless jaundice.

A. Arterial phase. A branch of the right hepatic artery is occluded (⟹). Collateral arteries bridge the occluded segment of hepatic artery. Several infiltrated arteries are present in the area. The findings, although subtle, are characteristic of cholangiocarcinoma.

B. Venous phase of a high-dose superior mesenteric angiogram. A concavity near the bifurcation of the portal vein (➡) corresponds to the area of arterial abnormalities.

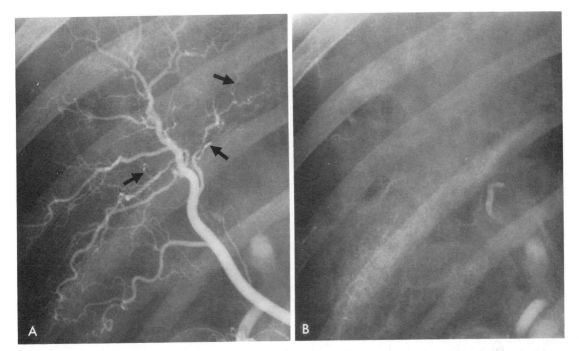

Figure 4–49. Diffuse cholangiocarcinoma. Right hepatic angiogram in a 53 year old man with a 6 month history of painless jaundice.

A. Arterial phase. There are diffuse areas of encasement and occlusion of hepatic artery branches throughout the right lobe of the liver (➡). These findings, although subtle, are characteristic of cholangiocarcinoma.

B. Parenchymal phase. The infiltrated arteries empty more slowly than the uninvolved branches. There is no increase in contrast accumulation through the tumor. The rounded, lucent areas in the central portion of the right lobe represent dilated bile ducts.

central portions of the tumors were hypo-vascular, perhaps related to the tendency of angiosarcomas to necrose.

GALLBLADDER CARCINOMA AND EXTRA-HEPATIC DUCTAL CARCINOMAS. The an-giographic appearance of carcinoma aris-ing in the gallbladder or extrahepatic bile ducts is the same as that of cholangiocar-cinoma. The primary angiographic abnor-mality is arterial invasion, and the amount of hypervascularity is proportional to the size of the tumor.

Carcinoma of the gallbladder rarely causes symptoms while still localized to the gallbladder unless it obstructs the cys-tic duct. It becomes symptomatic only after adjacent tissues have been invaded. While the tumors are small, the only artery which may be invaded is the cystic artery or one of its branches (Fig. 4–50). The cystic ar-teries have a relatively smooth, meandering course over the surface of the gallbladder, and any sharp angulation in the arteries should be suspect. When gallbladder car-

cinomas enlarge, they become hyper-vascular, with many tumor vessels and increased contrast accumulation. The cystic artery and other branches supplying such tumors dilate (Fig. 4–51).

Carcinomas of the extrahepatic biliary ducts and the ampulla of Vater cause the same angiographic abnormalities as other tumors of hepatic ductal origin. They are more difficult to diagnose, however, be-cause they cause jaundice while still small (Fig. 4–52). Because of their location near the head of the pancreas, they generally cannot be differentiated from small pan-creatic carcinomas.

DIFFERENTIAL DIAGNOSIS OF CARCIN-OMAS ARISING IN THE HEPATIC DUCTS. The major problem in the differential diag-nosis of cholangiocarcinomas is poorly vas-cularized hepatic metastases. Cholangio-carcinomas tend to be central in location, while metastases tend to be more periph-eral, more rounded and cause more hepatic vascular displacement. Also, invasion of

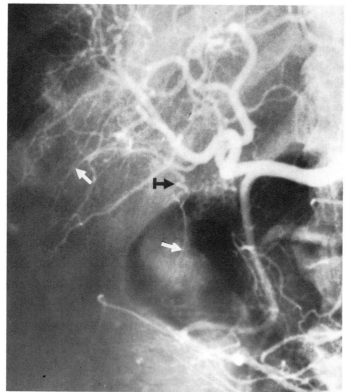

Figure 4–50. Cystic artery invasion by a gallbladder carcinoma. Arterial phase of a celiac angiogram in a 78 year old woman with a carcinoma still localized to the wall of the gallbladder. The cystic artery branches (⟹) are stretched around a distended gallbladder. The superficial branch is abruptly angulated in its proximal portion (➡). The normal course of cystic arteries is gently undulating, and any abrupt angulations in the course of these vessels must be suspect. (From Reuter, S. R., Redman, H. C., and Bookstein, J. J.: Angiography in carcinoma of the biliary tract. Brit. J. Radiol. *44*:638, 1971.)

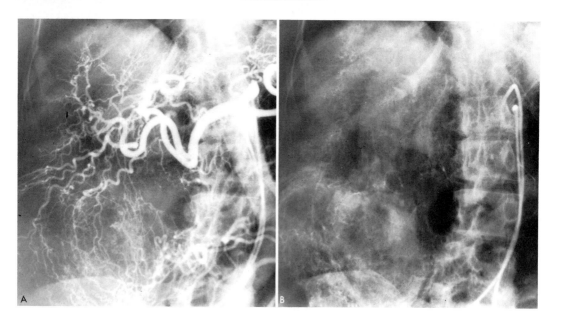

Figure 4–51. Dilated arterial supply to a large gallbladder carcinoma. Celiac angiogram in a 62 year old woman with carcinoma of the gallbladder which has invaded locally into the right lobe of the liver. A cholecystectomy had been performed several years previously, and carcinoma in situ had been found at that time.

A. Arterial phase. Several dilated arteries from hepatic artery branches supply numerous tumor vessels throughout the lesion.

B. Venous phase. There is only moderate, irregular increase in the contrast accumulation throughout the tumor.

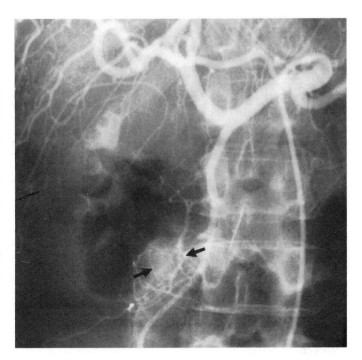

Figure 4-52. Carcinoma of the distal common duct. Arterial phase of a celiac angiogram in a 66 year old woman with obstructive jaundice. Branches of the anterior pancreaticoduodenal arcade are abruptly angulated through an area 2 cm in diameter (➡). This appearance could equally well represent carcinoma of the pancreas. The gallbladder is dilated, and the cystic artery branches are spread. (From Reuter, S. R., Redman, H. C., and Bookstein, J. J.: Angiography in carcinoma of the biliary tract. Brit. J. Radiol. *44*:638, 1971.)

hepatic artery branches by metastases is not common.

Another problem frequently occurring with large tumors in the region of the hilum of the liver, common duct or head of the pancreas is determination of the organ of origin. Did the tumor arise in the pancreas or common duct and spread toward the hilum of the liver or in the hilum of the liver and spread toward the head of the pancreas? Both carcinoma of the pancreas and carcinoma of the duodenum have histologic and angiographic appearances similar to that of biliary tract carcinoma. The differentiation has little practical significance, and tumors in this region could well be grouped as pancreaticoduodenobiliary carcinomas. Except for ampullary carcinomas, the prognosis is extremely poor, and even patients with resectable tumors are rarely cured.

Hepatic Metastases

Metastases are by far the most common malignant hepatic tumors, and the liver is the most common site for metastases from tumors of the gastrointestinal tract. The most common hepatic metastases come from the area drained by the portal vein: the stomach, the intestines and the pancre-

as. These are followed in frequency by metastases from breast carcinoma and, to a lesser extent, by metastasizing tumors from genitourinary organs. From an angiographic point of view, hepatic metastases fall into three groups: those that are hypervascular relative to the liver parenchyma, those that are hypovascular relative to the liver parenchyma and those having essentially the same vascularity as the liver parenchyma.

METASTASES THAT ARE HYPERVASCULAR RELATIVE TO THE HEPATIC PARENCHYMA. Hypervascular metastases stand out against the homogeneous capillary phase of the liver as rounded areas of increased contrast accumulation or, when larger, as areas with distinct tumor vessels and increased contrast accumulation. They may be solitary but generally are multiple. Such metastases can be identified when they are 0.5 to 1 cm in diameter. They tend to be round and have a peripheral location. Hepatic arteries are stretched and displaced by larger metastases. One of the most vascular metastases to the liver is from choriocarcinoma (Fig. 4-53). Such metastases tend to undergo necrosis, and hemorrhage is common. The liver metastases from hypernephroma are very vascular (Fig. 4-54) and may show arteriovenous shunting. In gen-

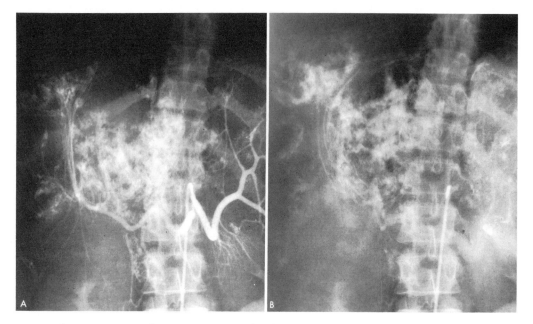

Figure 4–53. Hypervascular metastases to the liver. Celiac angiogram in a 23 year old woman with disseminated choriocarcinoma.

A. Arterial phase. Terminal hepatic artery branches are dilated and supply numerous abnormal vascular spaces throughout the liver. The centers of some of the metastases are necrotic.

B. Capillary phase. The contrast medium remains in the vascular spaces.

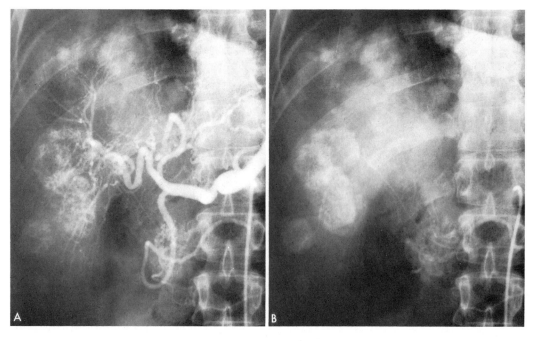

Figure 4–54. Hypervascular metastases to the liver. Celiac angiogram in a 55 year old man with metastatic hypernephroma.

A. Arterial phase. Dilated hepatic artery branches supply several hypervascular nodules. Some as small as 5 mm in diameter are well demonstrated.

B. Venous phase. The metastases retain the contrast medium. Some nodules have necrotic centers.

eral, hepatic metastases from endocrine carcinomas are hypervascular and multiple (Fig. 4–55).

Somewhat less vascular metastases, but generally still more vascular than the hepatic parenchyma, arise from malignant carcinoid tumor (Fig. 4–56) and leiomyosarcoma. These are also usually multifocal. Metastases from carcinoma of the alimentary tract may be hypervascular and may have areas of central necrosis. More frequently, however, these metastases fit into the hypovascular category or have the same vascularity as the liver parenchyma. Pancreatic carcinomas rarely have hypervascular metastases. Because of the accuracy of angiography in detecting small hypervascular hepatic metastases, a hepatic angiogram should be a part of all angiograms performed in evaluation of primary tumors.

METASTASES THAT ARE HYPOVASCULAR RELATIVE TO THE HEPATIC PARENCHYMA. These tumors may be identified by the presence of a filling defect in the capillary phase of the hepatic angiogram. If the metastases are multiple, the hepatogram will have a "Swiss cheese" appearance (Fig. 4–57). Hypovascular metastases must be approximately 2 to 3 cm or more in diameter to be identified by angiography. Displacement of intrahepatic arteries may be seen with larger lesions. Although angiography is more accurate than isotopic scanning in the detection of hypervascular metastases, scanning is as accurate or more accurate than angiography in the detection of hypovascular metastases. Hepatic metastases from carcinomas of the lung, the pancreas and the gastrointestinal tract are usually hypovascular.

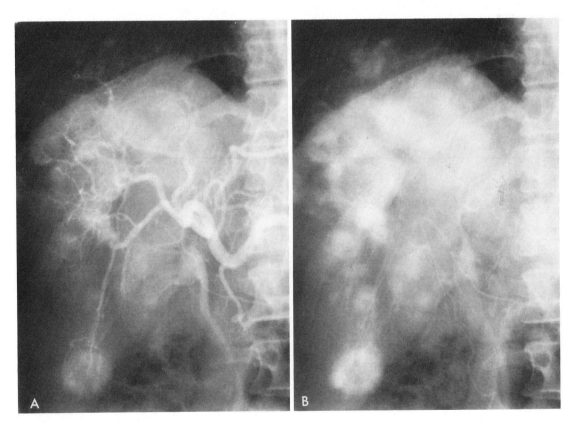

Figure 4–55. Hypervascular metastases to the liver from thyroid carcinoma. Celiac angiogram in a 53 year old woman.

A. The branches of the hepatic artery are slightly dilated and supply several rounded areas of increased contrast accumulation throughout the liver. Very few tumor vessels are seen in the metastatic nodules.

B. Parenchymal phase. The contrast accumulation within the nodules has increased. The central portions of the nodules are lucent, indicating necrosis.

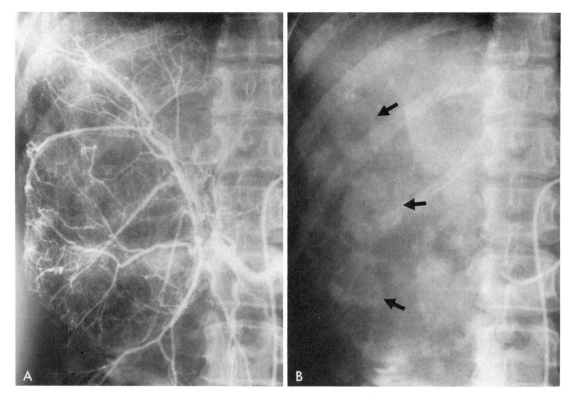

Figure 4–56. Hepatic metastases from a carcinoid tumor. Hepatic angiogram in a 37 year old woman with carcinoid syndrome.

A. Arterial phase. Several dilated hepatic artery branches are displaced around mass lesions. Tumor vessels are seen throughout the liver, particularly in the midportion.

B. Parenchymal phase. Scattered hypervascular metastases are present (➡). They stand out because the degree of contrast accumulation in the metastases is greater than in the surrounding liver parenchyma. Some of the hypervascular nodules have lucent centers, indicating necrosis.

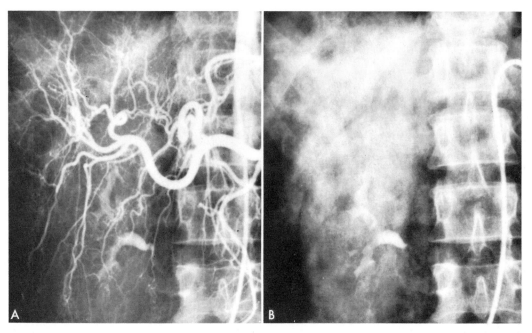

Figure 4–57. *See opposite page for legend.*

METASTASES WITH THE SAME DEGREE
OF VASCULARITY AS THE HEPATIC PAREN-
CHYMA. These metastases do not stand
out against the hepatic parenchyma in the
hepatogram phase as either areas of increased or decreased contrast accumulation
and are, therefore, the most difficult to
evaluate by angiography. The diagnosis
depends on invasion, displacement or compression of hepatic artery branches. If invasion of a hepatic artery is present, the
diagnosis is not particularly difficult, but
this is an unusual finding. More commonly,
the only finding is displacement of a hepatic artery branch. This is difficult to interpret because of the variation in the normal
branching pattern. Occasionally, a compressed arterial branch empties more
slowly than the other hepatic arteries.

Metastases to the right lobe of the liver
are more easily evaluated than those to the
left lobe, since the left lobe is partially obscured by the arteries and parenchyma of
the stomach and spleen and lies over the
spine. Therefore, if metastases to the left
lobe of the liver are suspected, selective
hepatic arteriography should be performed.
Occasionally, metastases in the left lobe
will displace the splenic artery and vein
downward (Fig. 4–58) or will spread the
two major left hepatic artery branches.

DIFFERENTIAL DIAGNOSIS OF LIVER ME-
TASTASES. In a liver diffusely involved by
metastases, it may be difficult to know if
the hypervascular or hypovascular areas
represent the metastases. Usually one or
the other area has a round configuration
and, if this is the case, the rounded areas
are the metastases.

The hypervascular form of metastasis is
generally quite distinct, and a differential
diagnostic problem occurs only if the metastasis is single and has rather indistinct
margins. It may then be confused with a
small hematoma or, rarely, an angioma.
Most metastases are multiple, and the diagnosis is easily established. More diagnostic
problems occur with metastases that have
essentially the same vascularity as the hepatic parenchyma or are hypovascular. Because of the diffuse distribution of lesions
throughout the liver, they may mimic hepatic parenchymal diseases, such as cirrhosis,
obstructive jaundice or cholangitis. This
differentiation can be extremely difficult.
The diagnosis of hepatic metastases must
also be made with circumspection in patients with obstructive jaundice secondary
to carcinoma of the head of the pancreas or
ampulla of Vater. The dilated bile ducts
resulting from common duct obstruction
can become quite large and appear the
same as multiple filling defects in the liver,
demonstrating the typical "Swiss cheese"
pattern. Unless there are large holes and
associated arterial displacement, invasion
or some other sign of metastasis, hepatic
metastases should not be diagnosed dog-
matically in the presence of obstructive
jaundice (Bree and Reuter, 1974).

The demonstration of metastases can be
enhanced by the slow injection of large
amounts of contrast medium into the hepatic artery. Approximately 50 cc of contrast
medium injected for 10 seconds into the
hepatic artery (Wirtanen, 1973) results in
increased accumulation of contrast medium
in the metastases and makes them stand
out to a greater degree. Also, the redistribution of blood flow that occurs with the use
of pharmacologic agents such as epinephrine or angiotensin may improve the
visualization of hepatic metastases. To date
this approach has given inconsistent results. However, the improvement is sometimes dramatic.

Figure 4–57. Hypovascular metastases to the liver. Celiac angiogram in a 65 year old woman
with carcinoma of the tail of the pancreas. She did not have obstructive jaundice.

A. Arterial phase. The hepatic artery branches are increased in number, but they are not distorted
or invaded.

B. Venous phase. Several areas of decreased contrast accumulation are present, giving a "Swiss
cheese" appearance. (From Reuter, S. R.: Angiography in the diagnosis of gastrointestinal cancer.
Proc. Nat. Cancer Conf. p. 452, 1968.)

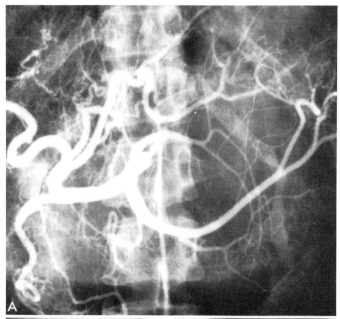

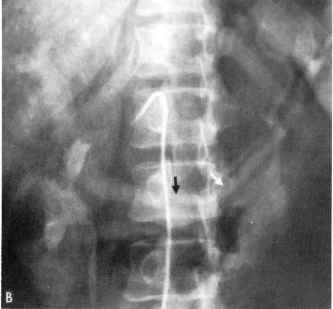

Figure 4-58. Hypovascular metastasis to the left lobe of the liver from carcinoma of the colon. Celiac angiogram in a 36 year old woman with an epigastric mass.

A. Arterial phase. The splenic artery is stretched downward.

B. Venous phase. The splenic vein (➡) is also displaced downward, stretched and slightly angulated.

LYMPHOMA. The hepatic lymphomas that have been reported have occurred in patients with Hodgkin's disease (Chuang et al., 1974; Jonsson and Lunderquist, 1974). Angiographic abnormalities have consisted primarily of displacement of hepatic arteries around single or multiple intrahepatic masses. The hepatic artery branches supplying the tumor do not dilate. Some tumors have a moderate number of tumor vessels (Fig. 4–59) and some have few tumor vessels (Fig. 4–60). In the venous phase the tumors are hypovascular relative to the surrounding liver parenchyma and stand out as filling defects in the hepatogram. The appearance is similar to that of lymphoma of the gastrointestinal tract. Occasionally, the liver is diffusely involved by

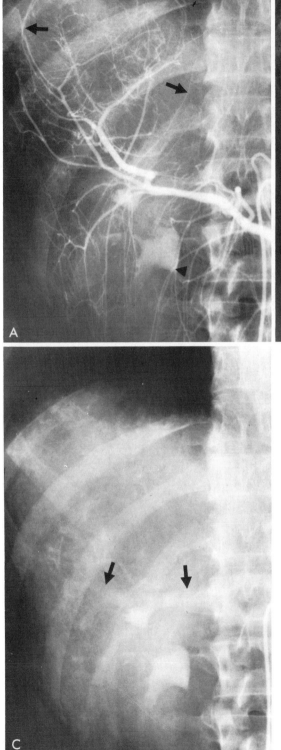

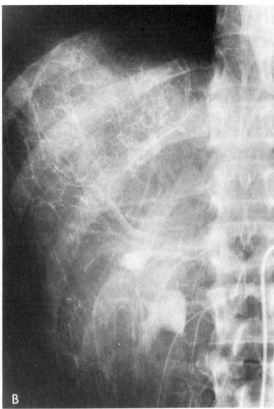

Figure 4-59. Hepatic Hodgkin's disease. Celiac angiogram in a 48 year old man.

A. Hepatic artery branches in the upper portion of the right lobe of the liver are stretched around a mildly hypervascular tumor mass (➡). In addition, a second mass is present in the region of the porta hepatis, also stretching the right hepatic artery branches to that area (▶).

B. Parenchymal phase. A moderate number of tumor vessels are present throughout the tumor of the upper right lobe, but the tumor in the porta hepatis is avascular.

C. The portal vein (➡) is displaced downward and is stretched between the two areas of tumor involvement.

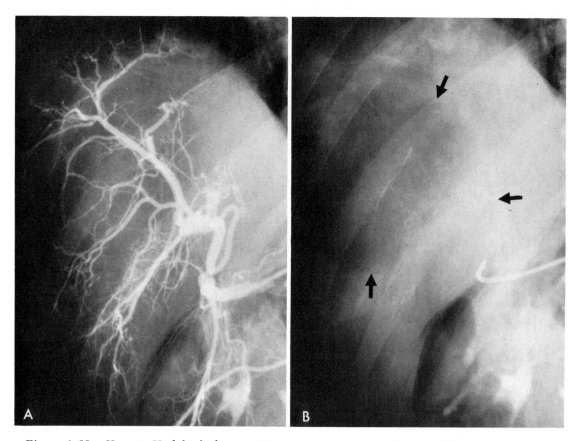

Figure 4-60. Hepatic Hodgkin's disease. Hepatic angiogram in a 38 year old woman.
A. Arterial phase. Branches of the hepatic artery in the midportion of the right lobe of the liver are displaced around a mass. Very few tumor vessels are present.
B. Parenchymal phase. The tumor stands out as a filling defect in the hepatogram phase (➡).

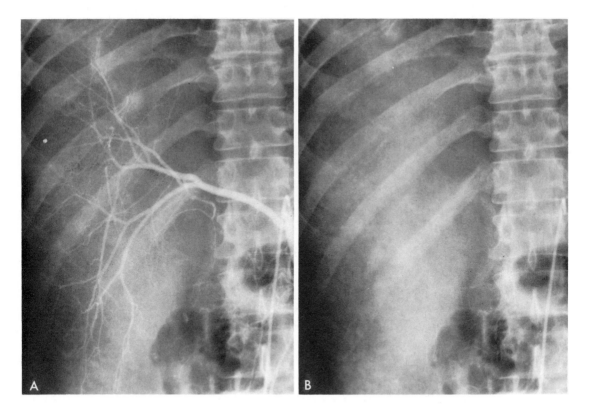

Figure 4-61. Diffuse involvement of the liver by Hodgkin's disease. Superior mesenteric angiogram in a 42 year old man.

A. The right hepatic artery is replaced to the superior mesenteric artery. Its branches through the enlarged right lobe of the liver are stretched but are of normal caliber. No tumor vessels are seen.

B. Parenchymal phase. The accumulation of contrast medium through the liver in the hepatogram phase is homogeneous. No tumor vessels or other signs of tumor are present.

Hodgkin's disease. In this case, the liver is enlarged, and the hepatic arteries are spread, but little else is seen (Fig. 4-61).

Pancreatic Neoplasms

The pancreas, like the liver, is difficult to examine by the usual radiographic techniques. Angiography, therefore, has maintained a central role in the evaluation of suspected pancreatic tumors. Gastrointestinal barium examinations, particularly hypotonic duodenography, ultrasound and computerized tomography are screening procedures generally done prior to angiography. Frequently these procedures provide the diagnosis. In a number of patients with pancreatic carcinoma, however, these diagnostic examinations are normal, or the findings are equivocal.

In these patients careful angiographic examinations should be performed to establish the diagnosis. Even when the diagnosis has been established, the surgeon may want an angiogram to obtain more information about the extent of the tumor, an estimation of its resectability and the presence of vascular variations which may complicate an already difficult surgical procedure. In fact, in recent years, the assessment of resectability and curability of carcinoma has become one of the most important uses of pancreatic angiography.

Angiography also plays a central role in the diagnosis and location of islet cell adenomas, since these rarely produce abnormalities on the barium examination. Islet cell adenomas are frequently small when they cause symptoms and are difficult to locate at operation. An accurate preoperative knowledge of their location allows the surgeon to perform a limited resection without attempting a complete pancreatic exploration.

Another uncommon pancreatic tumor which is well demonstrated by angiography is cystadenoma. Other tumors of the pancreas are rare, though metastases to the pancreatic bed are common.

Technique

Angiographic technique in the examination of the pancreas must be meticulous. The first angiographic procedures should be celiac and superior mesenteric angiography. In the past, a combined study was done using two catheters. However, the increased reliance on superselective catheterization for diagnosis of pancreatic lesions and the importance of demonstrating the veins around the pancreas to assess the resectability and curability of pancreatic carcinomas have led to the use of sequential celiac and superior mesenteric angiograms. The celiac angiogram is performed in the anteroposterior projection using 50 to 60 cc of contrast medium with filming up to 23 seconds to see the splenic vein. The liver is included in this study so that metastases can be seen. The superior mesenteric angiogram is done in a slight right posterior oblique projection. Approximately 70 cc of contrast medium is injected, frequently following the administration of 50 mg of tolazoline (Priscoline) (see Chapter 10). The large dose of contrast medium is used to visualize the superior mesenteric vein as it passes through the pancreas, and the slight obliquity is used to project both the superior mesenteric vein and the inferior portions of the pancreaticoduodenal arcades off of the spine. The remainder of the examination is done with superselective injections, generally combined with magnification technique.

Injections into the gastroduodenal, dorsal pancreatic and splenic arteries have four distinct advantages over conventional celiac or superior mesenteric angiograms. First, the pancreatic arteries are better filled with contrast medium of higher concentration. Second, overlying left gastric and jejunal artery branches are not filled. Third, injection into the gastroduodenal artery slightly distends the pancreaticoduodenal arcades, and to a lesser degree their branches, so that fixed, nondistensible irregularities in a lumen become more apparent. Finally, a selective injection of a large dose of contrast medium into the splenic artery results in excellent filling of the splenic and portal veins so that venous narrowing and occlusion can more easily be evaluated. With superselective angiography of the pancreas, vascular abnormalities are better defined and more easily interpreted correctly. The diagnosis of pancreatic carcinoma has been made on the basis of subtle but definite changes in the pancreaticoduodenal arcades or their branches at superselective injection when the diagnosis was not possible utilizing the conventional celiac–superior mesenteric angiogram. Such examinations also aid in the diagnosis of islet cell adenomas.

Excellent demonstration of the pancreatic arteries can usually be obtained by injecting the gastroduodenal and splenic arteries (Fig. 4–62). With a gastroduodenal injection, contrast medium is pushed through the widely anastomosing branches of the arcades to the dorsal pancreatic artery and even into the tail of the pancreas in about two thirds of the patients. This almost always allows complete evaluation of the head and body of the pancreas. The splenic artery injection demonstrates branches in the distal tail, as well as in the more proximal branches which are often filled by the gastroduodenal artery injection. Also, the injection of a large amount of contrast medium into the splenic artery provides an excellent demonstration of the splenic vein. If the dorsal pancreatic artery is entered during the catheterization of either the splenic or gastroduodenal artery, an injection can be made into this vessel. The origin of this artery is so variable, however, that it is rarely searched for. The dorsal pancreatic artery has wide anastomoses throughout the pancreas, and injection of this vessel results in excellent filling of the branches in the head and body of the pancreas, and frequently in the tail as well (Fig. 4–63). The injection volume should be kept small, and the catheter should not be wedged. The inferior pancreaticoduodenal artery is not used except as a last resort, since the inferior portions of the pancreaticoduodenal arcades usually have several anastomoses with the superior mesenteric artery, and an injection of any one of these results in incomplete pancreatic

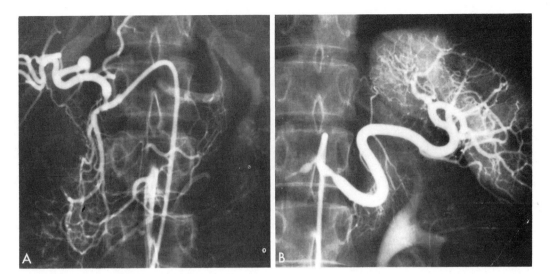

Figure 4-62. Superselective injections of the gastroduodenal and splenic arteries in a 31 year old woman with pancreatitis.
A. Arterial phase of a gastroduodenal angiogram. The pancreaticoduodenal arcades are well demonstrated, and contrast medium refluxes through the inferior pancreaticoduodenal artery to the superior mesenteric artery. Branches in the tail are also filled.
B. Arterial phase of a splenic angiogram. The pancreatic rami of the splenic artery are well demonstrated. (From Reuter, S. R.: Superselective pancreatic angiography. Radiology 92:84, 1969.)

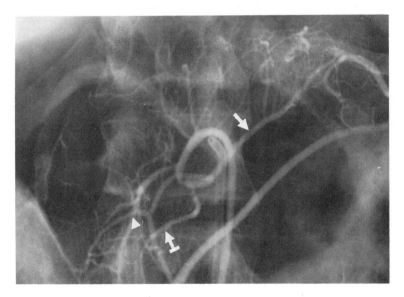

Figure 4-63. Arterial phase of a selective dorsal pancreatic angiogram in a 48 year old man with chronic pancreatitis. The transverse pancreatic branch (⟹) of the dorsal pancreatic artery extends toward the patient's left and supplies several small branches through the tail of the pancreas. The anastomotic branches (▷) pass toward the right to anastomose with the pancreaticoduodenal arcades. The most inferior branch (⟹) extends downward to supply the uncinate process.

filling. The amounts of contrast medium which are injected into the individual pancreatic arteries are as follows:

Gastroduodenal	6 to 8 cc per second for 2 seconds
Splenic	8 to 10 cc per second for 2 to 6 seconds
Dorsal pancreatic	2 to 5 cc per second for 2 seconds
Inferior pancreaticoduodenal	4 to 6 cc per second for 2 seconds

Carcinoma

Pancreatic adenocarcinoma is a scirrhous, infiltrating lesion similar to other adenocarcinomas of the gastrointestinal tract. The angiographic abnormalities that are caused by the tumor reflect the poorly vascularized, infiltrating nature of the lesion.

The primary angiographic abnormality is invasion of arteries in or around the pancreas. This invasion ranges from the characteristic serrated or serpiginous encasement to a nonspecific smooth encasement. The characteristic encasement varies somewhat, depending upon the diameter of the vessel invaded by the tumor. If the vessel is a major artery such as the splenic, hepatic, superior mesenteric or gastroduodenal artery, it will have a saw-toothed margin that the authors describe as serrated encasement (Figs. 4–1, 4–2 and 4–64). If the artery is an intrapancreatic branch, the entire vessel becomes saw-toothed, resulting in abrupt angulations in the course and caliber of the vessel which we refer to as serpiginous encasement (Figs. 4–1, 4–3 and 4–65). Frequently both types of encasement occur together. If the characteristic type of arterial invasion is present, it is quite certain that the changes are caused by a pancreatic carcinoma; however, if the encasement is smooth, further evidence of carcinoma must be sought.

Tumor vessels can be demonstrated in about 60 per cent of carcinomas of the pancreas (Fig. 4–66). The ability to demonstrate tumor vessels is directly proportional to the quality of the examination; we have seen these vessels more frequently since instituting superselective angiography.

The third major sign of pancreatic carcinoma is venous invasion (Fig. 4–67). Car-

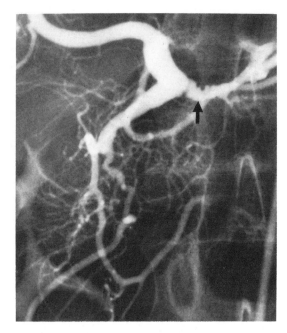

Figure 4–64. Serrated arterial encasement by carcinoma of the pancreas. Hepatic angiogram in a 61 year old woman. There is serrated encasement of the common hepatic artery (➡). The tumor also has invaded the distal gastroduodenal artery, causing marked angulation and changes in caliber.

cinomas of the head of the pancreas distort and occlude the superior mesenteric vein (Fig. 4–68), and those of the tail distort and occlude the splenic vein. The venous phases of the celiac and superior mesenteric angiograms should be carefully evaluated to be certain these veins are normal. Although Buranasiri and Baum (1972) have reported that almost all carcinomas of the head of the pancreas involve the superior mesenteric vein, our experience is that about 85 per cent do so.

It should be noted that three of the general characteristics of tumor are absent from this listing. These are arterial displacement, increased parenchymal accumulation of contrast medium and early venous drainage. One or more of these may be present in a pancreatic carcinoma but the occurrence of all three is unusual. Occasionally a pancreatic carcinoma is more vascular than usual, and, if a large number of tumor vessels are present, there may also be some increased contrast medium accumulation and displacement of arteries

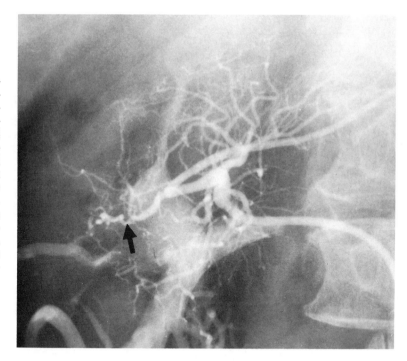

Figure 4-65. Serpiginous encasement in carcinoma of the pancreas. Arterial phase of a dorsal pancreatic angiogram in a 64 year old man with severe abdominal pain. The dorsal pancreatic artery arises from the superior surface of the superior mesenteric artery. The anastomotic branch is abruptly angulated and irregularly narrowed (➡). A few tumor vessels are seen in the region below the arterial encasement.

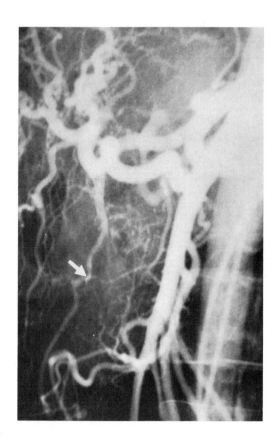

Figure 4-66. Tumor vessels in pancreatic carcinoma. Arterial phase of a celiac–superior mesenteric angiogram in a 51 year old man with carcinoma of the head of the pancreas. Numerous, short, serpiginous tumor vessels are seen throughout the head of the pancreas. In addition, the distal gastroduodenal artery (⟹) is invaded and angled by the carcinoma. (From Lindenauer, S. M., Reuter, S. R., and Joseph, R. R.: Carcinoma of the head of the pancreas presenting as duodenal obstruction without jaundice. Amer. J. Surg. *115*:707, 1968.)

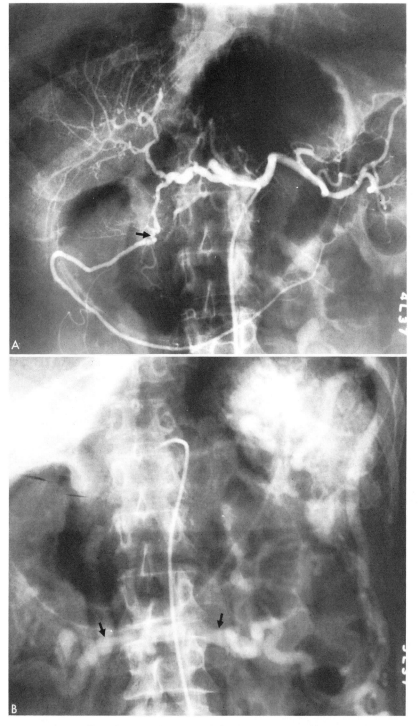

Figure 4–67. Venous occlusion in carcinoma of the pancreas. Celiac angiogram in a 79 year old woman with a large pancreatic carcinoma.

A. Arterial phase. The branches of the celiac artery are markedly atherosclerotic. There are some abrupt angulations in the distal gastroduodenal artery (➡), which are more severe than one would expect from atherosclerosis alone. A few tumor vessels are seen adjacent to the gastroduodenal artery invasion.

B. Venous phase. The splenic vein is occluded, and a collateral epiploic vein (➡) bypasses the occlusion and reconstitutes blood flow to the portal vein.

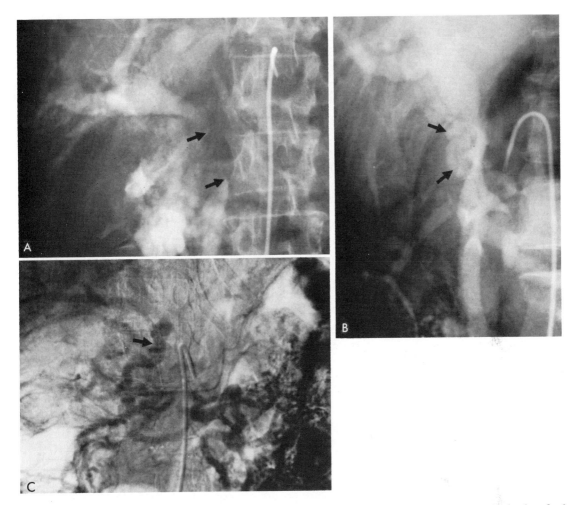

Figure 4–68. Superior mesenteric vein occlusion in three patients with carcinoma of the head of the pancreas.

A. Venous phase of a high-dose superior mesenteric angiogram following tolazoline injection in a 54 year old woman. The superior mesenteric vein is occluded for approximately 3 cm (➡), and the proximal portal vein is narrowed. The contrast medium from the superior mesenteric vein bypasses the occlusion over dilated collateral veins in the region of the pancreas and gallbladder.

B. Venous phase of a high-dose superior mesenteric arteriogram following tolazoline injection in a 64 year old woman. The superior mesenteric vein is occluded over a short segment, and collateral veins (➡) bypass the occlusion. Because a slightly oblique projection is used to visualize the superior mesenteric vein free of the spine, it frequently overlies the renal calices and pelvis, and these must be mentally subtracted in interpreting the venous phase of the angiogram.

C. Subtraction film of the venous phase of a high-dose superior mesenteric angiogram following tolazoline injection in a 60 year old woman. The superior mesenteric vein is occluded over a major segment, and collateral vessels from the jejunal veins bypass the occlusion via the pancreaticoduodenal veins (➡) to the distal portal veins. There is a great deal of stasis and dilatation in the jejunal veins.

around the tumor. However, it should be stressed that such lesions are rare. If the predominant findings are arterial displacement, a marked increase in contrast accumulation in the pancreas and early venous drainage, the disease is far more likely to be pancreatitis than carcinoma.

Differential Diagnosis of Pancreatic Carcinoma

The characteristic appearance of carcinoma of the pancreas occurs in approximately 70 per cent of patients (Bookstein et al., 1969). This appearance includes serpiginous or serrated encasement of arteries in and around the pancreas, tumor vessels and venous invasion. In the other 30 per cent of patients, the diagnosis is more difficult. Pancreatitis and atherosclerosis can simulate pancreatic carcinoma (Reuter et al., 1970). Other carcinomas invading the pancreas from the biliary ducts, stomach or peripancreatic lymph nodes can have findings similar to pancreatic carcinoma. Metastatic tumor to the pancreatic bed can also cause a problem in differential diagnosis. The differential diagnosis is not really important in these tumorous invasions of the pancreas; tumor can be correctly diagnosed by angiography and its general location and extent ascertained. Pancreatitis and atherosclerosis present more of a diagnostic problem because these diseases are far more common than carcinoma.

Clinical differentiation of patients with pancreatitis from those with carcinoma is difficult because of their similar symptoms — severe pain and occasional jaundice.

The angiographic abnormalities caused by pancreatitis are described in Chapter 7. In general, however, the characteristic changes of pancreatitis — hypervascularity with alternating dilatations and normal or narrowed segments of pancreatic arteries — do not occur in carcinoma. Pancreatitis usually involves a large segment of the pancreas, whereas the angiographic abnormalities in carcinoma are generally localized to a relatively small area. Also, carcinoma is only rarely hypervascular; a significant degree of hypervascularity leads one to the correct diagnosis of pancreatitis. Rarely, the diseases cannot be differentiated; however, experienced angiographers who have performed careful examinations of the pancreas, including superselective and magnification studies, can usually discriminate between the two diseases.

Atherosclerosis also causes a problem in differential diagnosis because of its frequent incidence in elderly patients, the same age group with the highest incidence of carci-

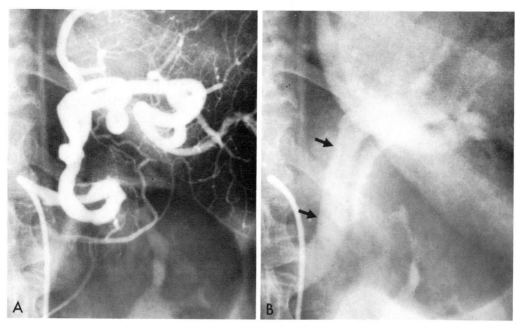

Figure 4-69. Normal splenic vein in a patient with severe atherosclerosis. Celiac angiogram in a 70 year old man in whom the clinical suspicion of carcinoma of the body of the pancreas was high.

A. Arterial phase. The splenic artery has many changes in caliber and some moderately abrupt angulations in course. These changes are marked, and it would be difficult to exclude carcinoma as their cause.

B. Venous phase. The splenic vein (➡) is perfectly normal. No pancreatic carcinoma responsible for the arterial changes would leave the adjacent splenic vein uninvolved.

noma. In general, however, the arterial changes of atherosclerosis consist of smooth, eccentric or circumferential narrowings of major arteries, occasionally with occlusions. Therefore, an atherosclerotic lesion will occasionally be overdiagnosed as representing carcinoma. Even if splenic artery atherosclerosis is severe, the splenic vein appears normal (Fig. 4–69). If pancreatic carcinoma involves the splenic artery, the splenic vein is almost always narrowed or occluded.

The diagnostic problems with pancreatitis and atherosclerosis usually result in the overdiagnosis of carcinoma. The authors' experience has indicated that a perfectly normal angiogram effectively excludes carcinoma of the pancreas. However, the large number of patients with pancreatitis and atherosclerosis who have been misdiagnosed as having pancreatic carcinoma can be reduced by eliminating smooth arterial encasement from the criteria for diagnosing pancreatic carcinoma. If smooth encasement is present, tumor vessels or venous invasion must also occur if a diagnosis of pancreatic carcinoma is to be made.

Finally, the importance of excellent angiographic technique in the evaluation of diseases of the pancreas must be stressed. This includes strict adherence to the principles of good radiographic technique, the use of superselective injections into pancreatic arteries and magnification angiograms. At the same time, the experience of the angiographer cannot be disregarded. Anyone who is beginning to perform pancreatic angiography should review the case material at an institution where a fair amount of angiographic experience has been accumulated. In this way a background in the various manifestations of pancreatic disease can be obtained.

Islet Cell Adenoma

Most tumors of the islets of Langerhans fall into two groups, insulinoma and Zollinger–Ellison adenoma. The former is a beta cell tumor causing hyperinsulinism; the latter is a nonbeta cell tumor causing overproduction of gastrin. A nonbeta cell tumor producing an unknown hormone which causes severe diarrhea and hypokalemia and an alpha cell tumor producing hyperglucagonism and diabetes are much less common. Occasionally, islet cell adenomas do not have endocrine function.

The accuracy of angiography in diagnosing islet cell adenomas has ranged from 33 per cent (Bookstein and Oberman, 1966) to 88 per cent (Boijsen and Samuelsson, 1970). The overall success rate is about 60 per cent. The angiographic abnormalities vary with the size of the tumor. In small lesions, the predominant finding is a well circumscribed, rounded area of increased contrast accumulation in the capillary and venous phases (Fig. 4–70). No tumor vessels or very few tumor vessels are seen within small tumors. As the adenomas become larger, more tumor vessels appear, and the arteries supplying the lesion dilate (Fig. 4–71).

Islet cell adenomas have similar appearances regardless of the hormones they produce. Although only a few adenomas producing unusual syndromes have been reported, both vascular and poorly vascularized tumors have been seen. Because nonfunctioning islet cell adenomas do not produce symptoms, they tend to become large before discovery (Fig. 4–72). For the same reason, they have a higher incidence of liver metastases than the functioning adenomas.

The angiographic findings in these tumors can be quite subtle, and superselective techniques aid in their diagnosis. The majority of islet cell adenomas occur in the tail of the pancreas, and a selective splenic injection should be a part of every angiographic search.

While poorly vascularized islet cell adenomas can be missed, the risk of a false positive diagnosis is also present. In some patients, the pancreas has an area of hypervascularity in the distal third portion supplied by the dorsal pancreatic or pancreatica magna arteries (Fig. 4–73). This area of increased contrast accumulation has a rounded appearance and covers the width of the pancreas. It is accentuated by superselective and subtraction techniques and has caused false positive diagnoses. Other causes of false positive diagnoses of islet cell adenomas are accessory spleens and hypervascular metastases to lymph nodes in the bed of the pancreas (Korobkin et al., 1971).

Angiographic abnormalities that differentiate between primary benign and malig-

Text continued on page 174.

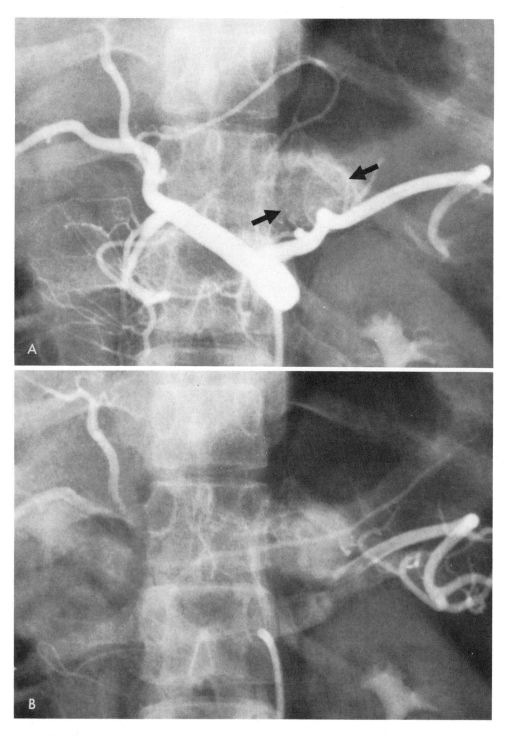

Figure 4-70. Islet cell adenoma. Celiac angiogram in a 49 year old woman with hyperinsulinism.
  A. Arterial phase. Dilated pancreatic rami supply a 2 cm in diameter nodule above the splenic artery (➡).
  B. Late arterial phase. Contrast accumulation throughout the adenoma is homogeneously increased.

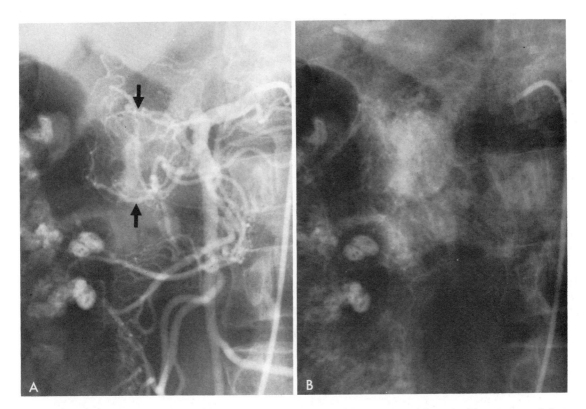

Figure 4–71.   Islet cell adenoma. Superior mesenteric angiogram in a 51 year old woman with hyperinsulinism.

A. Arterial phase. Several branches of the inferior pancreaticoduodenal artery supply a tumor approximately 3 cm in diameter (➡). The arteries in the head of the pancreas are displaced around the mass.

B. Parenchymal phase. There is an irregular increase in contrast accumulation throughout the tumor.

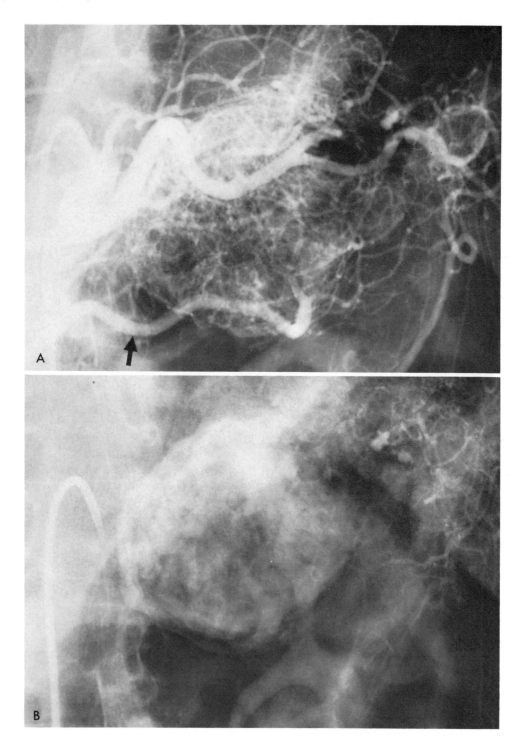

Figure 4–72. Nonfunctioning islet cell adenoma. Celiac and hepatic angiography in a 57 year old man.

A. Arterial phase of a celiac angiogram. The transverse pancreatic artery (➡) is dilated, and several branches from this vessel and the splenic artery supply a large hypervascular tumor in the body and tail of the pancreas. Many tumor vessels are present throughout the lesion.

B. Parenchymal phase. There is irregular, increased contrast accumulation throughout the adenoma. A vein can be seen draining from the inferior portion of the tumor.

Figure continued on opposite page.

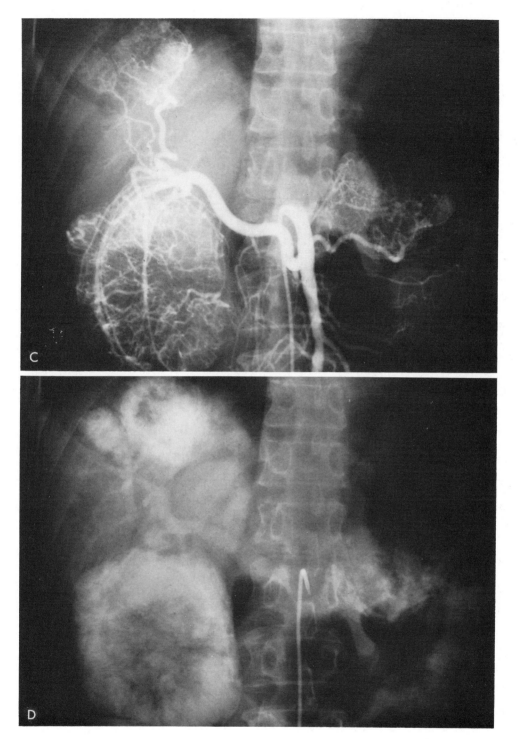

Figure 4–72 Continued. C. Arterial phase of a superior mesenteric angiogram. The right hepatic artery, replaced to the superior mesenteric artery, supplies several markedly hypervascular nodules of varying size throughout the right lobe of the liver. The transverse pancreatic artery supplying the primary tumor can be seen to the left of the superior mesenteric artery.

D. Venous phase. The metastatic nodules have lucent centers, indicating central necrosis.

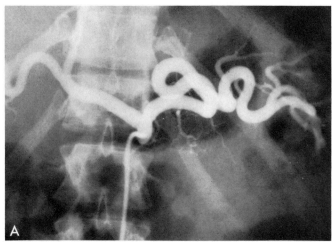

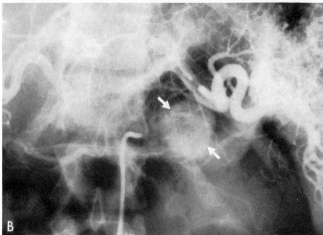

Figure 4–73. Hypervascularity in the distal third of the pancreas. Celiac angiogram in a 23 year old man with splenic trauma.

A. Early arterial phase. The pancreatica magna artery and its branches are well visualized.

B. Late arterial phase. There is an area of increased contrast accumulation at the distal third of the pancreas (⟹). This is homogeneous, round and extends across the entire width of the pancreas. (From Reuter, S. R.: Potential over-diagnosis of pancreatic islet cell adenomas. J. Canad. Ass. Radiol. 22:185, 1971.)

nant islet cell adenomas are nonexistent, but suspicion of malignancy should be higher when the tumors are large (in the range of 5 cm in diameter). In all patients with islet cell adenomas, the liver should be examined because the metastases of islet cell adenomas are quite hypervascular and are well demonstrated by angiography when they are 5 mm in diameter or larger.

Cystadenoma

Cystadenomas are rounded, coarsely lobulated pancreatic tumors which may be multiple. They are usually well encapsulated, have many cystic spaces and grow slowly. At angiography these lesions are generally hypervascular. In the arterial phase of the typical tumor, dilated arteries supply a large number of fine tumor vessels throughout the lesion, and contrast accumulation is increased (Fig. 4–74). The expansile growth usually causes displacement of arteries around the tumor. The angiographic appearance of cystadenomas in the capillary phase varies with the amount of cystic component present. The lesion shown in Figure 4–74 has very few cystic areas. If the tumor has a moderate number of cysts, a very typical appearance occurs in the capillary phase. The cysts stand out as areas of nonopacification in the overall increased contrast accumulation throughout the tumor (Fig. 4–75). This characteristic appearance becomes more apparent with superselective injections of contrast medium into the artery supplying the lesion. Occasionally, the cysts are large and the solid tumor tissue slight, resulting in poor demonstration by angiography. The latter lesions can be difficult to differentiate from pseudocysts of the pancreas.

Differentiation of benign and malignant cystadenomas is generally not possible,

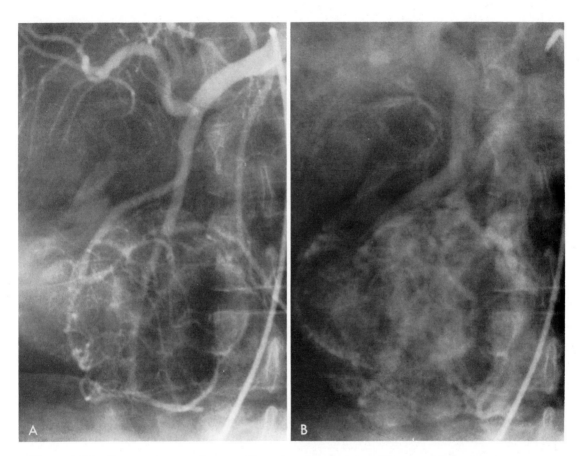

Figure 4–74. Pancreatic cystadenoma. Hepatic angiogram in a 59 year old woman.

A. The gastroduodenal artery and the pancreaticoduodenal arcades are dilated and supply numerous tumor vessels throughout a hypervascular mass in the head of the pancreas. Distribution of tumor vessels through the lesion is relatively homogeneous.

B. Venous phase. Dilated veins from all parts of the tumor drain to the pancreaticoduodenal and gastroepiploic veins. The filling of the veins with contrast medium is both early and dense. This tumor is primarily solid; few cystic spaces are present. Differentiation of solid cystadenomas from nonfunctioning islet cell tumors is difficult.

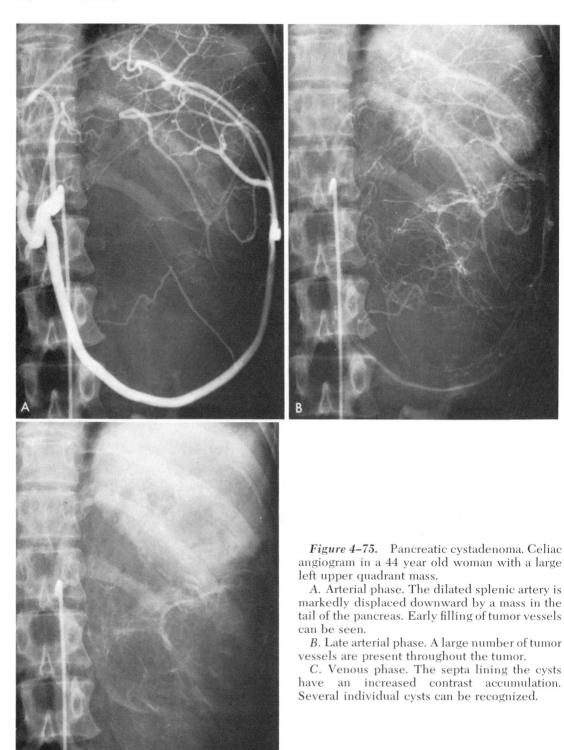

Figure 4–75. Pancreatic cystadenoma. Celiac angiogram in a 44 year old woman with a large left upper quadrant mass.

A. Arterial phase. The dilated splenic artery is markedly displaced downward by a mass in the tail of the pancreas. Early filling of tumor vessels can be seen.

B. Late arterial phase. A large number of tumor vessels are present throughout the tumor.

C. Venous phase. The septa lining the cysts have an increased contrast accumulation. Several individual cysts can be recognized.

although occasionally malignant lesions invade and occlude arteries. The hepatic metastases from these lesions tend to be hypervascular.

Splenic Neoplasms

Splenic tumors are rare; the angiographic appearances of only a few have been reported. The experience that any individual angiographer can accumulate with the various manifestations of splenic neoplasms, therefore, is small. Splenic tumors are found primarily during angiography performed to evaluate unexplained splenomegaly or during the evaluation of generalized neoplasms of reticuloendothelial origin.

Splenomegaly

Diffuse, symmetrical splenic enlargement is seen in such conditions as portal hypertension and in hematologic disorders. In generalized splenomegaly the homogeneous distribution of branches to the different parts of the spleen is maintained, and, although the branches sometimes have a straightened appearance, discrete displacement of the branches does not occur. In the capillary phase, the contrast accumulation through the spleen is homogeneous. As the spleen enlarges, the splenic artery is displaced medially and becomes tortuous. Dilatation of the splenic artery and vein may also occur with splenomegaly.

When the spleen is enlarged, the demonstration of the splenic and portal veins by high dose splenic artery injections may be difficult. The spleen soaks up the contrast medium in the large blood pool so that it becomes diluted.

Splenic Tumors

The benign tumors of the spleen are hemangioma, hamartoma and splenadenoma. All three may be the same entity. At least, the angiographic appearances are similar. They are characteristically hypervascular with a rich network of tumor vessels. Vascular lakes may be present (Fig. 4–76). The edges of the tumor tend to be well

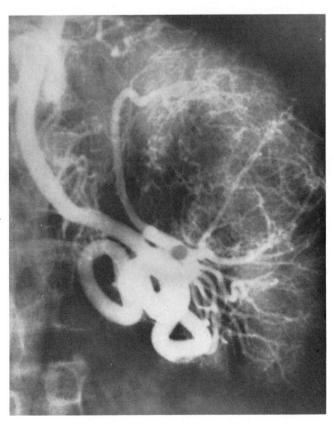

Figure 4–76. Splenadenoma. Arterial phase of a celiac angiogram in a 60 year old man. The branches of the splenic artery to the upper pole of the spleen are displaced around a hypervascular mass with many tumor vessels. (Courtesy of Dr. Josef Rösch. From Rösch, J.: Tumours of the spleen: The value of selective arteriography. Clin. Radiol. *17*:187, 1966.)

defined and cause a curvilinear displacement of adjacent arteries. In the capillary phase, the contrast accumulation may be increased, decreased or the same as the surrounding spleen.

The reticuloendothelial tumors are the most frequent malignant splenic lesions, and localized masses can occur in the spleen in both Hodgkin's disease and reticulum cell sarcoma. More frequently, however, the malignant tumors tend to be multifocal, poorly vascularized and have irregular, poorly defined borders. Splenic artery branches may be invaded. Castellino et al. (1971) have reported that the accuracy of angiography in assessing splenic involvement in patients with Hodgkin's disease is not good. The accuracy can be increased by using angiotomography.

The spleen can be involved by blood-borne metastases and generalized carcinomatosis (Fig. 4–77). Splenic metastases are especially common in disseminated malignant melanoma (Fig. 4–78). The appearance of blood-borne metastatic disease is the same as that of primary malignant tumors with multifocal, irregular, poorly vascularized areas in an enlarged spleen.

Most splenic metastases come from a direct extension of malignancies in adjacent organs, particularly the stomach, the pancreas and the kidneys. The appearance is the same as the primary lesion with a contiguous involvement of the adjacent spleen. Blood vessels from the organ of origin may supply the metastases. In the capillary phase, contrast accumulation is decreased in gastric and pancreatic carcinomas and increased in hypernephromas.

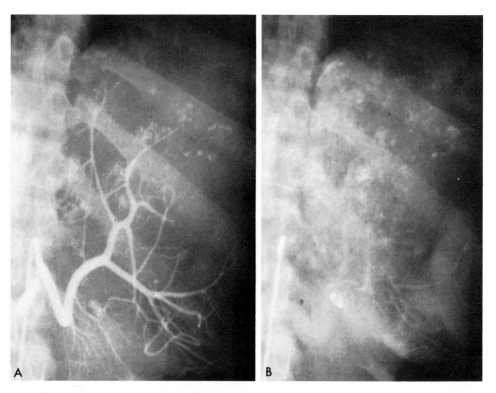

Figure 4–77.   Metastatic choriocarcinoma to the spleen. Celiac angiogram in a 23 year old woman with disseminated tumor (same patient as in Figures 4–27 and 4–53).

A. Multiple abnormal vascular spaces throughout the spleen fill from splenic artery branches.

B. Venous phase. The hypervascular nodules remain opacified. Some have central lucencies suggesting necrosis. The appearance of the mtastases is the same as those to the liver.

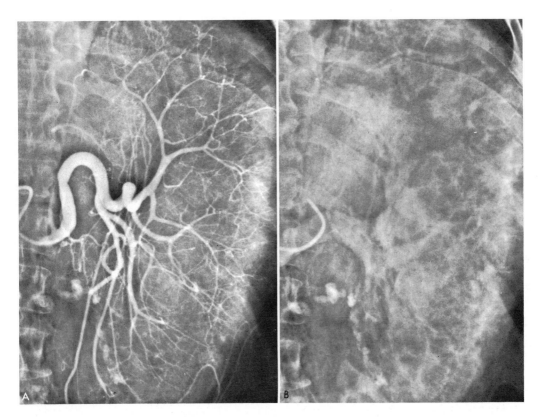

Figure 4–78. Metastatic melanosarcoma to the spleen. Splenic angiogram in a 63 year old man with a primary melanoma of the shoulder and abdominal pain.

A. Arterial phase. The splenic artery branches throughout the markedly enlarged spleen are stretched around multiple nodules. Some of the branches are flattened, and the angulation is increased at the branchings. Although a few tumor vessels are seen, most of the nodules are hypovascular.

B. Venous phase. Multiple avascular nodules are seen throughout the spleen, outlined by the remaining normal parenchyma. The splenic vein is markedly dilated. (Courtesy of Dr. Josef Rösch.)

CYSTS

Angiography is not frequently used to evaluate gastrointestinal cysts. Recently, the high accuracy of ultrasound in diagnosing cystic lesions has eliminated angiography from any role in their diagnosis. Occasionally, angiography may be used to clarify equivocal findings at ultrasound. Also, cysts may sometimes be examined by angiography to help determine the correct operative approach. Gastrointestinal cysts are congenital, posttraumatic or parasitic in nature. The latter two groups are discussed in Chapters 5 and 7.

General Angiographic Characteristics of Gastrointestinal Cysts

The angiographic characteristics of gastrointestinal cysts are the same as cysts anywhere in the body and consist of (1) displacement of arteries and veins, (2) avascularity in the capillary phase and (3) compression of adjacent normal parenchyma.

Displacement of Arteries and Veins

The primary angiographic abnormality caused by a cyst is displacement of the ar-

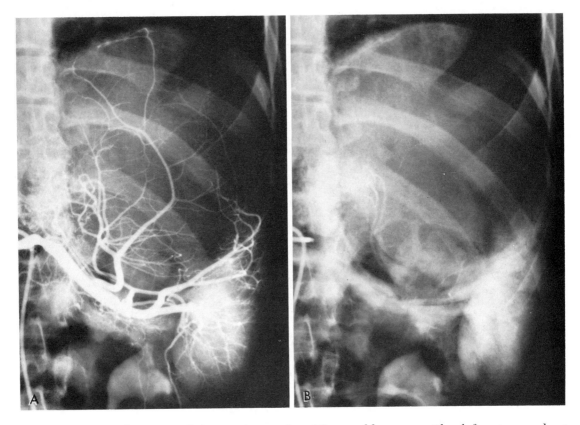

Figure 4–79. Splenic cyst. Celiac angiogram in a 35 year old woman with a left upper quadrant mass.

A. Arterial phase. The upper pole branches of the splenic artery are displaced around a large, avascular mass. The lower pole of the spleen has a normal appearance.

B. Parenchymal phase. Minimal residual splenic parenchyma can be seen superiorly and medially to the cyst. The cyst itself is avascular. The lower pole of the spleen appears normal.

teries and veins of the organ in which the cyst is located. The vessels appear stretched but maintain their normal smooth lumina (Fig. 4–79). The courses of the arteries and veins are circumlinear and regular, without angulation.

Avascularity in the Cyst in the Capillary Phase

The avascular nature of the cyst stands out as a defect in the parenchyma in the capillary phase. The size of the defect depends, of course, on the size of the cyst and the amount of parenchyma in front of and behind the cyst. Thus, a small cyst is more difficult to define in the liver than in the spleen. Frequently, the cyst, particularly a large cyst, has a sharply marginated border, and this generally makes the diagnosis easy.

Compression of Adjacent Normal Parenchyma

Some cysts compress the adjacent normal parenchyma as they expand, resulting in a zone of increased contrast accumulation around the cyst in the capillary phase.

Angiographic Abnormalities in Gastrointestinal Cysts

Hepatic Cysts

Hepatic cysts are not common in the United States, and most of those seen are caused by the parasite *Echinococcus granulosus*. Congenital cysts may be solitary but are generally multiple and are frequently associated with a congenital cystic

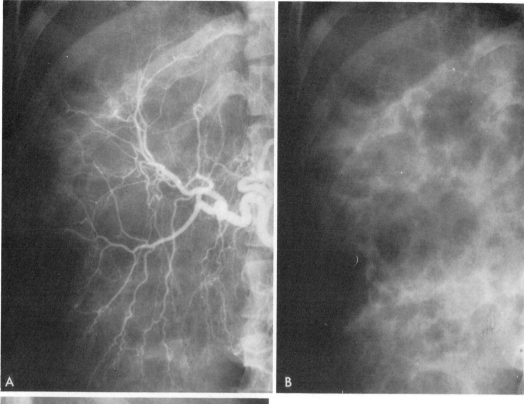

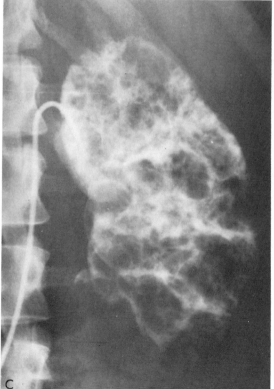

Figure 4-80. Polycystic disease of the liver. Hepatic and renal angiograms in a 33 year old woman.

A. Arterial phase of a celiac angiogram. The hepatic artery branches are slightly tortuous and slightly stretched.

B. Parenchymal phase. Multiple cysts of varying sizes are seen throughout the liver.

C. Parenchymal phase of a left renal angiogram. Multiple cysts of various sizes are seen throughout the kidney.

disease of the kidneys and other organs (Fig. 4–80). The cysts are generally small and located under the capsule, but occasionally congenital hepatic cysts become large (Fig. 4–81). At angiography they are seen as multiple peripheral filling defects and, therefore, present a diagnostic problem in differentiating between the cysts and avascular hepatic metastases. These two entities may be difficult to differentiate by angiography unless some other identi-

fying angiographic characteristic of metastases is present, such as invasion of hepatic artery branches around the lesion. However, the sharp margination of the cyst, along with the defect in the hepatogram, generally permits a diagnosis. As with *Echinococcus* and congenital cysts, posttraumatic cysts are rarely encountered. These are really pseudocysts resulting from the walling off and nonabsorption of a hepatic hematoma or infarct.

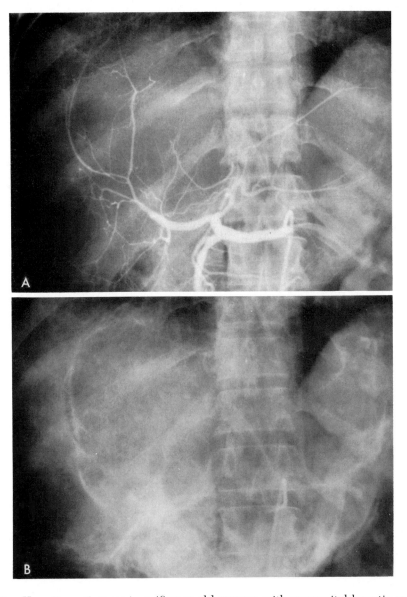

Figure 4–81. Hepatic angiogram in a 48 year old woman with congenital hepatic cysts.

A. Arterial phase. Several right hepatic artery branches are displaced around masses.

B. Parenchymal phase. Several large, lucent cysts are present in the right lobe of the liver. The cyst rims appear hypervascular because they compress the normal surrounding hepatic parenchyma.

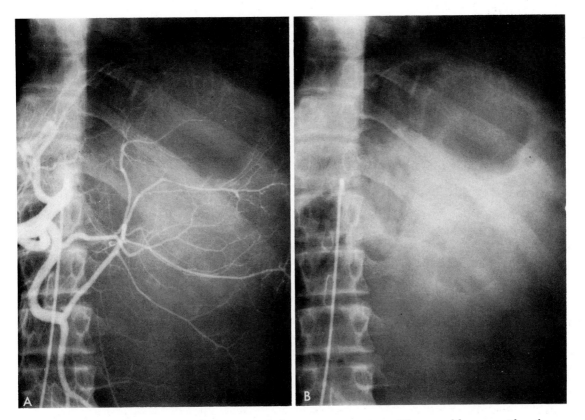

Figure 4–82. Multilocular splenic cyst. Celiac angiogram in a 17 year old man with a large, asymptomatic left upper quadrant mass.

A. Arterial phase. The spleen is markedly enlarged, and the splenic artery branches are stretched. The degree and direction of stretching vary throughout the spleen, in contrast to simple splenomegaly, in which the distribution of the stretched branches remains uniform and normal.

B. Parenchymal phase. Lucent areas represent splenic cysts. At operation, several large cysts were present throughout the spleen.

Splenic Cysts

Splenic cysts are rare. Almost all are posttraumatic and result from a subcapsular hematoma which has not ruptured. As the hematoma persists, the capsule around it becomes thickened and fibrotic. Rarely, splenic cysts are congenital. These are generally encountered during angiography, which is performed to evaluate an asymmetrically enlarged spleen. Splenic cysts are usually solitary and may be large. The angiographic appearance of these cysts is that of a rounded, avascular area surrounded by normal splenic parenchyma (Fig. 4–82). Splenic artery branches are stretched around the cyst, but no abnormal vessels are present. In the capillary phase, the margin between the normal splenic parenchyma and the cyst is sharp.

Pancreatic Cysts

Most pancreatic cysts result as complications of pancreatitis, either retention cysts caused by dilatation behind a duct obstruction or pseudocysts resulting from hemorrhage or necrosis. The angiographic findings in these cysts are described in Chapter 7. Congenital cysts of the pancreas are rare and are generally associated with cystic disease in the kidneys and the liver.

Mesenteric Cysts

Cysts may originate in any part of the mesentery, omentum or mesocolon. They grow slowly, and, since they do not produce symptoms until they become large, they generally present as large, mobile abdominal masses. These cysts may be chy-

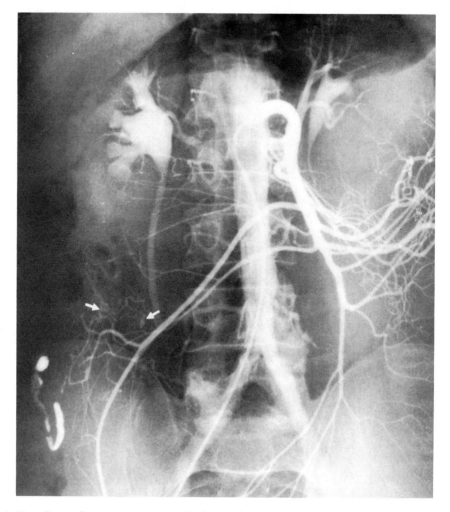

Figure 4-83. Cystic leiomyoma. Arterial phase of a superior mesenteric angiogram in a 63 year old man with a movable abdominal mass. The right colic, ileocolic and terminal superior mesenteric arteries are stretched around a large, avascular mass in the mesentery. A few dilated ileocolic branches supply tumor vessels (⟹) in the ascending colon. The tumor vessels justify the diagnosis of a cystic neoplasm. (Courtesy of Dr. Alan Hennessey.)

lous or serous. Not infrequently they are cystic tumors, such as a lymphangioendothelioma or a cystic leiomyoma. The angiographic abnormalities accompanying such cysts are stretching and displacement of branches of the mesenteric arteries, or in the case of omental tumors stretching and displacement of the gastroduodenal and epiploic arteries. If the cyst is neoplastic, abnormal tumor neovascularity may be identified (Fig. 4-83).

BIBLIOGRAPHY

Abrams, H. L.: The incidence of splenic metastasis of carcinoma. Calif. Med. 76:281, 1952.

Abrams, R. M., Beranbaum, E. R., Beranbaum, S. L., et al.: Angiographic studies of benign and malignant cystadenoma of the pancreas. Radiology 89:1028, 1967.

Abrams, R. M., Beranbaum, E. R., Santos, J. S., et al.: Angiographic features of cavernous hemangioma of liver. Radiology 92:308, 1969.

Abrams, R. M., Meng, C. H., Firooznia, H., et al.:

Angiographic demonstration of carcinoma of the gallbladder. Radiology 94:277, 1970.

Alfidi, R. J., Rastogi, H., Buonocore, E., et al.: Hepatic arteriography. Radiology 90:1136, 1968.

Almersjö, O., Bengmark, S., Hafström, L., et al.: Accuracy of diagnostic tools in malignant hepatic lesions. Amer. J. Surg., 127:663, 1974.

Ameriks, J. A., Thompson, N. W., Frey, C. F., et al.: Hepatic cell adenomas, spontaneous liver rupture, and oral contraceptives. Arch. Surg., 110:548, 1975.

Anacker, H.: Kritische Bewertung der Röntgenologischen Untersuchungsmethoden zur Pankreasdiagnostik. Radiologe (Berlin) 5:312, 1965.

Aronsen, K. F., Lunderquist, A., and Nylander, G.: The comparison of celiacography and direct portography in the diagnostic evaluation of liver diseases. Radiology 92:313, 1969.

Auerbach, R. C., and Koehler, R. P.: The many faces of islet cell tumors. Amer. J. Roentgenol. 119:133, 1973.

Baron, M. G., Mitty, H. A., and Wolf, B. S.: The arteriographic appearance of carcinoma of the uncinate process of the pancreas. Amer. J. Roentgenol. 101:649, 1967.

Bartley, O., Edlund, Y., and Helander, C. G.: Angiography in primary hepatic carcinoma. Acta Radiol. (Diagn.) (Stockh.) 6:81, 1967.

Baum, J. K., Holtz, F., Bookstein, J. J., et al.: Possible association between benign hepatomas and oral contraceptives. Lancet 2:926, 1973.

Baum, S.: Personal communication, 1971.

Baum, S., Roy, R., Finkelstein, A. K., et al.: Clinical application of selective celiac and superior mesenteric arteriography. Radiology 84:279, 1965.

Benkö, G.: Problems of differential diagnosis in angiography of the pancreas. Radiol. Clin. 39:334, 1970.

Bennet, J., and Bigot, R.: Arteriography in primary liver tumours. Aust. Radiol. 14:183, 1970.

Beranbaum, E. R., Beranbaum, S. L., and Abrams, R.: Correlation of barium studies with visceral angiography. Amer. J. Gastroent. 46:21, 1966.

Berdon, W. E., and Baker, D. H.: Giant hepatic hemangioma with cardiac failure in the newborn infant. Radiology 92:1523, 1969.

Berdon, W. E., Baker, D. H., and Casarella, W.: Liver disease in children: Portal hypertension, hepatic masses. Sem. Roentgenol. 10:207, 1975.

Bert, J. M., Lamarque, J. L., Balmes, J. L., et al.: La place de l'artériographie sélective dans l'identification des tumeurs digestives abdominales. Ann. Radiol. (Paris) 11:788, 1968.

Bieber, W. P., and Albo, R. J.: Cystadenoma of the pancreas: Its arteriographic diagnosis. Radiology 80:776, 1963.

Bjørn-Hansen, R., and Aakhus, T.: Angiography in intestinal carcinoid. Acta Radiol. (Diagn.) (Stockh.) 14:721, 1973.

Boijsen, E.: Angiographic diagnosis of pancreatic disease. T. Gastroent. 12:219, 1969.

Boijsen, E.: Inactive malignant endocrine tumors of the pancreas. Radiologe 15:177, 1975.

Boijsen, E.: Selective hepatic angiography in primary and secondary tumors of the liver. Rev. Int. Hépat. 15:385, 1965.

Boijsen, E., and Abrams, H. L.: Roentgenologic diagnosis of primary carcinoma of the liver. Acta Radiol. (Diagn.) (Stockh.) 3:257, 1965.

Boijsen, E., Kaude, J., and Tylén, U.: Radiologic diagnosis of ileal carcinoid tumours. Acta Radiol. (Diagn.) (Stockh.) 15:65, 1974.

Boijsen, E., and Reuter, S. R.: Combined percutaneous transhepatic cholangiography and angiography in the evaluation of obstructive jaundice. Amer. J. Roentgenol. 99:153, 1967.

Boijsen, E., and Reuter, S. R.: Mesenteric angiography in the evaluation of inflammatory and neoplastic disease of the intestine. Radiology 87:1028, 1966.

Boijsen, E., and Samuelsson, L.: Angiographic diagnosis of tumors arising from the pancreatic islets. Acta Radiol. (Diagn.) (Stockh.) 10:161, 1970.

Boijsen, E., Wallace, S., and Kanter, I. E.: Angiography in tumours of the stomach. Acta Radiol. (Diagn.) (Stockh.) 4:306, 1966.

Bookstein, J. J., and Oberman, H. A.: Appraisal of selective angiography in localizing islet-cell tumors of the pancreas. Radiology 86:682, 1966.

Bookstein, J. J., Reuter, S. R., and Martel, W.: Angiographic evaluation of pancreatic carcinoma. Radiology 93:757, 1969.

Bosniak, M. A., and Phanthumachinda, P.: Value of arteriography in the study of hepatic disease. Amer. J. Surg. 112:348, 1966.

Bree, R. L., and Reuter, S. R.: Angiographic findings in patients with cholelithiasis and obstructive jaundice. Radiology 112:291, 1974.

Buranasiri. S., and Baum, S.: The significance of the venous phase of celiac and superior mesenteric arteriography in evaluating pancreatic carcinoma. Radiology 102:11, 1972.

Capdeville, R., Bennet, J., Dubois, F., et al.: L'artériographie des tumeurs du grêle: A propos de 3 cas de schwannomes. Arch. Franc. Mal. Appar. Dig. 59:453, 1970.

Castaneda-Zuniga, W. R., and Amplatz, K.: Angiography of the liver in lymphoma. Radiology 122:679, 1977.

Castellino, R. A., Silverman, J. F., Glatstein, E., et al.: Splenic arteriography in Hodgkin's disease. Invest. Radiol. 6:341, 1971.

Castellino, R. A., Silverman, J. F., Glatstein, E., et al.: Splenic arteriography in Hodgkin's disease. Invest. Radiol. 6:341, 1971.

Chuang, V. P., and Lorman, J. G.: The paradoxical halo sign in hepatic pseudotumor. Radiology 123:315, 1977.

Chuang, V. P., Bree, R. L., and Bookstein, J. J.: Angiographic features of focal lymphoma of the liver. Radiology 111:53, 1974.

Clemett, A. R., and Park, W. M.: Arteriographic demonstration of pancreatic tumor in the Zollinger-Ellison syndrome. Radiology 88:32, 1967.

Clouse, M. E., Costello, P., Legg, M. A., et al.: Subselective angiography in localizing insulinomas of the pancreas. Amer. J. Roentgenol. 128:741, 1977.

Clouse, M. E., Gregg, J. A., and Sedgwick, C. E.: Angiography vs. pancreatography in diagnosis of carcinoma of the pancreas. Radiology 114:605, 1975.

Colapinto, R. F.: Arteriography in the diagnosis of liver tumours. Canad. Med. Ass. J. 99:1175, 1968.

Curry, J. L., Johnson, W. G., Feinberg, D. H., et al.: Thorium induced hepatic hemangioendothelioma. Amer. J. Roentgenol. 125:671, 1975.

Daird, F., Tavernier, J. Rabin, A., et al.: Radiologic aspects of primary malignant tumors of the bile ducts, with exclusion of Vater's ampulla tumors. J. Radiol. Electrol. Med. Nucl. 55:561, 1974.

Debray, C., Morin, D., Leymarios, J., et al.: Tumeurs de l'intestin grêle diagnostiquées exclusivement par l'artériographie selective de la mésenterique supérieure. Arch. Mal. Appar. Dig. 54:593, 1965.

de Lorimier, A. A., Simpson, E. B., Baum, R. S., et al.: Hepatic-artery ligation for hepatic hemangiomatosis. New Eng. J. Med. 277:333, 1967.

Deutch, V., Adar, R., Jacob, E. T., et al.: Angiographic diagnosis and differential diagnosis of islet-cell tumors. Amer. J. Roentgenol. 119:121, 1973.

Deutch, V., Adar, R., and Mozes, M.: Angiography of the greater omentum. Amer. J. Roentgenol. 113:174, 1971.

Diamond, A. B., Meng, C. H., and Goldin, R. R.: Arteriography of unusual mass lesions of the mesentery. Radiology 110:547, 1974.

Dijken, B. G., Hart, H. C., Imhof, J. W., et al.: Benign hemangioma of the liver: The significance of selective angiography. Radiol. Clin. (Basel) 40:50, 1971.

Efsen, F., and Fischerman, K.: Angiography in gastric tumours. Acta Radiol. (Diagn.) (Stockh.) 15:193, 1974.

Epstein, H. Y., Abrams, R. M., Beranbaum, E. R., et al.: Angiographic localization of insulinomas: High reported success rate and two additional cases. Ann. Surg. 169:349, 1969.

Filly, R. A., and Freimanis, A. K.: Echographic diagnosis of pancreatic lesions. Radiology 96:575, 1970.

Fredens, M.: Angiography in primary hepatic tumours in children. Acta Radiol. (Diagn.) (Stockh.) 8:193, 1969.

Fredens, M., Egeblad, M., and Holst-Nielsen, F.: The value of selective angiography in the diagnosis of tumors in pancreas and liver. Radiology 93:765, 1969.

Fulton, R. E., Sheedy, P. F., McIlrath, D. C., et al.: Preoperative angiographic localization of insulin producing tumors of the pancreas. Amer. J. Roentgenol. 123:367, 1975.

Gammill, S. L., Shipkey, F. H., Himmelfarb, E. H., et al.: Roentgenology-pathology correlative study of neovascularity. Amer. J. Roentgenol. 126:376, 1976.

Geindre, M., and Coulomb, M.: Aspects artériographiques des cancers secondaires du foie et confrontations anatomiques. Ann. Radiol. (Paris) 11:827, 1968.

Giacobazzi, P., and Passaro, E.: Preoperative angiography in the Zollinger-Ellison syndrome. Amer. J. Surg. 126:74, 1973.

Gold, R. P., Black, T. J., Rotterdam, H., et al.: Radiologic and pathologic charactistics of the WDHA syndrome. Amer. J. Roentgenol 127:397, 1976.

Goldstein, H. M., and Miller, M.: Angiographic evaluation of carcinoid tumors of the small intestine: The value of epinephrine. Radiology 114:23, 1975.

Goldstein, H. M., Neiman, H. L., Mena, E., et al.: Angiographic findings in benign liver cell tumors. Radiology 110:339, 1974.

Goldstein, H. M., Thaggard, A., Wallace, S., et al.: Priscoline-augmented hepatic angiography. Radiology 119:275, 1976.

Göthlin, J., Mansoor, M., and Tranberg, K. G.: Combined percutaneous cholangiography (PTC) and selective visceral angiography (SVA) in obstructive jaundice. Amer. J. Roentgenol. Radium Ther. Nucl. Med. 117:419, 1973.

Gould, H. R., Clemett, A. R., and Rossi, P.: Radiologic diagnosis of splenic metastasis. Amer. J. Roentgenol. 109:755, 1970.

Graham, J. C., Jr., Weidner, W. A., and Vinik, M.: The angiographic features or organizing splenic hematoma (? Hamartoma). Amer. J. Roentgenol. 107:430, 1969.

Gray, R. K., Rösch, J., and Grollman, J. H., Jr.: Arteriography in the diagnosis of islet-cell tumors. Radiology 97:39, 1970.

Gregg, F. P., Goldstein, H. M., Wallace, S., et al.: Arteriographic demonstration of intravenous tumor extension. Amer. J. Roentgenol. 123:100, 1975.

Grieco, R. V., and Bartone, N. F.: Roentgen visualization of phleboliths in hemangioma of the GI tract. Amer. J. Roentgenol. 101:406, 1967.

Gross, G., Goldberg, H. I. and Schrock, T. R.: Use of selective, intrahepatic, portal venogram and in vivo coloration in planning segmental hepatic resection. Amer. J. Roentgenol. 122:327, 1974.

Hardin, W. J., and Hardy, J. D.: Mesenteric cysts. Amer. J. Surg. 119:640, 1970.

Hatfield, P. M., and Pfister, R. C.: Adult polycystic disease of the kidneys (Potter Type 3). J.A.M.A. 222:1527, 1972.

Ishak, K. G., and Rabin, L.: Benign tumors of the liver. Med. Clin. N. Amer. 59:995, 1975.

Jonsson, K., and Lunderquist, A.: Angiography of the liver and spleen in Hodgkin's Disease. Amer. J. Roentgenol. 121:789, 1974.

Kaude, J., and Rian, R.: Cholangiocarcinoma. Radiology 100:573, 1971.

Kaude, J., Silseth, Ch., and Tylén, U.: Angiography in myomas of the gastrointestinal tract. Acta Radiol. (Diagn.) (Stockh.) 12:691, 1972.

Kido, C., Sasaki, T., and Kaneko, M.: Angiography of primary liver cancer. Amer. J. Roentgenol. 113:70, 1971.

Kim, D. K., McSweeney, J., Yeh, S. D. J., et al.: Tumors of the liver as demonstrated by angiography, scan, and laparotomy. Surg. Gynec. Obstet. 141:409, 1975.

Kishikawa, T., Numaguchi, Y., Tokunaga, M., et al.: Hemangiosarcoma of the spleen with liver metastases: angiographic manifestations. Radiology 123:31, 1977.

Korobkin, M. T., Palubinskas, A. J., and Glickman, M. G.: Pitfalls in arteriography of islet cell tumors of the pancreas. Radiology 100:319, 1971.

Leonidas, J. C., Strauss, L., and Beck, A. R.: Vascular tumors of the liver in newborns: A pediatric emergency. Amer. J. Dis. Children. 125:507, 1973.

Lerona, P. T., Go, R. T., and Cornell, S. H.: Limitations of angiography and scanning in diagnosis of liver masses. Radiology 112:139, 1974.

Levin, D. C., Gordon, D. H., Kinkhabwala, M., et al.: Arteriography of retroperitoneal lymphoma. Amer. J. Roentgenol. 126:368, 1976.

Ludin, H., Enderlin, F., Fahrländer, H. J., et al.: Failure to diagnose Zollinger-Ellison syndrome by pancreatic arteriography. Brit. J. Radiol. 39:494, 1966.

Lunderquist, A.: Angiography in carcinoma of the pancreas. Acta Radiol. (Suppl. 235), 1965.

Lunderquist, A., Lunderquist, A., Holmdahl, K. H.,

et al.: Selective superior mesenteric arteriography in reticulum-cell sarcoma of the small bowel. Radiology 98:113, 1971.

Madsen, B.: Demonstration of pancreatic insulomas by angiography. Brit. J. Radiol. 39:488, 1966.

McLoughlin, M. J.: Angiography in cavernous hemangioma of the liver. Amer. J. Roentgenol. 113:50, 1971.

McLoughlin, M. J., and Gilday, D. L.: Angiography and colloid scanning of benign mass lesions of the liver. Clin. Radiol. 23:377, 1972.

McLoughlin, M. J., and Phillips, M. J.: Angiographic findings in multiple bile duct hamartomas of the liver. Radiology 116:41, 1975.

McLoughlin, M. J., Colapinto, R. F., Gilday, D. L., et al.: Focal nodular hyperplasia of the liver: Angiography and radioisotope scanning. Radiology 107:257, 1973.

McMullen, C. T., and Montgomery, J. L.: Arteriographic findings of focal nodular hyperplasia of the liver and review of the literature. Amer. J. Roentgenol. 117:380, 1973.

Meyers, H. A., and King, M. C.: Leiomyosarcoma of the duodenum. Angiographic findings and report of a case. Radiology 91:788, 1968.

Miller, W. J., Reuter, S. R., and Redman, H. C.: Epinephrine effect in angiography of colonic carcinoma. An inconsistent aid in diagnosis. Invest. Radiol. 4:246, 1969.

Moss, A. A., Clark, R. E., Palubinskas, A. J., et al.: Angiographic appearance of benign and malignant hepatic tumors in infants and children. Amer. J. Roentgenol. 113:61, 1971.

Nakamura, T., Nakamura, S., Onodera, A., et al.: Hepatic venography in hepatic tumors. Tohoku J. Exp. Med. 99:281, 1969.

Nebesar, R. A., and Pollard, J. J.: A critical evaluation of selective celiac and superior mesenteric angiography in the diagnosis of pancreatic diseases, particularly malignant tumor: Facts and "artefacts." Radiology 89:1017, 1967.

Nebesar, R. A., Pollard, J. J., and Stone, D. L.: Angiographic diagnosis of malignant disease of the liver. Radiology 86:284, 1966.

Nebesar, R. A., Tefft, M., and Filler, R. M.: Correlation of angiography and isotope scanning in abdominal diseases of children. Amer. J. Roentgenol. 109:323, 1970.

Neiman, H. L., and Goldstein, H. M.: Angiography of benign and malignant hepatic masses. Sem. Roentgenol. 10:197, 1975.

Neiman, H. L., Goldstein, H. M., Silverman, P. J., et al.: Angiographic features of peripancreatic malignant lymphoma. Radiology 115:589, 1975.

Novy, S., Wallace, S., Medellin, H., et al.: Angiographic evaluation of primary malignant hepatocellular tumors in children. Amer. J. Roentgenol. 120:353, 1974.

Okuda, K., Musha, H., Yamasaki, T., et al.: Angiographic demonstration of intrahepatic arterioportal anastomoses in hepatocellular carcinoma. Radiology 122:53, 1977.

Okuda, K., Musha, H., Yoshida, T., et al.: Demonstration of growing casts of hepatocellular carcinoma in the portal vein by celiac angiography: The thread and streaks sign. Radiology 117:303, 1975.

Okuda, K., Obata, H., Jinnouchi, S., et al.: Angiographic assessment of gross anatomy of hepatocellular carcinoma: Comparison of celiac angiograms and liver pathology in 100 cases. Radiology 123:21, 1977.

Olsson, O.: Angiographie bei Pankreastumoren. Radiologe (Berlin) 5:281, 1965.

Olsson, O.: Angiographie in drei Fällen von Insuloma Pancreatis. Radiologe (Berlin) 5:286, 1965.

Olsson, O.: Angiography in duodenal carcinoma. Acta Radiol. 11:177, 1971.

Olsson, O.: Angiography in the diagnosis of duodenal lesions—I. Differentiation between primary duodenal carcinoma and carcinoma of the head of the pancreas involving the duodenum. Acta Radiol. 12:49, 1972.

Olsson, O.: Angiography in the diagnosis of duodenal lesions. II. Benign tumours, ulceration, and inflammatory and vascular lesions. Acta Radiol. (Diagn.) (Stockh.) 12:164, 1972.

Olsson, O., and Tylén, U.: Angiography in carcinoma at the ampulla of Vater. Acta Radiol. (Diagn.) (Stockh.) 12:375, 1972.

Palubinskas, A. J., Baldwin, J., and McCormack, K. R.: Liver-cell adenoma. Angiographic findings and report of a case. Radiology 89:444, 1967.

Pettersson, H.: Carcinoma of the gallbladder. Acta Radiol. (Diagn.) (Stockh.) 15:225, 1974.

Plachta, A.: Calcified cavernous hemangioma of the liver. Radiology 79:783, 1962.

Pollard, J. J., Nebesar, R. A., and Mattoso, L. F.: Angiographic diagnosis of benign diseases of the liver. Radiology 86:276, 1966.

Poller, S., and Wholey, M. H.: Splenic cysts: Confirmation by selective visceral angiography. Amer. J. Roentgenol. 96:418, 1966.

Pressman, B. D., Asch, T., and Casarella, W. J.: Cystadenoma of the pancreas: A reappraisal of angiographic findings. Amer. J. Roentgenol. 119:115, 1973.

Rabinowitz, J. G., Kinkabwala, M., and Ulreich, S.: Macro-regenerating nodule in the cirrhotic liver. Amer. J. Roentgenol. 121:140, 1974.

Raffucci, F. L., and Ramirez-Schon, G.: Management of tumors of the liver. Surg. Gynec. Obstet. 130:371, 1970.

Ramer, M., Mitty, H. A., and Baron, M. G.: Angiography in leiomyomatous neoplasms of the small bowel. Amer. J. Roentgenol. 113:263, 1971.

Ranninger, K., and Saldino, R. M.: Arteriographic diagnosis of pancreatic lesions. Radiology 86:470, 1966.

Reuter, S. R.: Angiography in the diagnosis of gastrointestinal cancer. Proc. Nat. Cancer Conf., 6:447, 1970.

Reuter, S. R.: Potential over-diagnosis of pancreatic islet cell adenomas. J. Can. Ass. Radiol. 22:184, 1971.

Reuter, S. R.: Superselective pancreatic angiography. Radiology 92:74, 1969.

Reuter, S. R., and Boijsen, E.: Angiographic findings in two ileal carcinoid tumors. Radiology 87:836, 1966.

Reuter, S. R., Redman, H. C., and Bookstein, J. J.: Angiography in carcinoma of the biliary tract. Brit. J. Radiol. 44:636, 1971.

Reuter, S. R., Redman, H. C., and Bookstein, J. J.: Differential problems in the angiographic diagnosis of carcinoma of the pancreas. Radiology 96:93, 1970.

Reuter, S. R., Redman, H. C., and Siders, D. B.: The spectrum of angiographic findings in hepatoma. Radiology 94:89, 1970.

Riba, P. O., and Lunderquist. A.: Angiographic findings in villous tumors of the colon. Amer. J. Roentgenol. 117:287, 1973.

Rizk, G. K., Tayyarah, K. A., and Ghandur-Mnaymneh, L.: The angiographic changes in hydatid cysts of the liver and spleen. Radiology 99:303, 1971.

Robins, J. M., Bookstein, J. J., Oberman, H. A., et al.: Selective angiography in localizing islet-cell tumours of the pancreas. A further appraisal. Radiology 106:525, 1973.

Rösch, J.: Tumors of the spleen: The value of selective arteriography. Clin. Radiol. 17:183, 1966.

Rösch, J., and Bret, J.: Arteriography of the pancreas. Amer. J. Roentgenol. 94:182, 1965.

Rösch, J., Grollman, J. H., Jr., and Steckel, R. J.: Arteriography in the diagnosis of gallbladder disease. Radiology 92:1485, 1969.

Rossi, P., and Gould, H. R.: Angiography and scanning in liver disease. Radiology 96:553, 1970.

Rossi, P., and Ruzicka, F. F., Jr.: Differentiation of intrahepatic and extrahepatic masses by arteriography. Radiology 93:771, 1969.

Sato, T., Watanabe, K., Saitoh, Y., et al.: Selective arteriography for gallbladder diseases. Arch. Surg. 99:598, 1969.

Shanser, J. D., Glickman, M. G., and Palubinskas, A. J.: Pitfalls in the arteriographic differentiation of intrahepatic and extrahepatic masses. Amer. J. Roentgenol. 121:420, 1974.

Shanser, J. D., Moss, A. A., Clark, R. E., et al.: Angiographic evaluation of cystic lesions of the spleen. Amer. J. Roentgenol. 119:166, 1973.

Sherlock, S.: Hepatic adenomas and oral contraceptives. Gut 16:753, 1975.

Shibata, S., and Iwasaki, N.: Angiographic findings in diseases of the stomach. Amer. J. Roentgenol. 110:322, 1970.

Slovis, T. L., Berdon, W. E., Haller, J. O., et al.: Hemangiomas of the liver in infants. Amer. J. Roentgenol. 123:791, 1975.

Sprayregen, S.: Parasitic blood supply of neoplasms: Mechanisms and significance. Radiology 106:529, 1973.

Sprayregen, S., and Messinger, N. H.: Angiography of the jaundiced patient. Amer. J. Roentgenol. 122:335, 1974.

Sprayregen, S., and Messinger, N. H.: Carcinoma of the gallbladder: Diagnosis and evaluation of renal spread by angiography. Amer. J. Roentgenol. 116:382, 1972.

Strasberg, Z., Hyland, J., Salem, S., et al.: The role of angiography in the management of intestinal carcinoid. Angiology 26:573, 1975.

Ström, B. G., and Winberg, T.: Percutaneous selective angiography of the inferior mesenteric artery. Acta Radiol. (Diagn.) (Stockh.) 57:401, 1962.

Sundgren, R.: Selective angiography of the left gastric artery. Acta Radiol. (Diagn.) (Suppl 299), (Stockh.), 1970.

Suzuki, T., Karatsuka, H., Uchida, K., et al.: Carcinoma of the pancreas arising in the region of the uncinate process. Cancer 30:796, 1972.

Suzuki, T., Kawabe, K., Imamura, M., et al.: Survival of patients with cancer of the pancreas in relation to findings on arteriography. Ann. Surg. 176:37, 1972.

Suzuki, T., Kitagawa, S., and Honjo, I.: Role of splenic arteriography in the evaluation of malignant tumors in the body of the pancreas. Surg. Gynecol. Obstet. 139:509, 1974.

Suzuki, T., Tani, T., and Honjo, I.: Appraisal of arteriography for assessment of operability in periampullary carcinoma. Ann. Surg. 182:66, 1975.

Swanson, G. E.: A case of cystadenoma of the pancreas studied by selective angiography. Radiology 81:592, 1963.

Teates, C. D., Seales, D. L., and Allen, M. S.: Hamartoma of the spleen. Amer. J. Roentgenol. 116:419, 1972.

Tentoya, E.: Angiography in liver hemangioma. Amer. J. Roentgenol. 104:874, 1968.

Thomas, M. L., Lamb, G. H. R., and Barraclough, M. A.: Angiographic demonstration of a pancreatic "vipoma" in the WDHA syndrome. Amer. J. Roentgenol. 127:1037, 1976.

Tylén, U.: Accuracy of angiography in the diagnosis of carcinoma of the pancreas. Acta Radiol. (Diagn.) (Stockh.) 14:449, 1973.

Tylén, U.: Angiographic differentiation between inflammatory disease and carcinoma of the pancreas. Acta Radiol. (Diagn.) (Stockh.) 14:257, 1973.

Viamonte, M., Jr., Warren, W. D., Fomon, J. J., et al.: Angiographic investigations in portal hypertension. Surg. Gynec. Obstet. 130:37, 1970.

Walter, J. F., Bookstein, J. J., and Bouffard, E. V.: Newer angiographic observations in cholangiocarcinoma. Radiology 118:19, 1976.

Wexler, L., and Abrams, H. L.: Hamartoma of the spleen; Angiographic observations. Amer. J. Roentgenol. 92:1150, 1964.

Whelan, J. G., Jr., Creech, J. L., and Tamburro, C. H.: Angiographic and radionuclide characteristics of hepatic angiosarcoma found in vinyl chloride workers. Radiology 118:549, 1976.

Wholey, M. H., Bron, K. M., and Haller, J. D.: Selective angiography of the colon. Surg. Clin. N. Amer. 45:1283, 1965.

Winograd, J., and Palubinskas, A. J.: Arterial-portal venous shunting in cavernous hemangioma of the liver. Radiology 122:331, 1977.

Wirtanen, G. W.: A new angiographic technique in the diagnosis of liver tumor. Radiology 108:51, 1973.

Yü, C.: Primary carcinoma of the liver (hepatoma). Its diagnosis by selective celiac arteriography. Amer. J. Roentgenol. 99:142, 1967.

Zollinger, R. M.: Islet cell tumors and the alimentary tract. Amer. J. Roentgenol. 126:933, 1976.

Chapter 5

TRAUMA

GENERAL INDICATIONS FOR ANGIOGRAPHY IN ABDOMINAL TRAUMA

Abdominal trauma can be divided into two broad categories, penetrating and blunt. Penetrating trauma, regardless of the cause, is generally treated by exploratory laparotomy if there is any suggestion that the peritoneum has been entered. Therefore, angiography is seldom used in the initial evaluation of penetrating trauma. However, angiography has been very useful in evaluating the presence and severity of blunt abdominal trauma.

Childhood injuries and automobile accidents account for most civilian blunt trauma. The patients can be divided into six general categories, depending on the severity of injury. The first group is dead on arrival at the emergency room. The second is severely injured and generally is in shock. Surgery must be performed immediately, and there is no time for angiography. When the patient's condition becomes stable, angiography may be performed while the patient is still under anesthesia or in the immediate postoperative period. Angiography is most commonly needed in such patients when the initial operation corrected a neurologic or thoracic injury and did not include an abdominal exploration. The third group of patients arrives at the emergency room in relatively stable condi-

tion, perhaps with injuries to several areas, including clinical signs of significant abdominal trauma, and having a positive paracentesis or strongly positive peritoneal lavage. These patients also undergo an exploratory celiotomy without angiography. However, if associated injuries such as aortic laceration or subdural hematoma are evaluated by angiography, suspected visceral injury can be evaluated at the same time. The fourth group of patients has no life-threatening injury and has little clinical evidence of abdominal trauma. However, they have a positive peritoneal lavage. Angiography should be used to exclude any significant visceral injury in these patients, thus preventing unnecessary exploratory surgery. Since these patients are in stable condition, the angiography does not need to be done as an emergency procedure. If no injury is demonstrated by angiography, the patient can be treated for his other injuries and simply observed for any progressing abdominal symptoms. The fifth group has equivocal signs of visceral injury, but peritoneal lavage is negative. Since a positive peritoneal lavage requires less than 5 cc of intraperitoneal blood, significant trauma in the absence of a positive lavage is unlikely (Olsen, 1971). Therefore, these patients do not need angiography.

Finally, some trauma will seem insignificant to the patient, and medical advice will

189

be sought only when symptoms occur days or weeks after the incident. Such trauma may not even be remembered. In minor childhood accidents, such as falling off a bicycle or running into a tree, visceral injury may not be apparent initially. In these patients, angiography can define the presence and extent of visceral trauma.

Although the clinical findings may indicate injury to only one organ, multiple injuries are not uncommon. An abdominal aortogram in the anteroposterior projection should be the initial angiographic examination. The radiographic field should be centered on the midline and should include the diaphragm. This survey will reveal any major arterial damage, such as amputation or occlusion of a renal artery or an aortic intimal tear. In most patients, the renal arteries and parenchyma will be demonstrated well enough to exclude major renal artery injury, and, in the absence of hematuria, the renal arteries need not be catheterized selectively. If the aortogram suggests renal injury, however, the appropriate selective examination should be done. The celiac artery injections must be filmed in two or more projections to obtain an adequate study of both the liver and the spleen. The superior mesenteric artery should be injected to look for mesenteric tears and small bowel or colonic injury. It is rarely necessary to study the inferior mesenteric artery unless there has been a specific left lower quadrant injury.

Visceral injury caused by percutaneous liver biopsy, splenoportography or surgery can also be evaluated and followed by angiography. Arteriovenous fistulas, aneurysms or vascular occlusions may occur secondary to these procedures.

SPLENIC TRAUMA

The spleen is the intraabdominal organ most commonly injured by blunt trauma (Perry, 1965). Plain films of patients with splenic injury may show an enlarged spleen or a left upper quadrant mass, free abdominal fluid, displacement of the stomach or colon to the right and inferiorly, left lower rib fractures, displacement of the left kidney, obliteration of the left psoas margin and elevation of the left hemidiaphragm (Cimmino, 1964; Norell, 1957). However, none of these findings can be considered specific for splenic injury, and abdominal radiographs may be normal in the presence of splenic rupture. If splenic injury is suspected, angiography should be performed. This procedure is as valuable in avoiding unnecessary exploratory celiotomies in patients without injury as it is in confirming the presence of rupture.

A serious complication of even mild splenic trauma is delayed rupture, which occurs from 48 hours to 2 or more weeks following an injury to the left upper quadrant (Shirkey et al., 1964). The cause of these delayed ruptures is not entirely clear. Patients may be asymptomatic during the latent period, or they may have mild but increasing anemia, a left upper quadrant mass, splinting of the left hemidiaphragm or evidence of peritoneal irritation (Bollinger and Fowler, 1966). Delayed ruptures usually cause massive bleeding so that the patients with suspected splenic trauma must be carefully observed for at least 2 weeks if exploratory laparotomy is not performed. Splenic angiography in these patients can shorten the length of hospitalization.

Technique

Celiac or splenic angiography must be performed for evaluation of splenic injury. Aortography is not adequate. Filming must cover at least 20 seconds, including the arterial, capillary and venous phases. The volume of contrast medium used must be adequate to ensure good capillary and venous phases. Celiac studies should be performed with 30 to 40 cc of 75 to 76 per cent contrast medium injected at a rate of 10 to 12 cc per second. When splenic artery injections are made, 30 to 40 cc of 75 to 76 per cent contrast medium should be injected at a rate of 8 to 10 cc per second. If the gastric vessels or wall overlies the spleen, the stomach can be distended with 300 to 400 cc of air to change the positions of these structures and help identify them. Filming in the left posterior oblique position will also help to separate the overlying stomach and the left lobe of the liver from the spleen.

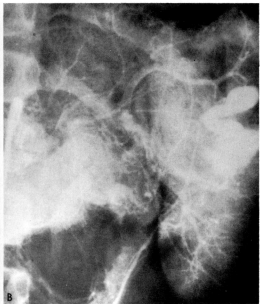

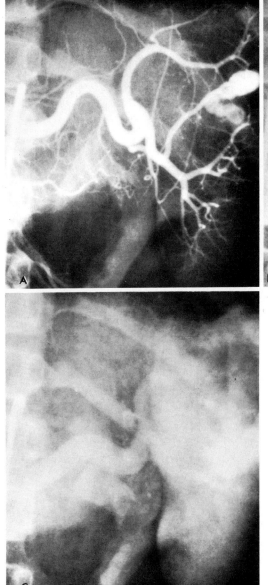

Figure 5-1. Splenic rupture with arterial extravasation of contrast medium. Splenic angiogram in an 8 year old boy who fell and hit his left side on the curb. Splenic rupture was confirmed at surgery.

A. Arterial phase. Contrast medium has extravasated into the splenic laceration.

B. Later arterial phase. The contrast medium has diffused throughout the splenic tear. No early venous drainage is present.

C. Venous phase. The splenic vein is normal, but extravasated contrast medium persists. (From Redman, H. C., Reuter, S. R., and Bookstein, J. J.: Angiography in abdominal trauma. Ann. Surg. *169*:57, 1969.)

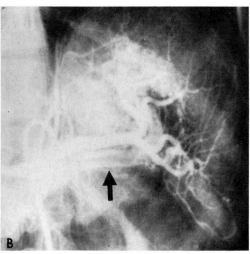

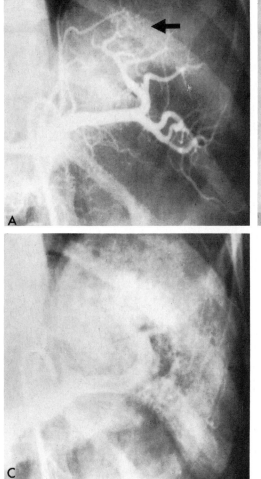

Figure 5–2. Splenic rupture with early venous drainage. Celiac angiogram in a 7 year old girl who fell off a bicycle, hitting her left side. At operation, a 3 cm laceration and contusion of the upper pole were found.

A. Arterial phase. Patchy areas of contrast medium pool at the upper pole (➡).

B. The splenic vein (➡) is opacified 1 second later.

C. Parenchymal phase. Irregular collections of contrast medium are present in the upper half of the spleen. (From Redman, H. C., Reuter, S. R., and Bookstein, J. J.: Angiography in abdominal trauma. Ann. Surg. *169:* 57, 1969.)

Angiographic Findings

The results of significant blunt trauma to the spleen are rupture, subcapsular hematoma, or both. The angiographic appearance varies, depending on what has occurred.

In splenic rupture, the angiographic findings include one or more of the following: active leakage of contrast medium from the splenic arteries into the splenic pulp (Fig. 5–1), early filling of the splenic vein during the arterial phase (Fig. 5–2), displacement or occlusion of intrasplenic arterial branches (Fig. 5–3), irregular accumulation of contrast medium (Fig. 5–3) and irregular or ill-defined areas of absent contrast accumulation representing infarcts (Fig. 5–3).

When rupture occurs without a subcapsular hematoma, the spleen is usually normal in size, although it may be slightly enlarged. If it is enlarged, the splenic artery is displaced medially.

Subcapsular hematoma leads to splenic enlargement and medial displacement of the splenic artery and vein (Fig. 5–4). The intrasplenic arteries are stretched and displaced medially, and the capsular branches are spread around a large, avascular mass. In the capillary phase, the splenic pulp is displaced medially and compressed by the hematoma, frequently assuming a crescent shape if the hematoma is seen in profile. The margin between the splenic parenchyma and the hematoma may be sharply defined but is more frequently indistinct and slightly irregular.

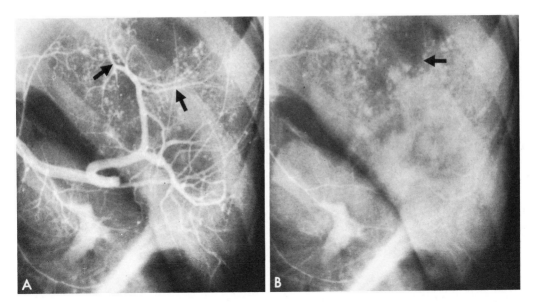

Figure 5–3. Splenic rupture with displacement of intrasplenic arterial branches. Splenic angiogram in an 11 year old boy who had been in an automobile accident. At operation the laceration was filled with clot.

A. Arterial phase. The intrasplenic arteries to the upper pole are spread (➡), and there is patchy, irregular extravasation of contrast medium.

B. Parenchymal phase. The extravasated contrast medium persists, and a triangular defect caused by the laceration is present (➡).

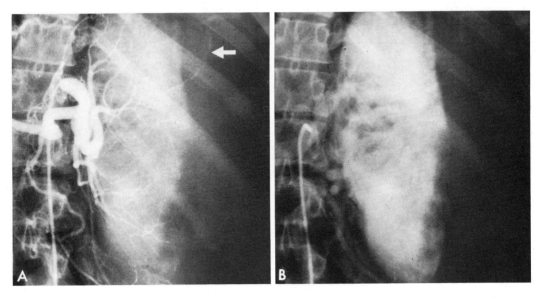

Figure 5–4. Splenic subcapsular hematoma. Celiac angiogram in a 49 year old woman who had fallen down stairs 2 weeks earlier.

A. Arterial phase. The splenic artery is displaced to the right by the enlarged spleen. The intrasplenic branches are stretched, and the splenic parenchyma is displaced medially by an avascular mass. Capsular arteries pass around this mass (⇨).

B. Venous phase. The splenic vein is compressed to the right. The splenic parenchyma has a crescentic shape and a moderately indistinct margin. The indistinct, transverse lucencies represent multiple small transverse lacerations.

Occasionally, none of these findings of significant splenic injury are present, but there is an irregular, unhomogeneous capillary phase in a localized area of the spleen. This is the appearance of splenic contusion, which may occur without a capsular tear or subcapsular hematoma. Patients with contusion do not need to be explored if they remain stable. They may be followed with ultrasound to detect a change in splenic size if clinical concern persists.

Splenic cysts have an angiographic appearance similar to subcapsular hematomas. In fact, many cysts are old subcapsular hematomas which have not proceeded to rupture. For example, one patient, a young alcoholic injured in a fight had had several previous traumatic incidents. A large spleen was demonstrated on plain films. The angiogram revealed a large subcapsular hematoma (Fig. 5–5), but at operation a well encapsulated chocolate cyst with a fibrotic wall approximately 2 cm thick was encountered. There also had been recent bleeding.

The angiographic diagnosis of splenic rupture is generally neither difficult nor subtle. One or more of the findings of rupture or subcapsular hematoma are almost invariably present. The few difficulties that occur in the angiographic evaluation of splenic trauma are caused by overdiagnosis of normal variations in the position and contour of the spleen or overinterpretation

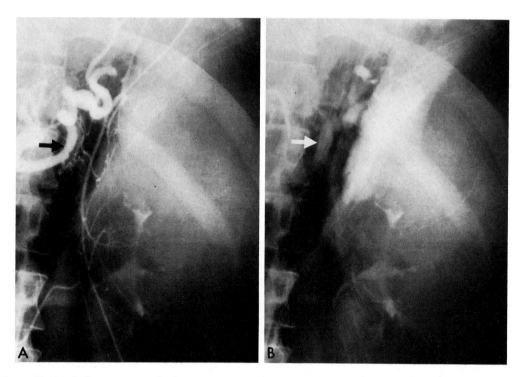

Figure 5–5. Splenic cyst. Splenic angiogram in a 24 year old alcoholic with repeated episodes of trauma. A splenic cyst with evidence of recent bleeding was found at celiotomy. There was fibrosis along the splenic pedicle surrounding the splenic artery and vein.

A. Arterial phase. The splenic artery is irregular (➡) and is displaced to the right by the enlarged spleen. The intrasplenic branches are spread around a large avascular mass.

B. Late parenchymal phase. The splenic parenchyma has been displaced by the subcapsular cyst, and the capsular arteries empty slowly. The splenic vein (⇨) is irregular in contour and is displaced to the right. (From Redman, H. C., Reuter, S. R., and Bookstein, J. J.: Angiography in abdominal trauma. Ann. Surg. *169*:57, 1969.)

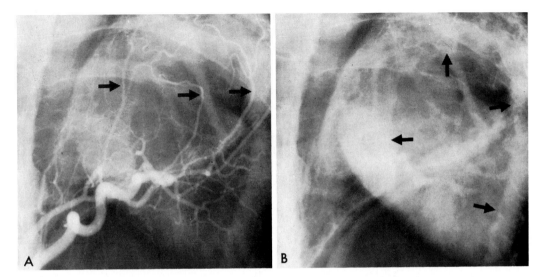

Figure 5-6. Gastric arteries simulating a splenic subcapsular hematoma. Celiac angiogram in a 27 year old man who had a positive paracentesis for blood following an automobile accident. At operation the spleen was normal.

A. Arterial phase. Both the left gastric and splenic arteries are demonstrated. Several gastric arteries (➡) appear to arise from the splenic artery and surround an avascular mass, suggesting a subcapsular hematoma.

B. Venous phase. The superior splenic contour is indistinct, a rather common normal variation. Contrast medium accumulates in the gastric wall (➡). Distention of the stomach with air changed the position of the gastric arteries, allowing their correct identification.

of confluent images in the capillary phase. The distance of the spleen from the diaphragm is normally variable and should not be considered a factor in the diagnosis of subcapsular hematoma. Short gastric arteries arise from the distal splenic artery, and these may be stretched if the stomach is distended with air (Fig. 5–6). They should not be confused with stretched splenic capsular branches.

The spleen often has prominent fetal lobulations (Fig. 5–7); these must be distinguished from lacerations. A left posterior oblique projection generally demonstrates that these irregularities in the contour are simply lobulations. They occur on the anterolateral edge of the spleen and are sharply defined. The parenchymal contrast accumulation adjacent to these lobulations is homogeneous and smooth. Accessory spleens may also simulate irregular contrast accumulation (Fig. 5–8), but their sharp margination makes the differentiation of accessory spleens and parenchymal contusion possible.

Superimposition of arteries of other organs occasionally suggests splenic injury. Both the stomach and liver generally overlie a portion of the spleen in the anteroposterior projection. Use of the left posterior oblique projection and distention of the stomach with air help to distinguish the arteries of these organs from splenic arteries. Omentum adherent to the left upper quadrant can also mimic irregular splenic accumulation of contrast medium (Fig. 5–9). In our experience with more than 100 patients with suspected blunt splenic trauma, no known false negative diagnoses have been made. False positive diagnoses can be avoided by careful attention to these pitfalls.

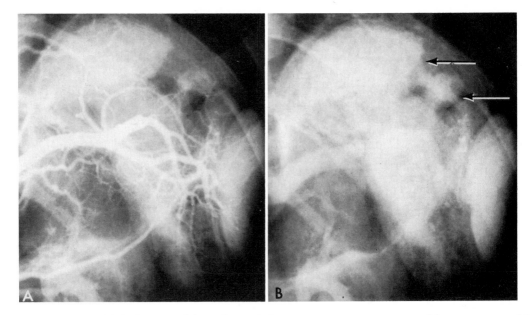

Figure 5–7. Fetal lobulations of the spleen. Celiac angiogram in a 22 year old man examined following an automobile accident. Autopsy confirmed marked fetal lobulation in a normal spleen.

  A. Arterial phase. The lateral margin of the spleen is markedly irregular, but the intrasplenic arteries are normal.

  B. Venous phase. Sharply defined defects are present laterally in the splenic parenchyma (➡), representing fetal lobulations. Emptying of contrast medium from the gastric arteries is delayed.

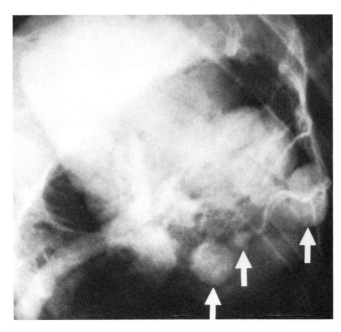

Figure 5–8. Accessory spleens. Venous phase of a splenic angiogram in a 47 year old man. Three accessory spleens (⟹) are superimposed on the lower pole of the spleen. In addition, there are prominent fetal lobulations on the lateral splenic margin.

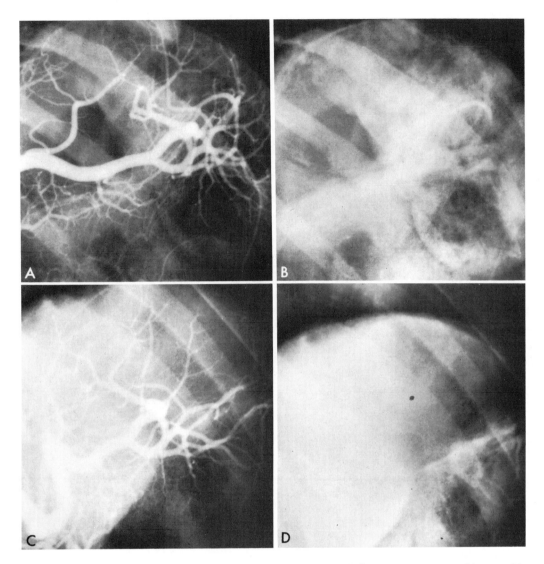

Figure 5-9. Adherent omentum simulating splenic rupture. Celiac angiogram in a 22 year old man examined following an automobile accident. At operation omentum was adherent to the spleen, which was normal. Identification of extravasated contrast medium should be made in two or more projections to be considered positive.

A. Arterial phase in the anteroposterior projection. The findings are normal.

B. Parenchymal phase. The overlying stomach and colon cause a mottled appearance, but no specific abnormalities are seen.

C. Arterial phase in the left posterior oblique projection. The findings are normal.

D. Parenchymal phase. A rather discrete, linear accumulation of contrast medium suggests a splenic laceration.

Other Types of Splenic Trauma

Penetrating trauma to the spleen will almost always lead to immediate surgical exploration and splenectomy. However, if an angiogram is performed, the angiographic findings may be normal or may be similar to those of blunt trauma. A high velocity penetrating injury is more likely to demonstrate the findings of blunt trauma than a stab wound or other low velocity penetrating trauma.

Splenoportography, a type of penetrating trauma, may cause intrasplenic arterial aneurysms (Boijsen and Efsing, 1967) and arteriovenous fistulas. The fistulas probably close within days of their formation. The aneurysms occur along the needle track, and their distribution helps distinguish them from the aneurysms that sometimes accompany splenomegaly and portal hypertension.

HEPATIC TRAUMA

Liver injury occurs in about 10 per cent of patients with blunt abdominal trauma, about one half as often as the occurrence of splenic injury (McCort, 1962). Specific clinical signs of liver trauma are often lacking, and misdiagnosis carries a high morbidity. Chest and abdominal films show right rib fractures, blood in the right pleural space, elevation of the right hemidiaphragm, intraabdominal fluid and hepatic enlargement. None of these signs are specific, however, and angiography is frequently important in evaluating the presence and extent of liver injury.

Liver trauma takes several forms. Frequently the capsule and liver parenchyma are lacerated superficially. These lesions may stop bleeding spontaneously and require little or no surgical therapy (McClelland, 1965). However, many liver lacerations extend more deeply into the liver substance. In the adult, the liver becomes harder in consistency, and injury may cause a fracture pattern running into the liver parenchyma. Such fracturing lesions are hard to define fully at operation, and a residual deep injury may lead to delayed bleeding, bile leakage, hemobilia or abscess. In children, the liver is softer, and trauma may cause a central disruption and hematoma without capsular laceration; this may be very difficult to detect at operation. Complications similar to those of an overlooked deep laceration may occur. Finally, a superficial liver injury without a tear in Glisson's capsule may lead to subcapsular hematoma.

The majority of patients with liver lacerations who arrive at the emergency room alive are in shock, have a positive peritoneal lavage and require an immediate operation to control the hemorrhage. Angiography has no role in the immediate evaluation of such patients. Less severe liver trauma is frequently difficult to evalu-

ate clinically and at operation, and angiography performed prior to exploration has been helpful to the surgeon. Occasionally, the presence of hepatic damage is missed in the initial clinical evaluation of the patient, either because few symptoms are present or because the severity of other trauma masks it. Such patients may later have jaundice, hemobilia, an enlarging liver or fever of uncertain origin. Clinical evaluation of these problems is difficult, and angiography has a central role in defining the delayed complications of liver trauma.

Technique

Angiography for hepatic trauma must cover the entire hepatic blood supply. Celiac or common hepatic arterial injections should be made in each patient, and, in addition, replaced hepatic arteries from the superior mesenteric artery or left gastric artery must be injected. The filming sequence should cover at least 20 seconds. Thirty to 50 cc of 75 to 76 per cent contrast medium should be injected over 3 to 4 seconds for a celiac injection, while slightly less can be injected for a common hepatic arterial study. Two projections may be needed to localize the abnormalities in liver trauma adequately.

Angiographic Findings

The angiographic findings in patients with liver trauma are similar to those of splenic trauma. The common hepatic artery and its extrahepatic branches may be displaced downward and to the left. The intrahepatic arteries may be displaced around an intrahepatic mass or may be compressed together and stretched by a subcapsular hematoma (Figs. 5–10 and 5–11). Tearing injuries to the liver can lead to pseudoaneurysms and disruption of small arterial branches (Fig. 5–12). In addition, contrast medium may leak into a liver laceration (Fig. 5–13). When an arteriovenous fistula forms, it is almost always between the hepatic artery and the portal vein (Fig. 5–14), probably because of the proximity of these two vessels in the portal spaces. Rarely, contrast medium may pass into the biliary

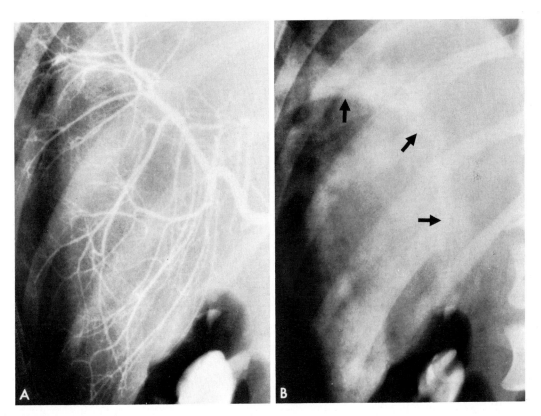

Figure 5–10. Hepatic subcapsular hematoma. Hepatic angiogram in a 12 year old girl examined following a fall.

A. Arterial phase. The intrahepatic arteries are stretched around an avascular peripheral mass. No abnormal arteries are present.

B. Parenchymal phase. The normal hepatic parenchyma has been compressed to the left by the subcapsular hematoma (➡). The compressed parenchyma forms a sharp border with the lucent hematoma (➡). (From Redman, H. C., Reuter, S. R., and Bookstein, J. J., Angiography in abdominal trauma. Ann. Surg. *169*:57, 1969.)

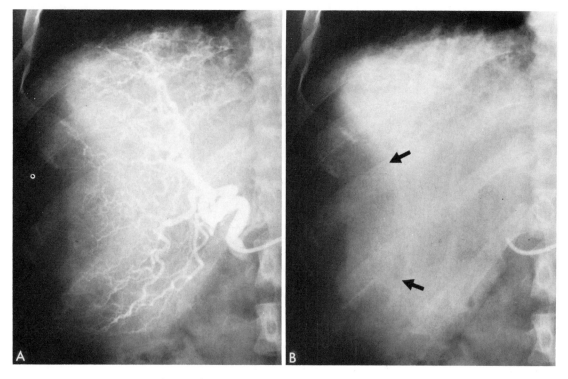

Figure 5–11. Hepatic subcapsular hematoma. Hepatic angiogram in a 38 year old man following an automobile accident.

A. Arterial phase. The intrahepatic arteries are stretched around an avascular, lateral peripheral mass. The arteries throughout the liver are somewhat tortuous, consistent with the patient's alcoholic history, but no abnormal vessels are present.

B. Parenchymal phase. There is a crescentic defect in the lateral margin of the liver (➡) caused by the subcapsular hematoma.

system, identifying the site of hemobilia (Fig. 5–15).

In the parenchymal phase of the angiogram, liver contusion causes mottled accumulation of contrast medium with irregular and somewhat delayed arterial emptying (Fig. 5–16). Arterial collaterals may bypass arterial occlusions and fill branches peripheral to lacerations. Subcapsular hematomas compress normal parenchyma and may appear as a sharply defined lucent defect against the increased contrast accumulation in the compressed parenchyma (Figs. 5–10 and 5–11). Discrete lacerations may also appear as lucent defects; intrahepatic hematomas are more poorly defined lucent defects.

The venous phase generally provides no further information, though confirmation of parenchymal defects may be obtained. Arteriovenous shunting is apparent in the arterial or early parenchymal phases. However, peripheral portal venous filling during the venous phase may be unusually well demonstrated in the presence of contusion (Boijsen et al., 1966).

One or more of these findings are almost always present on angiograms performed shortly following blunt hepatic trauma. Angiograms performed several days after the trauma are more difficult to interpret. Subcapsular hematomas, occluded arteries, intraparenchymal hematomas and hemobilia can be demonstrated if present. Clots tend to form in lacerations, however, and active leakage of contrast medium into the lacerations ceases, making them more difficult to detect by angiography. Traumatic arteriovenous fistulas and aneurysms frequently regress with time.

Angiography performed following liver resection for trauma often shows vascular changes in addition to absence of the resected portion of the liver. These operations are generally performed rapidly under adverse conditions, and the surgeon is often forced to make a nonanatomic resection. Hemostasis is the major concern,

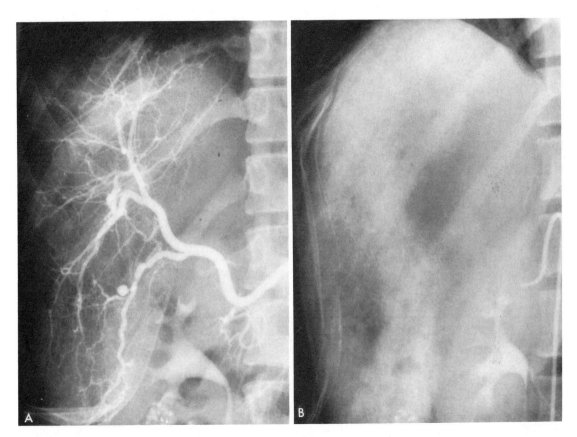

Figure 5–12. Hepatic trauma with pseudoaneurysm formation. Hepatic angiogram in a 20 year old woman examined 1 week following abdominal trauma.

A. Arterial phase. A small pseudoaneurysm is present in the lower right lobe of the liver.

B. Capillary phase. There is irregular contrast accumulation through the lower portion of the right lobe of the liver with a mottled, bubbly appearing area of decreased contrast accumulation representing an abscess.

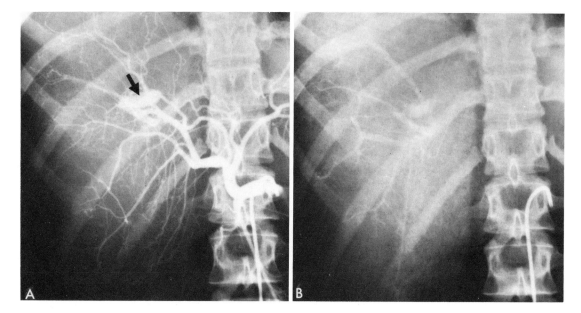

Figure 5–13. Hepatic laceration with extravasation of contrast medium and arterioportal shunting. Hepatic angiogram in a 16 year old girl following an automobile accident.

A. Arterial phase. Contrast medium has extravasated from a lacerated right hepatic artery branch into the midportion of the right lobe of the liver (➡) and immediately fills a right portal vein radicle. In addition, the arterial branches are stretched around an intrahepatic hematoma.

B. Parenchymal phase. Portal vein radicles stretched around the hematoma fill from the arterioportal fistula. They drain in their normal, peripheral direction.

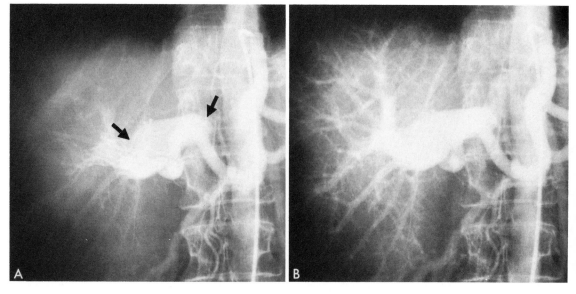

Figure 5–14. Massive arterioportal shunt. Celiac angiogram in a 58 year old woman 6 months following blunt abdominal trauma.

A. Early arterial phase. The hepatic artery is dilated, and contrast medium shunts immediately to an aneurysmally dilated portal vein (➡).

B. Midarterial phase. The portal vein radicles are opacified throughout the liver.

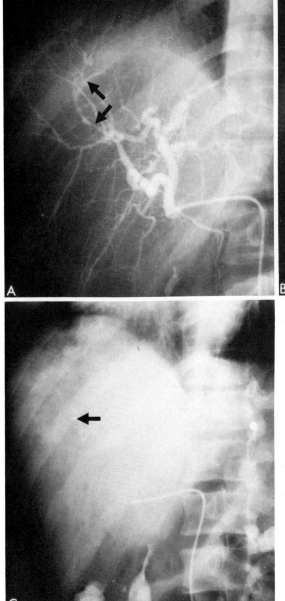

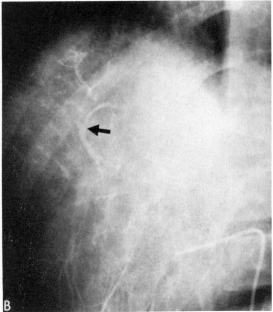

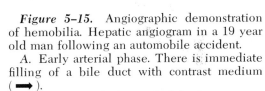

Figure 5-15. Angiographic demonstration of hemobilia. Hepatic angiogram in a 19 year old man following an automobile accident.

A. Early arterial phase. There is immediate filling of a bile duct with contrast medium (➡).

B. Late arterial phase. The bile duct remains filled with contrast medium (➡). The hepatic artery branches through the right lobe of the liver empty irregularly, indicating contusion.

C. Parenchymal phase. Contrast medium can still be seen in the bile duct (➡).

At operation, the biliary tract was filled with blood. Although a T-tube was positioned in the common duct, repeated blood clots formed in the hepatic ducts, and the patient eventually developed an abscess.

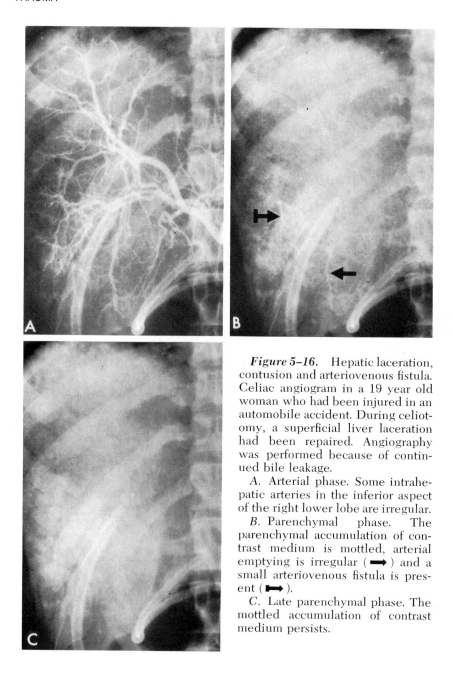

Figure 5–16. Hepatic laceration, contusion and arteriovenous fistula. Celiac angiogram in a 19 year old woman who had been injured in an automobile accident. During celiotomy, a superficial liver laceration had been repaired. Angiography was performed because of continued bile leakage.

A. Arterial phase. Some intrahepatic arteries in the inferior aspect of the right lower lobe are irregular.

B. Parenchymal phase. The parenchymal accumulation of contrast medium is mottled, arterial emptying is irregular (➡) and a small arteriovenous fistula is present (➡).

C. Late parenchymal phase. The mottled accumulation of contrast medium persists.

and angiography following a large resection may show ligation of major hepatic artery branches (Fig. 5–17). Collateral vessels supply the liver distal to the ligation. Portions of the liver thought to be resected sometimes remain. In addition, residual areas of traumatized liver, such as intrahepatic hematomas, arteriovenous fistulas or pseudoaneurysms, may occasionally be present. Subcapsular hematomas are found infrequently in the postoperative period.

Following a major liver resection, the remaining liver enlarges, and the supplying arteries dilate and spread as liver regeneration occurs (Fig. 5–18; also see Fig. 4–40). In addition, the spleen may also be enlarged in the early postoperative period because of the proliferation of splenic reticuloendothelial tissue and the portal hypertension caused by the decreased volume of liver parenchyma and trauma to the remaining liver.

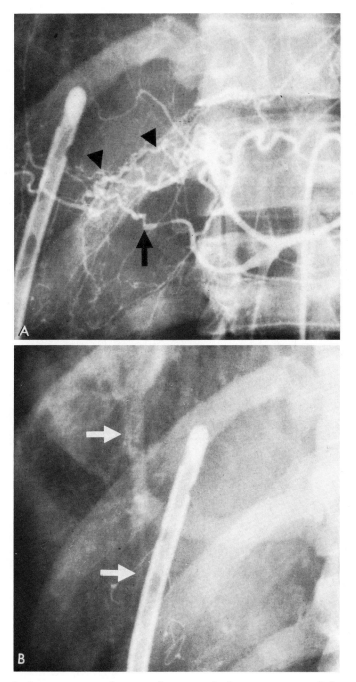

Figure 5–17. Right hepatic artery ligation during right liver resection. Celiac angiogram in a 41 year old man who had been in an automobile accident. Massive bleeding led to a nonanatomic resection, although the surgeons believed they had removed the entire right lobe.

A. Arterial phase. The hepatic arteries are small, and the right hepatic artery is occluded just distal to an area of severe stenosis (➡). Collateral arteries (▶) from the left and proximal right hepatic arteries supply the distal right hepatic artery branches.

B. Venous phase. Portal veins are seen in the residual right lobe of the liver (⇒).

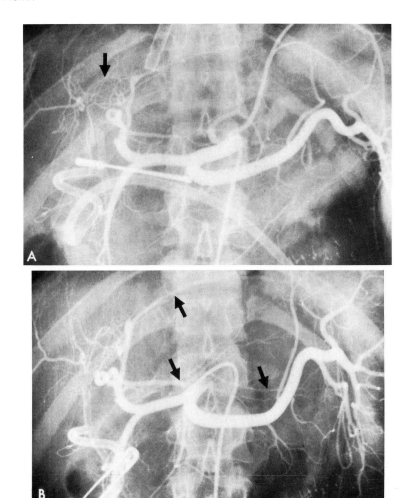

Figure 5–18. Partial right hepatic resection. Celiac angiography was performed both 3 days and 2 weeks after liver resection in an 18 year old man who had been in an automobile accident.

   A. Angiogram at 3 days postresection, arterial phase. Many left hepatic to right hepatic arterial collaterals (➡) are filled. The left hepatic artery and its branches are small. Few, small right hepatic branches are seen.

   B. Angiogram at 2 weeks, arterial phase. The collateral arteries are larger, and the left hepatic arteries (➡) are dilated and are spread. These changes are secondary to compensatory enlargement of the left lobe. The spleen has also enlarged.

Other Types of Hepatic Trauma

The initial therapy of choice in penetrating trauma to the liver is generally operative intervention. Occasionally, associated injuries, to the aorta or kidneys, for example, will necessitate angiography, and in such patients the liver should also be evaluated. High velocity bullet injuries can cause lacerations at a distance from their course. They also tend to cause burst injuries with distant contusion and parenchymal disruption. All the angiographic findings of blunt trauma, including arteriovenous shunting (Fig. 5–19), displaced arteries, mottled or decreased parenchymal accumulation, subcapsular hematomas and false aneurysms (Fig. 5–20) can be seen in these patients. Angiography can also be of use in detecting complications developing late in the postoperative course of such a patient. These complications would generally be the same as those that occur following blunt trauma.

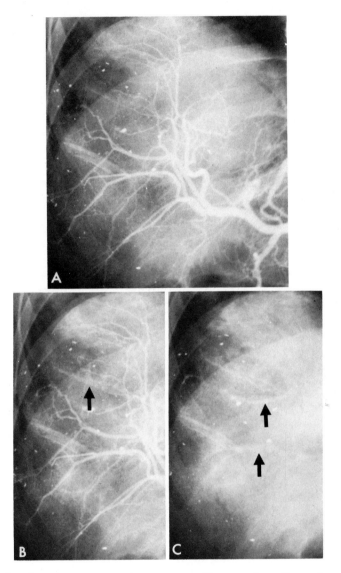

Figure 5-19.   High velocity penetrating liver trauma. Common hepatic angiogram in a 22 year old man who had been shot in the right flank, injuring his right kidney and the right lobe of the liver. Marked right hepatic parenchymal disruption and several lacerations were found at celiotomy.

   A. Early arterial phase. The peripheral right hepatic artery branches are irregular and displaced.

   B. Late arterial phase. Some contrast medium has extravasated into the liver parenchyma (➡), and the irregular, displaced arteries are still filled.

   C. Parenchymal phase. The accumulation of contrast medium is irregular and several portal veins are filled (➡).

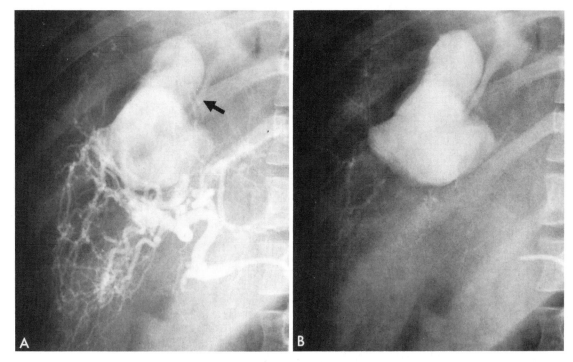

Figure 5–20. Large false aneurysm and hepatic artery–hepatic vein fistula. Hepatic angiogram in a 36 year old woman 1 month following a right upper quadrant gunshot wound.

A. Arterial phase. A large bilobed false aneurysm fills with contrast medium. There is immediate shunting of blood to a hepatic vein (➡).

B. Parenchymal phase. The aneurysm remains filled with contrast medium. The arteriovenous fistula can be better visualized.

Low velocity penetrating wounds to the liver, such as stab wounds or liver biopsy, can lead to two types of intrahepatic complications—arterial aneurysms, either true or false, and arteriovenous fistulas (Fig. 5–21) (Preger, 1967). Both are uncommon, and little is known about the natural course of such lesions, but arteriovenous fistulas have been observed to close spontaneously. Rarely, liver biopsies may cause intrahepatic hematomas. Any hepatic operation can lead to arterial occlusions, arteriovenous fistulas or pseudoaneurysms, but such problems occur more often during difficult gallbladder or common duct surgery. Angiography can be used to demonstrate or follow the course of these lesions.

STOMACH AND BOWEL TRAUMA

Significant injury to the stomach or intestine occurs in less than 10 per cent of patients with blunt abdominal trauma (Solheim, 1963). These injuries are frequently associated with other serious injuries. Although survival depends upon an accurate, early diagnosis, this is often difficult (Perry, 1965). Plain films of the abdomen may reveal free intraabdominal air if a viscus has been perforated. Dilated and edematous loops of bowel may be seen. Free intraabdominal fluid and generalized or localized ileus may be present. If recognition of the injury is delayed, peritonitis may occur. The radiographic signs are obviously not specific. Angiographic experience and application in these areas are limited, since the multiple injuries usually lead to immediate exploratory laparotomy. However, the following angiographic abnormalities may be present. Slowed arterial blood flow to the stomach or bowel can occur in the presence of contusion. In these cases, the vessels empty slowly and irregularly. This may be associated with arteriovenous shunting, seen as dense and early venous drainage (Fig. 5–22). The arteries may be distorted, irregular or apparently in spasm (Fig. 5–23). Arterial occlusions may be present and can represent transection of the bowel or the mesentery. Contrast medium may leak into the gut or gut wall during angiography if free bleeding occurs (Figs. 5–24 and 5–25). If intramural bleeding is great enough, arteries may be stretched or displaced around the hematoma. These angiographic abnormalities may be subtle, and survey angiograms performed for blunt abdominal trauma should be evaluated with extreme care.

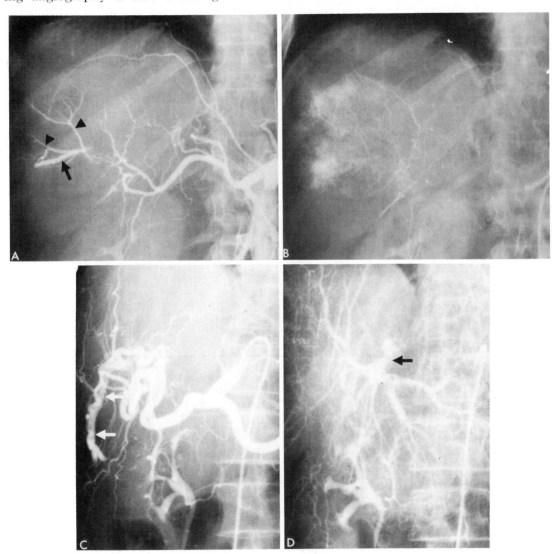

Figure 5–21. Arteriovenous fistulas following percutaneous liver biopsy.

A. Celiac angiogram 1 week following liver biopsy in a 36 year old woman with early cirrhosis. Arterial phase. The needle track (➡) fills with contrast medium early in the arterial phase, and portal veins (▶) fill simultaneously.

B. Late arterial phase. Terminal portal vein radicles are filled. The patchy areas of increased contrast density in the lateral right portion of the liver represent groups of sinusoids that fill from the portal vein radicles to which contrast medium has been shunted.

C. Celiac angiogram in a 42 year old man 1 week after percutaneous liver biopsy. Early arterial phase. A peripheral right hepatic artery is dilated and communicates directly with a peripheral portal vein (⟹).

D. Late arterial phase. The contrast medium fills the portal vein of the right lobe as far as the right portal vein (➡). The shunt closed spontaneously. A celiac angiogram performed several months after the first examination was normal.

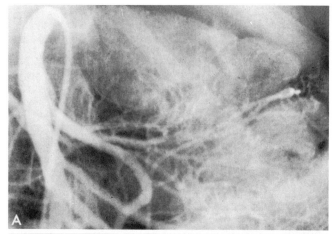

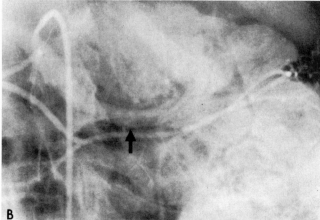

Figure 5–22. Arteriovenous shunting associated with mesenteric laceration. Superior mesenteric angiogram in a 22 year old man examined following an automobile accident. At operation a mesenteric laceration and hematoma were found. The jejunum was contused but viable.

A. Early arterial phase. Two seconds following the start of contrast medium injection, a dense accumulation of contrast medium occurs in the wall of the proximal jejunum.

B. Late arterial phase. One-half second later veins draining this area are opacified (➡). Some arteries are still filled with contrast medium. Venous drainage from the remainder of the small bowel appeared 5 seconds later when venous opacification from this area was diminishing.

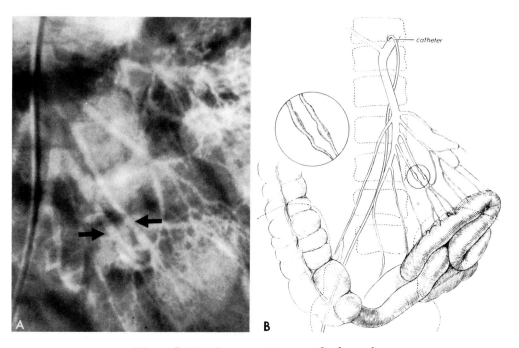

Figure 5–23. *See opposite page for legend.*

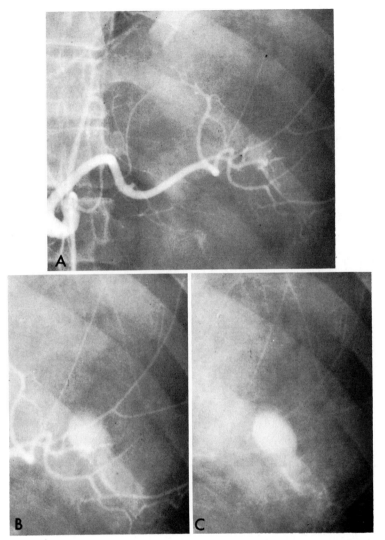

Figure 5–24. Intramural bleeding into the gastric wall. Celiac angiogram in a 34 year old man examined following an abdominal gunshot wound. At operation a greater curvature intramural hematoma was found. The spleen was normal.

 A. Early arterial phase. No abnormalities are present.

 B. Midarterial phase. Contrast medium has extravasated outside the arterial bed.

 C. Late arterial phase. A discrete accumulation of contrast medium is present. Bleeding was thought to have come from a short gastric artery.

Figure 5–23. Mesenteric laceration. Superior mesenteric angiogram in a 7 year old girl examined following an automobile accident. At celiotomy, a mesenteric tear and hematoma were found.

 A. Arterial phase, subtraction technique. Two mesenteric arterial branches have an irregular caliber (➡). Emptying of these arteries was slightly delayed.

 B. Line drawing of the irregular arterial branches.

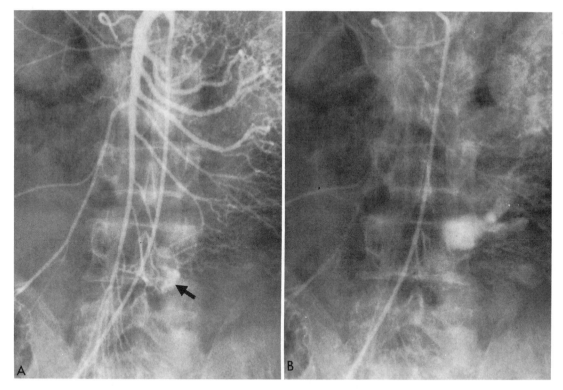

Figure 5–25. Mesenteric laceration. Superior mesenteric angiogram in a 42 year old man following an automobile accident.

A. Arterial phase. Contrast medium extravasates from a proximal ileal artery (➡).

B. Late arterial phase. The extravasating contrast medium spreads. At exploration the mesentery was found to be torn.

DIAPHRAGMATIC RUPTURE

Diaphragmatic rupture may accompany blunt abdominal trauma, particularly that caused by seat belts. When the left hemidiaphragm is ruptured, the diagnosis is usually apparent on the chest film, since the air-filled stomach or jejunum herniates into the left hemithorax. A ruptured spleen may also pass through the diaphragmatic rent, and the intrathoracic hemorrhage which then occurs may obscure the plain film findings. If angiography is done, the small bowel and spleen can be identified above the diaphragm (Fig. 5–26).

Rupture of the right hemidiaphragm is more difficult to diagnose on plain films. Generally the only organ herniating on the right is the liver, and the dome of the herniated liver may simulate an elevated right hemidiaphragm. The angiographic appearance of a herniated liver is characteristic. Besides the intrahepatic vascular changes of liver trauma, an indentation of the lateral portion of the diaphragmatic tear into the lateral margin of the liver may be identified on the angiogram (Fig. 5–27).

RETROPERITONEAL TRAUMA

Blunt trauma frequently causes injury to the retroperitoneal structures, with renal injury the most common occurrence. The genitourinary tract is outside the scope of this book, but when angiography is performed for blunt trauma to the abdomen, investigation of the kidneys must be included if hematuria is present. Over one third of patients with significant blunt abdominal trauma will have some renal injury.

Blunt trauma to the pancreas is uncommon, occurring in 2.2 per cent of patients (Solheim, 1963). Pancreatic injury is most common with multiple severe injuries, and few patients ever require angiography. We have examined three patients with pan-

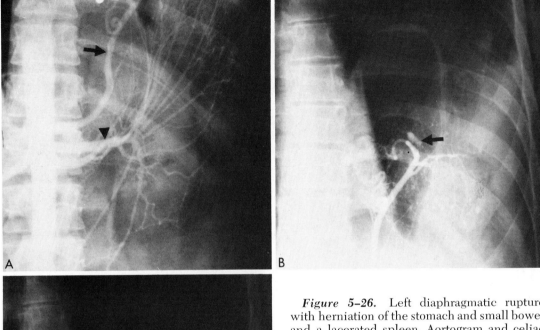

Figure 5–26. Left diaphragmatic rupture with herniation of the stomach and small bowel and a lacerated spleen. Aortogram and celiac angiogram in a 25 year old man following an automobile accident.

A. Aortogram. The splenic (➡) artery extends through the left hemidiaphragm. The main portion of the superior mesenteric artery is elevated (▶), and jejunal branches also pass to the left chest.

B. Arterial phase of a celiac angiogram. The air-filled stomach and spleen are in the left hemithorax. Extravasation of contrast medium (➡) indicates splenic rupture.

C. Venous phase. The splenic vein passes back through the tear. The extravasated contrast medium persists.

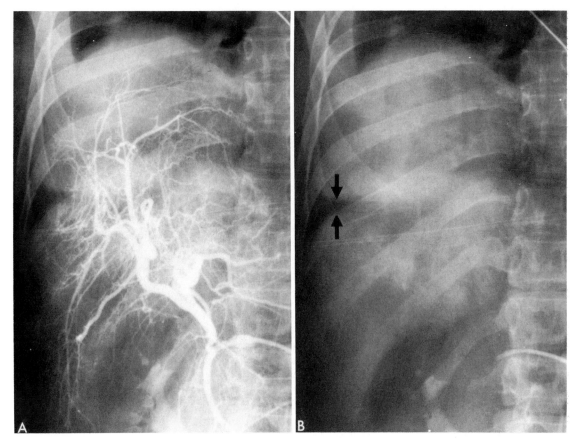

Figure 5–27. Right diaphragmatic rupture with herniation of the liver. Hepatic angiogram in a 25 year old woman following an automobile accident 1 week earlier.

A. Arterial phase. The intrahepatic artery branches are diffusely distorted, indicating contusion. No hematoma or extravasation of contrast medium is seen. The upper portion of the right lobe of the liver extends well into the right thoracic cavity, and a hemothorax is present along the upper right thoracic wall.

B. Parenchymal phase. The hepatogram is reasonably homogeneous. A notch is present in the mid-lateral portion of the right lobe where the liver is compressed by the edge of the diaphragmatic tear (➡).

creatic trauma. One, who had a complete transection of the pancreas, had no angiographic abnormalities in or around the pancreas. The second had a traumatic pseudocyst, which was demonstrated by angiography (Fig. 5–28). The third had a hematoma of the tail of the pancreas, in addition to a splenic laceration. No abnormal angiographic findings were present in the pancreas.

VASCULAR TRAUMA

Intraabdominal arterial injury may accompany both penetrating and blunt trauma, although it is more common in penetrating trauma. Most injuries causing bleeding are found during exploratory laparotomy, but occasionally some are overlooked. Some vascular injuries, especially in the retroperitoneum, do not cause free bleeding and are, therefore, difficult to detect during operation.

Penetrating trauma causes three types of arterial injuries—complete transection, partial transection and nonpenetrating arterial wall damage. In complete and partial transections, free leakage of contrast medium may be seen, or thrombosis may occur at the injury so that arterial occlusion is the only finding. Partial transection may lead to a hematoma or pseudoaneurysm, especially when the involved artery lies in relatively firm tissue. Transection injuries can also lead to arteriovenous fistulas (Fig. 5–29).

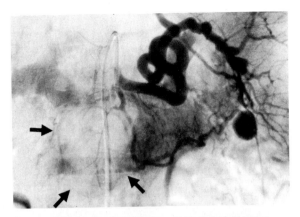

Figure 5-28. Traumatic pancreatic pseudocyst and pseudoaneurysm. Splenic angiogram in a 35 year old woman following an automobile accident.

Late arterial phase. Subtraction technique. Arteries in the neck and body of the pancreas are bowed around a 4 cm in diameter pseudocyst (➡), which has no parenchymal accumulation of contrast medium. A 1 cm false aneurysm of a small pancreatic artery in the tail is filled. Early portal vein filling is demonstrated.

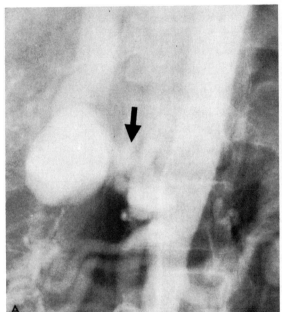

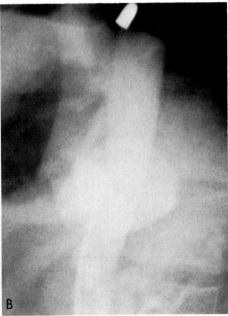

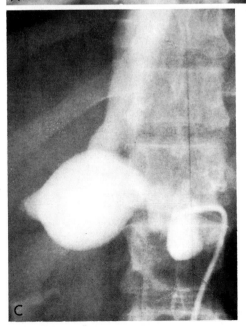

Figure 5-29. Aortocaval fistula. Aortography in a 35 year old man examined 2 months following a left upper quadrant gunshot wound. Immediately after the injury, a lacerated spleen was removed, but no other injuries were found. The patient was rehospitalized with an abdominal bruit. At operation, a communication was found between the aorta and the inferior vena cava lateral and slightly inferior to the origin of the celiac artery. A venous aneurysm was present at the junction of the fistula with the inferior vena cava.

A. Anteroposterior aortogram. A communication (➡) between the aorta and inferior vena cava is demonstrated. The inferior vena cava is aneurysmally dilated at its junction with the fistula.

B. Lateral lumbar aortogram.

C. Selective injection of the fistula. No visceral vessels fill from the fistulous tract.

Arterial contusion can be caused by penetrating or blunt trauma producing intimal damage. The arterial lumen may be slightly narrowed, and a fine, lucent line representing an intimal flap is present. Such lesions may progress to thrombosis, stricture or aneurysm. Occasionally, vascular dissection may occur.

BIBLIOGRAPHY

Aakhus, T., and Enge, I.: Angiography in rupture of the liver. Acta Radiol. (Diagn.) (Stockh.) 11:353, 1971.

Adams, J. T., Elebute, E. A., and Schwartz, S. I.: Isolated injury to the pancreas from nonpenetrating trauma in children. J. Trauma 6:86, 1966.

Aronsen, K. F., Ericsson, B., Nosslin, B., et al.: Evaluation of hepatic regeneration by scintillation scanning, cholangiography and angiography in man. Ann. Surg. 171:567, 1970.

Berk, R. N., and Wholey, M. H.: The application of splenic arteriography in the diagnosis of rupture of the spleen. Amer. J. Roentgenol. 104:662, 1968.

Blackwell, T. L., and Whelan, T. J.: Arteriovenous fistula as a complication of gastrectomy. Amer. J. Surg. 109:197, 1965.

Boijsen, E., and Efsing, H. O.: Intrasplenic arterial aneurysms following splenoportal phlebography. Acta Radiol. (Diagn.) (Stockh.) 6:487, 1967.

Boijsen, E., Judkins, M. P., and Simay, A.: Angiographic diagnosis of hepatic rupture. Radiology 86:66, 1966.

Boijsen, E., Kaude, J., and Tylén, U.: Angiography in hepatic rupture. Acta Radiol. (Diagn.) (Stockh.) 11:363, 1971.

Bollinger, J. A., and Fowler, E. F.: Traumatic rupture of the spleen, with special reference to delayed splenic rupture. Amer. J. Surg. 91:561, 1966.

Brindle, M. J.: Arteriography and minor splenic injury. Clin. Radiol. 23:174, 1972.

Burke, W. F., and Madigan, J. P.: The roentgenologic diagnosis of rupture of the liver and spleen as visualized by thorotrast. Radiology 21:580, 1933.

Bushkin, F. L., MacGregor, A. M., Hawkins, I. E., Jr., et al.: Hepatic artery dissection as a result of abdominal trauma. Surg. Gynec. Obstet. 135:721, 1972.

Campbell, D. K., and Austin, R. F.: Seat-belt injury: Injury of the abdominal aorta. Radiology 92:123, 1969.

Chisholm, T. P., and Lenio, P. T.: Traumatic injuries of the portal vein. Amer. J. Surg. 124:770, 1972.

Cimmino, C. V.: Ruptured spleen: Some refinements in its roentgenologic diagnosis. Radiology 82:57, 1964.

Foley, W. J., Turcotte, J. G., Hoskins, P. A., et al.: Intrahepatic arteriovenous fistulas between the hepatic artery and portal vein. Amer. Surg. 174:849, 1971.

Freeark, R. J., Carley, R. D., Norcross, W. J., et al.: Unusual aspects of pancreatoduodenal trauma. J. Trauma 6:482, 1966.

Fulton, R. L., and Wolfel, D. A.: Hepatic artery-portal vein arteriovenous fistula. Arch. Surg. 100:307, 1970.

Gold, R. E. and Redman, H. C.: Splenic trauma: Assessment of problems in diagnosis. Amer. J. Roentgenol. 116:413, 1972.

Graham, J. C., Jr., Weidner, W. A., and Vinik, M.: The angiographic features of organizing splenic hematoma (Hamartoma). Amer. J. Roentgenol. 107:430, 1969.

Haertel, M., and Fuchs, W. A.: Angiography in pancreatic trauma. Brit. J. Radiol. 47:641, 1974.

Hawes, D. R., Franken, E. A., Jr., Fitzgerald, J. F., et al.: Traumatic hemobilia. Angiographic diagnosis. Amer. J. Dis. Child. 125:130, 1973.

Hermann, R. E., and Hoerr, S. O.: Aids in the diagnosis of traumatic hemobilia. Surg. Gynec. Obstet. 125:55, 1967.

Horns, J. W., and Barnes, R. A.: Arteriography in occult splenic rupture. Surg. Gynec. Obstet. 137:227, 1973.

Kahn, P. C.: Iatrogenic diseases of the arteries. Seminars Roentgenol. 5:284, 1970.

Katz, M. C., and Meng, C. H.: Angiographic evaluation of traumatic intrahepatic pseudoaneurysm and hemobilia. Radiology 94:95, 1970.

Kaude, J., Dudgeon, D. L., and Talbert, J. L.: The role of selective angiography in the diagnosis and treatment of hepatoportal arteriovenous fistula. Radiology 92:1271, 1969.

King, M. C., Glick, B. W., and Freed, A.: The diagnosis of splenic cysts. Surg. Gynec. Obstet. 127:509, 1968.

Lang, E. K.: Arteriographic assessment of viability of bowel after perforating abdominal injury. J. Indiana Med. Ass. 62:1322, 1969.

Lepasoon, J., and Olin, T.: Angiographic diagnosis of splenic lesions following blunt abdominal trauma. Acta Radiol. (Diagn.) (Stockh.) 11:257, 1971.

Levin, D. C., Watson, R. C., Sos, T. A., et al.: Angiography in blunt hepatic trauma. Amer. J. Roentgenol. 119:95, 1973.

Lewis, M. L., and Pirruccello, R.: Use of angiography to diagnose subcapsular hematoma of the spleen before delayed rupture. Amer. Surg. 39:587, 1973.

Longmire, W. P.: Hepatic surgery: Trauma, tumors and cysts. Ann. Surg. 161:1, 1965.

Love, L.: Arterial trauma. Seminars Roentgenol. 5:267, 1970.

Love, L., Greenfield, G. B., Braun, T. W., et al.: Arteriography of splenic trauma. Radiology 91:96, 1968.

Lundström, B.: Angiographic demonstration of rupture of the spleen. Acta Radiol. (Diagn.) (Stockh.) 10:145, 1970.

McClelland, R. N., and Shires, T.: Management of liver trauma in 259 consecutive patients. Ann. Surg. 161:248, 1965.

McCort, J. J.: Rupture or laceration of the liver by non-penetrating trauma. Radiology 78:49, 1962.

Nahum, H., and Levesque, M.: Arteriography in hepatic trauma. Radiology 109:557, 1973.

Norell, H. G.: Traumatic rupture of the spleen diagnosed by abdominal aortography. Acta Radiol. (Diagn.) (Stockh.) 48:449, 1957.

Olsen, W. R., Redman, H. C., and Hildreth, D. H.: Quantitative peritoneal lavage in blunt abdominal trauma. Arch. Surg. 104:536, 1972.

Osborn, D. J., Glickman, M. G., Grnja, V., et al.: The

role of angiography in abdominal nonrenal trauma. Radiol. Clin. North Amer. *11*:579, 1973.

Parrish, R. A., Edmondson, H. T., and Moretz, W. H.: Duodenal and biliary obstruction secondary to intramural hematoma. Amer. J. Surg. *108*:428, 1964.

Perry, J. F., Jr.: A five-year survey of 152 acute abdominal injuries. J. Trauma *5*:53, 1965.

Pollard, J. J., and Nebesar, R. A.: Splenic rupture demonstrated by selective splenic artery angiogram. J.A.M.A. *187*:994, 1964.

Preger, L.: Hepatic arteriovenous fistula after percutaneous liver biopsy. Amer. J. Roentgenol. *101*:619, 1967.

Redman, H. C., Reuter, S. R., and Bookstein, J. J.: Angiography in abdominal trauma. Ann. Surg. *169*:57, 1969.

Robb, H. J., Akamine, F., and Moggi, L.: Bursting injuries of the liver. J. Trauma *1*:555, 1961.

Scatliff, J. H., Fisher, O. N., Guilford, W. B., et al.: The "starry night" angiogram: Contrast material opacification of the Malpighian body marginal sinus circulation in spleen trauma. Amer. J. Roentgenol. *125*:91, 1975.

Schreiber, M. H., Wolma, F. J., Mankse, A. O., et al.: Experimental visceral arteriography in blunt abdominal trauma. Amer. J. Roentgenol. *104*:732, 1968.

Seltzer, R. A., Rossiter, S. B., Cooperman, L. R., et al.: Hemobilia following needle biopsy of the liver. Amer. J. Roentgenol. *127*:1035, 1976.

Shirkey, A. L., Wukasch, D. C., Beall, A. C., Jr., et al.: Surgical management of splenic injuries. Amer. J. Surg. *108*:630, 1964.

Solheim, K.: Closed abdominal injuries. Acta Chir. Scand. *126*:579, 1963.

Solheim, K., and Evensen, K. A.: Subcapsular rupture of the spleen and the liver. The value of selective angiography. Acta Chir. Scand. *139*:523, 1973.

Stein, H. L.: The diagnosis of traumatic laceration of the spleen by selective arteriography, direct serial magnification angiography, and intra-arterial epinephrine. Radiology *93*:367, 1969.

Steinberg, I., Tillotson, P. M., and Halpern, M.: Roentgenography of systemic (congenital and traumatic) arteriovenous fistulas. Amer. J. Roentgenol. *89*:343, 1963.

Stone, H. H., Jordan, W. D., Acker, J. J., et al.: Portal arteriovenous fistulas. Amer. J. Surg. *109*:191, 1965.

Terry, J. H., Self, M. M., and Howard, J. M.: Injuries of the spleen. Surgery *40*:615, 1956.

Thompson, D. P., Shultz, E. H., and Benfeld, J. R.: Celiac angiography in the management of splenic trauma. Arch. Surg. *99*:494, 1969.

Westcott, J. L., and Smith, J. R. V.: Mesentery and colon injuries secondary to blunt trauma. Radiology *114*:597, 1975.

Whelan, T. J., and Gillespie, J. T.: Treatment of traumatic hemobilia. Ann. Surg. *162*:920, 1965.

Williams, J. S., Lies, B. A., Jr., and Hale, H. W., Jr.: The automotive safety belt: In saving a life may produce intra-abdominal injuries. J. Trauma *6*:303, 1961.

Williams, L. F., Jr., and Byrne, J. J.: Trauma to the liver at the Boston City Hospital from 1955 to 1965. Amer. J. Surg. *112*:368, 1966.

Chapter 6

GASTROINTESTINAL BLEEDING

In recent years, angiography has assumed a central role in the diagnosis and treatment of gastrointestinal bleeding. In 1959, Rastelli et al. showed experimentally that contrast medium extravasating into the lumen of the bowel in the presence of active gastrointestinal hemorrhage could be demonstrated radiographically. The following year, Margulis et al. (1960) showed active gastrointestinal bleeding in one patient with colonic carcinoma by using operative mesenteric angiography. They also demonstrated multiple vascular malformations in another patient. In 1963, Nusbaum and Baum determined that contrast medium leaking into the lumen of the gastrointestinal tract of a dog at a rate of 0.5 cc per minute could be identified on selective serial angiograms. In 1965, Baum et al. reported finding an active bleeding site in four of the first eight patients they examined by angiography. This success led other angiographers to use the method, and in the intervening years a large volume of experience has accumulated concerning the use of angiography for the diagnosis and treatment of gastrointestinal bleeding.

Since the reports in 1971 by Rösch et al. and Baum and Nusbaum that arterial gastrointestinal bleeding could be controlled by the selective arterial infusion of vasoconstrictive drugs, the angiographic control of bleeding has been increasingly emphasized. The infusion of vasopressin has also been used to control bleeding from esophageal varices, and recently, several authors have reported controlling arterial bleeding with selectively injected emboli.

ANGIOGRAPHIC DIAGNOSIS OF GASTROINTESTINAL BLEEDING

Massive Arterial Upper Gastrointestinal Bleeding

The primary diagnostic procedure in patients with massive upper gastrointestinal bleeding should generally be endoscopy. Barium examinations are rarely useful. Diagnostic angiography should be used only when endoscopy fails to reveal the bleeding site. Even when the bleeding site has been identified by endoscopy, however, the patient may be referred for angiographic therapy.

The majority of healthy, young patients with upper gastrointestinal hemorrhage respond to bed rest and conservative medical management. In elderly patients and in patients with cirrhosis or other diseases that interfere with blood clotting mechanisms, however, spontaneous cessation of the bleeding is less frequent. In general, angiography should not be used until the patient has failed to respond to conservative management, and three to four units of blood replacement have been required.

Immediately prior to angiography the rate of bleeding should be assessed, since angiography is useless if the bleeding has ceased. In patients with upper gastrointestinal bleeding, this is most simply done by using a wide bore nasogastric tube, such as an Ewald tube. After most of the major clots have been removed from the stomach, continued rinsing with saline gives a good indication of the rate of bleeding. If the nasogastric return is clear or consists of coffee-ground material, the patient is generally not bleeding enough to demonstrate the bleeding site and should not have angiography until there is evidence of active bleeding. However, if the nasogastric return is deep pink, red or dark red, a good chance exists that the angiogram will reveal the bleeding site. If a nasogastric tube cannot be placed, the clinician's impression must be relied upon. Hematemesis and melenic stools are good indicators of brisk bleeding. However, most clinicians overestimate the rate of bleeding based on a falling hematocrit level because of the normal hemodilution which follows blood loss.

When the nasogastric return indicates acute upper gastrointestinal bleeding, the first procedure should be an anteroposterior celiac angiogram. If extravasation is seen, the catheter is advanced into the bleeding artery (the left gastric or gastroduodenal artery, or the splenic artery for short gastric artery extravasations) to confirm the bleeding site and in preparation for angiographic therapy to control the hemorrhage. If a bleeding site is not demonstrated on the celiac angiogram, an injection is made into the superior mesenteric artery. Finally, sequential selective injections should be made into the left gastric and gastroduodenal arteries if a bleeding site has not been identified. These studies generally reveal the site of active arterial bleeding. When extravasation is not seen after any of the injections, the rate of bleeding must be reassessed. If it is determined that the patient is still bleeding actively,

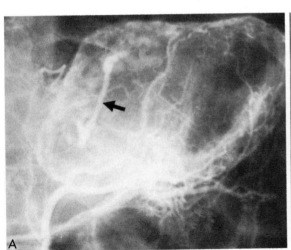 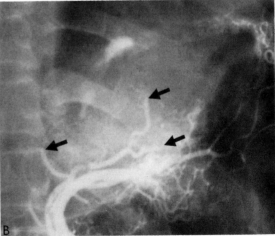

Figure 6–1. Typical appearance of massive gastrointestinal bleeding. Left gastric angiogram in a 48 year old man with massive bleeding from an ulcer high on the lesser curvature.

A. Arterial phase. Contrast medium extravasating near the cardioesophageal junction runs along a mucosal fold to the most dependent portion of the fundus, where it collects. This results in the appearance of a "pseudovein" (➡).

B. Left gastric angiogram following embolization with 0.5 cc autogenous blood clot. Several left gastric artery branches are occluded (➡). The pool of contrast medium in the fundus remains from the preembolization angiogram. Emboli have also spilled over into the splenic artery, and splenic artery branches are also occluded. The bleeding was controlled and did not recur.

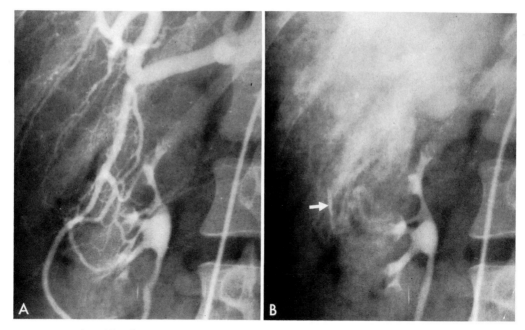

Figure 6–2. Slow bleeding from a stress ulcer. Celiac angiogram in a 27 year old man with a stress ulcer in the second portion of the duodenum.

A. Arterial phase. The gastroduodenal artery and its branches are well visualized, and no extravasation has occurred.

B. Venous phase. As the contrast medium empties from the arteries, a subtle but definite linear accumulation of contrast medium (⇒) is seen in the lumen of the duodenum. This was present in both anteroposterior and right posterior oblique projections.

even without angiographic demonstration of a bleeding site, or if the endoscopist saw hemorrhagic gastritis, the catheter is placed in the left gastric artery for vasopressin infusion. If the endoscopist saw varices, the catheter is placed in the superior mesenteric artery for vasopressin infusion or a systemic vasopressin infusion is begun.

The general angiographic appearance of acute arterial upper gastrointestinal bleeding is extravasation of contrast medium of arterial density at the bleeding site. The specific appearance depends on the rate and location of the bleeding. The more rapid the bleeding, the denser the collection of contrast medium at the bleeding site. The extravasating contrast medium frequently runs toward the most dependent part of the viscus, creating the "pseudovein" appearance (Fig. 6–1) described by Ring et al. (1974). If the bleeding is slight, the diagnosis may be difficult, and the concentration of the extravasated contrast me-

dium may be only slightly greater than the normal density of the mucosa itself (Fig. 6–2). In such a situation, confirmation of active bleeding may require a second projection.

Mallory-Weiss Lacerations

Bleeding from Mallory-Weiss lacerations appears as extravasation in the region of the cardioesophageal junction. Contrast medium may either run cephalad in the esophagus, outlining the esophageal mucosa (Fig. 6–3), or run toward the dependent fundus of the stomach (Fig. 6–4). Rarely, when the tear is along the posterior surface, a linear collection of contrast medium may be seen in the laceration. It is difficult to differentiate between Mallory-Weiss lacerations and high lesser curvature gastric erosions or ulcers by angiography alone.

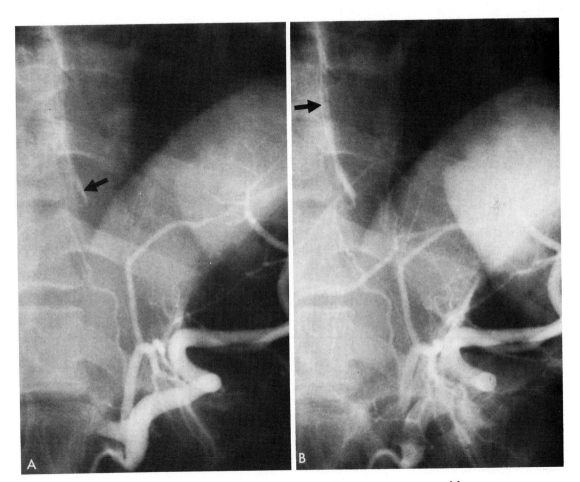

Figure 6–3. Mallory-Weiss laceration. Left gastric angiogram in a 39 year old man.

A. Early arterial phase. Contrast medium extravasates from a branch of the left gastric artery supplying the distal esophagus (➡).

B. Late arterial phase. Contrast medium collects at the site of the laceration and runs cephalad, outlining the esophageal mucosa (➡).

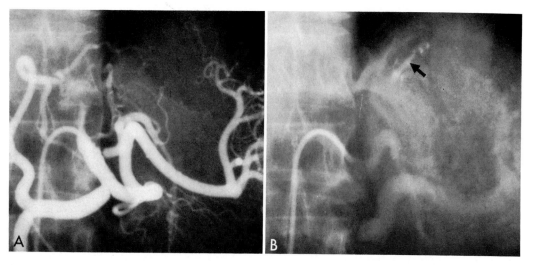

Figure 6–4. Massive upper gastrointestinal bleeding from a Mallory-Weiss tear. Celiac angiogram in a 48 year old man with portal hypertension being evaluated for an emergency portacaval shunt.

A. Arterial phase. The branches of the left gastric artery are well visualized, but no contrast medium has yet extravasated. The bleeding in this patient is not as massive as that in the patient in Figure 6–3, and the actual hemorrhage from the artery is not apparent.

B. Parenchymal phase. The linear accumulation of contrast medium (➡) on the mucosa of the stomach can be appreciated. Its position at the cardioesophageal junction indicates a Mallory-Weiss tear.

Gastric Ulcer

The appearance of bleeding from gastric ulcers depends upon the position of both the ulcer and the patient. When the patient is in the supine position, bleeding from a posterior wall ulcer appears as a localized collection of contrast medium which may run toward a more dependent portion of the posterior gastric wall (Fig. 6–5). The collection is easy to see and may be demonstrated when the bleeding is slow. If, however, the ulcer is on the anterior wall of the stomach, the contrast medium spreads out as soon as it extravasates, and a localized collection is not seen unless it is held in place by blood clot or by a collapsed stomach. Therefore, the bleeding must be brisk to be demonstrated and may be seen only as a curvilinear streak of contrast medium along the lesser curvature (Figs. 6–6 and 6–7). Occasionally, the bleeding artery is a branch of a short gastric or accessory gastric artery arising from the splenic artery. The bleeding may be seen on the celiac angiogram, but when an injection is made in the left gastric artery, no extravasation is seen. This indicates the possibility of short gastric artery bleeding, and a splenic angiogram will then reveal the bleeding artery (Figs. 6–7 and 6–8). Some ulcers erode both left gastric and short gastric artery branches, and injection of either artery will demonstrate the bleeding site.

Duodenal Bleeding

Bleeding into the duodenum appears as extravasation (Fig. 6–9) which may remain localized (Fig. 6–10) or may spread through the duodenum, outlining the mucosa (Fig. 6–11). Identification of the exact portion of the duodenum that is bleeding may be difficult. Bleeding from proximal branches of the posterior pancreaticoduodenal arcade is generally into the duodenal bulb. Bleeding into the bulb may also be identified by increased contrast accumulation in the mucosa of the bulb (Fig. 6–9; also see Fig. 6–39).

Text continued on page 229

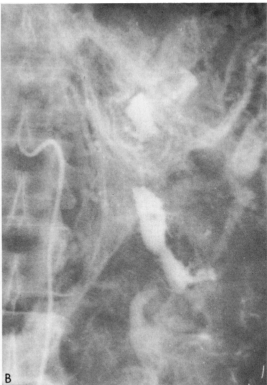

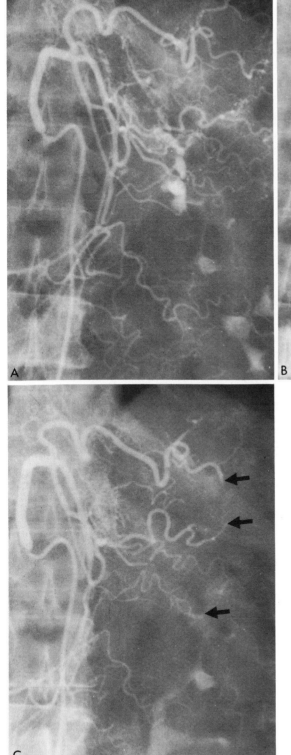

Figure 6–5. Posterior wall gastric ulcerations. Left gastric angiogram in a 54 year old woman with chronic alcoholism.

A. Arterial phase. Three separate areas of extravasating contrast medium are present in the upper body of the stomach.

B. Venous phase. The contrast medium collects at the point of extravasation on the posterior wall and spreads to slightly more dependent portions of the stomach. The density and quantity of the extravasated contrast medium indicate a massive hemorrhage.

C. Left gastric angiogram following selective embolization of the left gastric artery with 0.5 cc autogenous blood clot. Most of the branches crossing to the greater curvature are occluded (➡). No contrast medium extravasates. The nasogastric rinses became clear over the subsequent 15 minutes, indicating control of the bleeding.

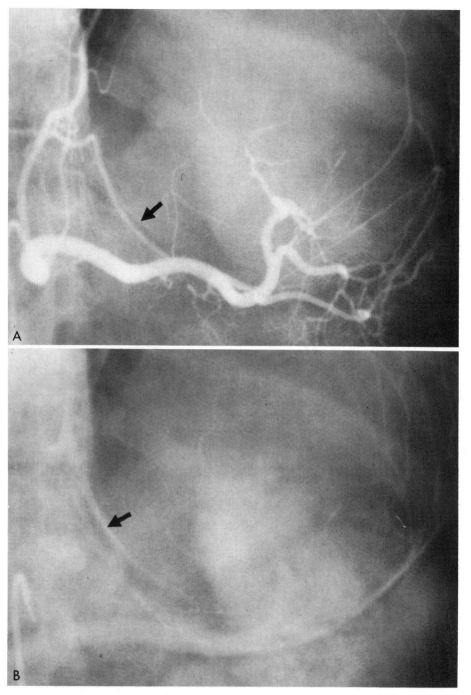

Figure 6-6. Anterior wall gastric bleeding. Celiac angiogram in a 55 year old man with chronic alcoholism.

A. Arterial phase. The splenic and left gastric arteries have a common, separate origin from the aorta. The left gastric artery branches are stretched around a stomach markedly distended by blood. Minimal early extravasation of contrast medium can be seen (➡). Note also how a markedly distended stomach compresses the upper pole of the spleen and causes irregular filling of the upper pole splenic artery branches.

B. The curvilinear streak of contrast medium can be seen along the high lesser curvature (➡). The diagnosis of bleeding is more difficult in this patient than in the patient shown in Figure 6–7 because the density of the contrast medium is not as great. Note the irregular parenchymal phase of the spleen, which appears similar to small infarcts. This is caused by the pressure of the distended stomach.

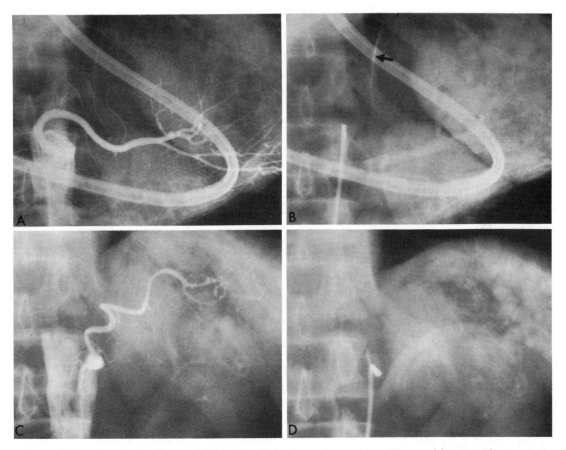

Figure 6–7. Anterior wall gastric bleeding. Splenic angiogram in a 62 year old man with an anterior wall gastric ulcer which has eroded the short gastric artery branches.

A. Arterial phase. Minimal early extravasation of contrast medium can be seen.

B. A curvilinear streak of contrast medium has developed along the high lesser curvature (➡). This occurs because the stomach is distended by blood and air, and the extravasated contrast medium runs along the lesser curvature towards the posterior wall.

C. Arterial phase of a splenic angiogram following a selective infusion of 0.2 pressor unit of vasopressin per minute for 20 minutes. The splenic artery and its branches are markedly constricted. The short gastric arteries are not seen.

D. Venous phase. No extravasated contrast medium is apparent along the high lesser curvature, indicating control of the bleeding by the infusion. The infusion was continued for another 12 hours. The dosage was then reduced to 0.1 pressor unit per minute and the infusion continued an additional 12 hours. Bleeding did not recur.

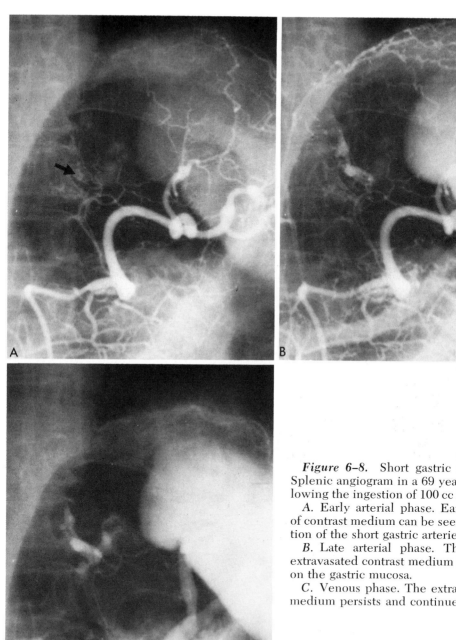

Figure 6–8. Short gastric artery bleeding. Splenic angiogram in a 69 year old woman following the ingestion of 100 cc formaldehyde.

A. Early arterial phase. Early extravasation of contrast medium can be seen in the distribution of the short gastric arteries (➡).

B. Late arterial phase. The collection of extravasated contrast medium begins to spread on the gastric mucosa.

C. Venous phase. The extravasated contrast medium persists and continues to spread.

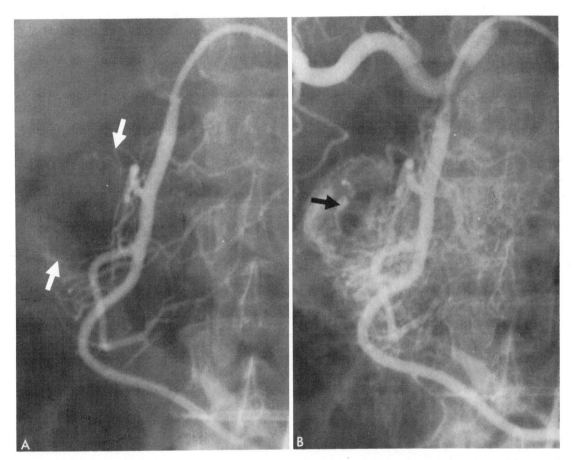

Figure 6-9. Bleeding into the duodenal bulb. Gastroduodenal angiogram in a 62 year old woman.
 A. Early arterial phase. The duodenal branches of the gastroduodenal artery pass around the duodenal bulb (⟹).
 B. Contrast medium of arterial density has extravasated into the bulb (➡). The accumulation of contrast medium in the mucosa of the bulb is increased. This is commonly seen in patients with inflammatory disease of the duodenum or pancreas.

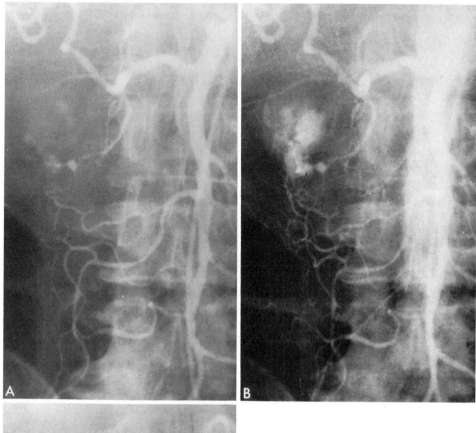

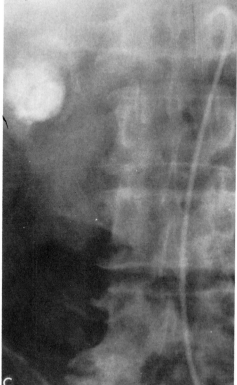

Figure 6–10. Massive bleeding into the duodenum. Superior mesenteric angiogram in a 75 year old man with a duodenal ulcer.

A. Early arterial phase. The right hepatic artery is replaced to the superior mesenteric artery, and the gastroduodenal artery arises from the right hepatic artery. A rounded collection of extravasated contrast medium is present in the region of the duodenal bulb. The gastroduodenal artery is markedly constricted because the patient is in shock.

B. Late arterial phase. The blood flow in the superior mesenteric artery and its branches is slowed because of the vasoconstriction, and there is moderate reflux of contrast medium into the aorta. The extravasating contrast medium collects in the duodenal bulb. The density and rate of accumulation indicate a massive hemorrhage.

C. The rounded collection of contrast medium persists in the duodenal bulb after the arteries and veins have cleared.

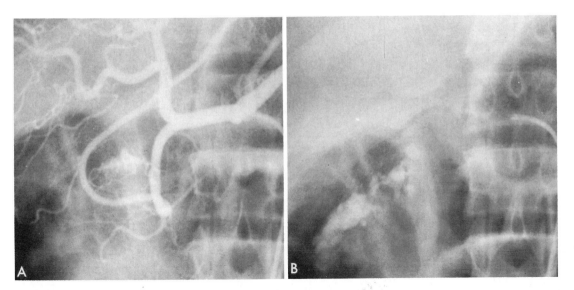

Figure 6–11. Duodenal bleeding producing a mucosal pattern. Celiac angiogram in a 48 year old man with a duodenal ulcer.
   A. Arterial phase. Contrast medium extravasating from duodenal branches of the pancreatico-duodenal arcade collects in the duodenum.
   B. The contrast medium spreads in the duodenum, outlining the mucosal pattern.

Hemorrhagic Gastritis

Hemorrhagic gastritis causes a diffuse, fine, irregular hypervascularity throughout the stomach (Fig. 6–12). Mucosal accumulation of contrast medium is increased, and the very small gastric arteries are irregular. This appearance is presumptive evidence of hemorrhagic gastritis in a patient with massive upper gastrointestinal bleeding without localized extravasation of contrast medium. One or more areas of active extravasation of contrast medium may be superimposed on the hypervascular pattern. Multiple bleeding sites are also seen in stress ulcerations of the stomach in patients on cortisone therapy or postoperatively, but the mucosa is not as diffusely hypervascular as in gastritis. With the use of endoscopy, the presence of gastritis is generally known prior to angiography. Angiography is then done to exclude localized massive extravasation superimposed upon the diffuse gastritis and is usually directed more toward therapy of the gastritis than toward diagnosis.

High lesser curvature bleeding must be differentiated from the normal appearance of the left adrenal gland. The adrenal gland is seen as a dense area of contrast accumulation on most celiac angiograms, especially if the inferior phrenic artery is well filled with contrast medium (Fig. 6–13). This configuration has been misinterpreted as extravasation of contrast medium. However, the adrenal gland can generally be recognized because the cortex appears as two almost parallel lines which diverge slightly inferiorly.

Hiatus hernias can be recognized by the arcuate extension of left gastric artery branches above the diaphragm. Bleeding from an erosion in a hiatus hernia is therefore seen over the spine at or above the level of the diaphragm (Fig. 6–14).

Occasionally, an aneurysm ruptures into the upper gastrointestinal tract, causing massive bleeding. Boijsen et al. (1969) found a number of aneurysms among their actively bleeding patients. They therefore include a previous hepatic rupture or pancreatitis in their list of indications for angiography in patients with gastrointestinal bleeding, since abscesses accompanying these two conditions predispose the surrounding arteries to aneurysm formation.

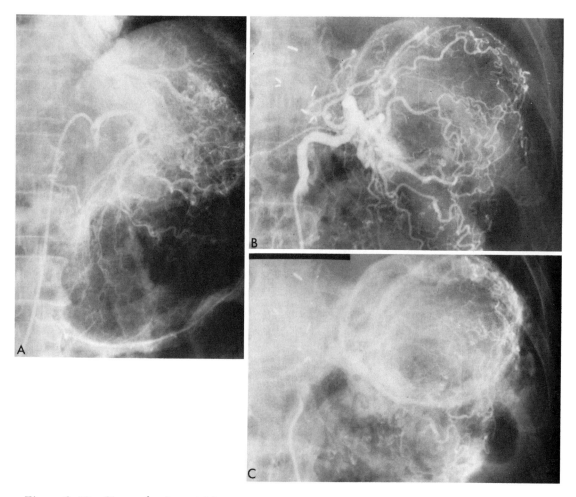

Figure 6–12. Hemorrhagic gastritis.

A. Left gastric angiogram in a 38 year old woman with chronic alcoholism. The left gastric artery branches are dilated and tortuous, and there is a fuzzy, indistinct hypervascularity throughout the stomach. Veins fill with contrast medium in the arterial phase.

B. Left gastric angiogram in a 47 year old man with chronic alcoholism and massive upper gastrointestinal bleeding. The branches of the left gastric artery are dilated and irregular, and blood flow to the body and fundus of the stomach is increased. There is a suffusion of dilated small gastric artery branches through the stomach.

C. Parenchymal phase. Mucosal accumulation of contrast medium is increased. No extravasation of contrast medium is seen.

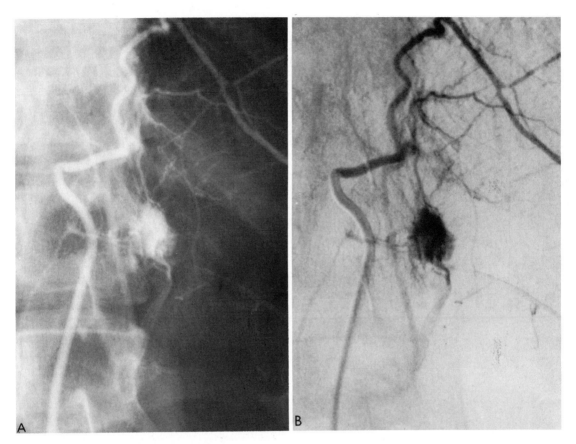

Figure 6-13. Normal left adrenal gland. Left inferior phrenic angiogram in a 23 year old woman.
A. Arterial phase. Superior adrenal arteries from the inferior phrenic artery supply the left adrenal gland. The accumulation of contrast medium is dense and simulates the appearance of lesser curvature gastric bleeding.
B. Subtraction film of A.

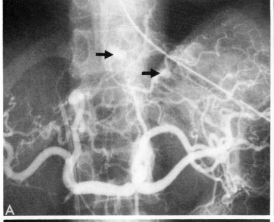
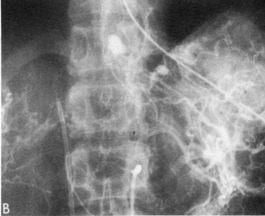
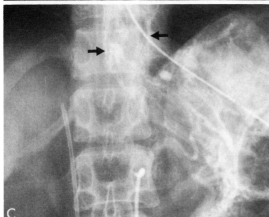

Figure 6-14. Bleeding into a hiatus hernia. Celiac angiogram in a 34 year old woman in whom endoscopy had revealed erosions in a hiatus hernia.

A. Midarterial phase. The branches of the left gastric artery extend above the diaphragm just to the left of the midline, and two rounded areas of extravasated contrast medium can be seen (➡).

B. Late arterial phase. The collections of extravasated contrast medium have become denser.

C. Venous phase. With time, the collections of contrast medium fade. The contrast accumulation in the gastric mucosa outlines the hiatus hernia (➡).

Suspected Esophageal Varices

When a patient has a history of chronic alcoholism, cirrhosis or abnormal liver function studies, esophageal variceal bleeding must be considered as a cause of massive upper gastrointestinal hemorrhage. The severity of the cirrhosis can be assessed by angiographic criteria (Chapter 8). In patients with advanced cirrhosis the celiac angiogram reveals a cirrhotic arterial pattern in the liver. In the venous phase portal–systemic collateral veins may be seen. These collaterals are best demonstrated by the use of arterial portography or percutaneous transhepatic portography. Wedged hepatic venography reveals an elevated portal pressure and a cirrhotic venous drainage pattern. However, about 20 per cent of patients with massive gastrointestinal bleeding and known portal hypertension and cirrhosis bleed from sources other than the varices (McCray et al., 1969).

Suspicion of a nonvariceal source of hemorrhage should be particularly high when the wedged hepatic venous or transhepatic portal pressure is less than 250 mm of saline.

Extravasation of contrast medium from bleeding varices is rarely seen at angiography. This is due in part to the poor concentration of contrast medium that reaches the varices, even from a high dose left gastric artery injection. Even with transhepatic portal venography or splenoportography, extravasated contrast medium is demonstrated infrequently.

Rarely, varices cause massive lower gastrointestinal bleeding. Such varices occur most commonly in the duodenum or rectum. The latter is a particularly susceptible site because of the portal–systemic communications between the inferior mesenteric vein and the internal iliac veins. Very rarely, varices in other parts of the colon or small bowel are the cause of massive gastrointestinal bleeding (Fig. 6–15).

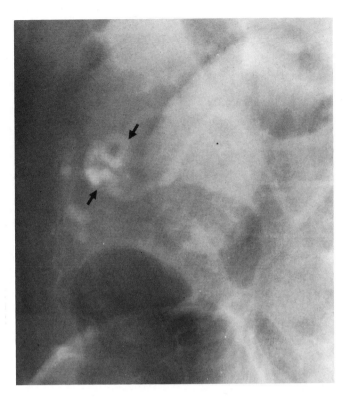

Figure 6–15. Colonic varices. Venous phase of a superior mesenteric angiogram in a 78 year old man with massive lower gastrointestinal bleeding. The dilated, tortuous varices (➡) can be seen along the right and transverse colons. The patient expired, and both colonic and esophageal varices were present at autopsy. (Courtesy of Dr. Leo Sheiner.)

Acute Lower Gastrointestinal Bleeding

From a diagnostic point of view, angiography is far more important in the evaluation of lower gastrointestinal hemorrhage than upper gastrointestinal hemorrhage. Although the early results with the use of colonoscopy have been encouraging, the site of lower gastrointestinal bleeding may still be extremely difficult to find. Barium examinations have little use. At operation, the major problem encountered in lower gastrointestinal bleeding is that blood spreads through the bowel in both directions and be present throughout the small bowel and colon. In patients with small bowel hemorrhage, the surgeon must isolate one segment of bowel after another to pinpoint the bleeding site, frequently without success. Angiographers have had the experience of hearing from the sigmoidoscopist that the blood is coming from above 15 cm, only to find a site of active extravasation near the rectosigmoid. Therefore, angiography should be used early in evaluating patients with massive lower gastrointestinal bleeding. Also, the determination of the rate of bleeding in patients with lower gastrointestinal hemorrhage is more difficult than in patients with upper gastrointestinal bleeding. In patients with rapidly dropping hematocrit levels and bright red stools, angiography will certainly reveal a bleeding site. However, many patients do not have such obvious signs, and the bleeding may have stopped by the time the angiogram is performed. Nevertheless, all patients with signs of massive lower gastrointestinal bleeding should have angiograms as soon as possible after hospitalization, since angiography may be the only means of locating the bleeding site.

In patients with lower gastrointestinal bleeding, the inferior mesenteric artery should be injected first so that the rectosigmoid area can be seen free of the bladder, which rapidly fills with contrast medium (Fig. 6–16). This examination is generally done in a slight left posterior oblique projection to separate the loops of the sigmoid colon. If no bleeding site is demonstrated, a superior mesenteric angiogram is then done in the anteroposterior projection. If the patient is bleeding actively from the lower gastrointestinal tract, these examinations usually reveal the bleeding site.

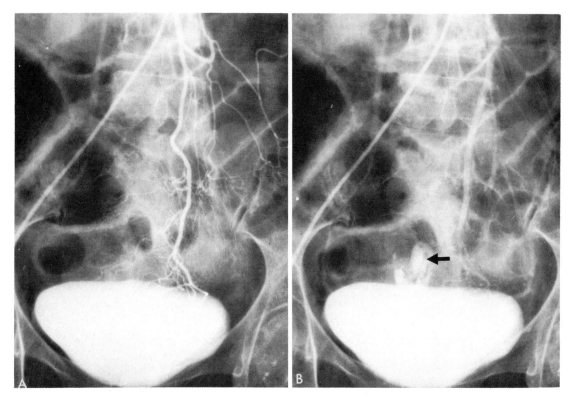

Figure 6–16. Rectosigmoid bleeding partially obscured by a bladder filled with contrast medium. Inferior mesenteric angiogram in a 54 year old woman with rectal bleeding. A superior mesenteric angiogram had been done prior to the inferior mesenteric angiogram because the sigmoidoscopist reported that the bleeding was coming from above 15 cm.

A. Arterial phase. The branches of the superior hemorrhoidal artery are obscured by the contrast-filled bladder. Early extravasation cannot be demonstrated.

B. The extravasating contrast medium becomes apparent as it collects on the mucosa and runs towards the sigmoid (➡). At operation the bleeding was found to be from a diverticulum in the region of the rectosigmoid.

However, if no bleeding is demonstrated, a celiac angiogram should be done because of the rare occurrence of duodenal bleeding with clear nasogastric lavage.

Following identification of the bleeding site, the catheter is placed in the artery to be infused. For left colonic bleeding, the inferior mesenteric artery is used. For small bowel and right colonic bleeding, the superior mesenteric artery is usually infused, although the infusion may be made directly into a specific superior mesenteric artery branch.

The angiographic appearance of massive bleeding from all parts of the small bowel is similar. Contrast medium extravasating at the bleeding site appears in the early to midarterial phase (Figs. 6–17 and 6–18). As

Figure 6–18. Distal ileal bleeding. Superior mesenteric angiogram in a 16 year old boy with regional enteritis.

A. Early arterial phase. Contrast medium extravasates from vasa recta near the junction of the terminal superior mesenteric artery and ileocolic artery. The vasa recta of the terminal ileum and the ascending colon are stretched around the distended bowel.

B. Venous phase. The extravasated contrast medium collects on the mucosa.

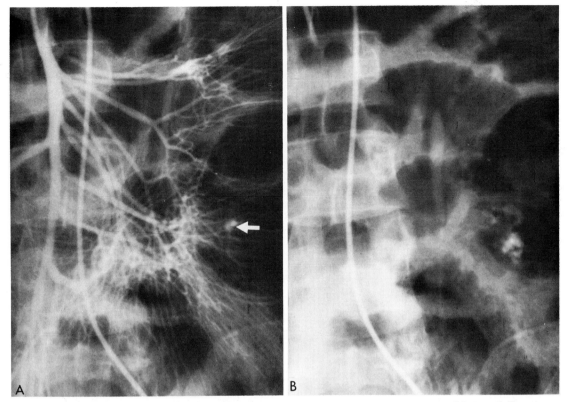

Figure 6–17. Ileal hemorrhage. Superior mesenteric angiogram in a 20 year old man following a gunshot wound.

A. Arterial phase. Extravasating contrast medium can be seen near the junction of the jejunum and ileum (⟹). The exact artery that is bleeding cannot be identified. The vasa recta are elongated, indicating bowel distention.

B. Venous phase. The contrast medium collects at the bleeding site and spreads over the mucosa.

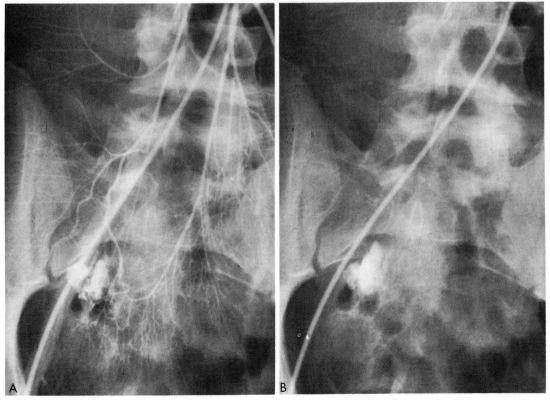

Figure 6–18. See opposite page for legend

the collection increases, it frequently spreads out, producing a mucosal pattern (Fig. 6–19). Occasionally, the disease causing the bleeding, such as tumor (Fig. 6–20), regional enteritis or a Meckel's diverticulum, may be recognized by its angiographic characteristics. Descriptions of the angiographic findings in tumor and regional enteritis are found in Chapters 4 and 7 respectively. Meckel's diverticulum is a common cause of small bowel bleeding in young patients. Occasionally, the diverticulum can be recognized in the capillary phase by the presence of contrast accumulation in its wall, adjacent to the site of the active extravasation (Fig. 6–21). Also, irregular arteries, the remnants of the vitelline arteries, may be seen in the wall of the diverticulum.

In colonic bleeding, the extravasated contrast medium runs toward the dependent portion of the colon (Fig. 6–22). In bleeding diverticula, an aneurysm-like collection of contrast medium is present on the mesenteric side of the bowel (Fig. 6–23). The contrast medium may remain localized to the diverticulum or may spread over the mucosa. Right-sided colonic diverticula bleed more frequently than left-sided colonic diverticula. Since diverticula occur much more often on the left, some unknown mechanism must be responsible for the higher incidence of right-sided bleeding.

Aneurysms on terminal branches of the superior and inferior mesenteric arteries may also rupture into the bowel, causing massive bleeding. Although such aneurysms occasionally occur in elderly patients, some of those reported in the literature as occurring in actively bleeding patients may actually be bleeding diverticula.

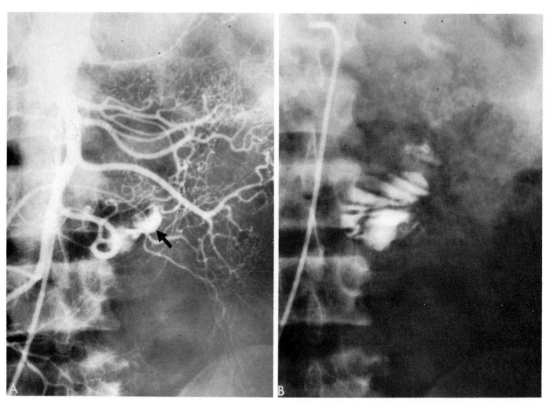

Figure 6–19. Mucosa demonstrated by massive gastrointestinal bleeding. Superior mesenteric angiogram in a 49 year old man with massive gastrointestinal bleeding caused by uremic ulcerations in the jejunum.

A. Arterial phase. Some extravasation of contrast medium into the jejunum has already begun. The bleeding vessel ($\Longrightarrow$) is a distal jejunal branch.

B. Venous phase. The extravasating contrast medium spreads out, producing a mucosal pattern. (From Frey, C. F., Reuter, S. R., and Bookstein, J. J.: Localization of gastrointestinal hemorrhage by selective angiography. Surgery 67:551, 1970.)

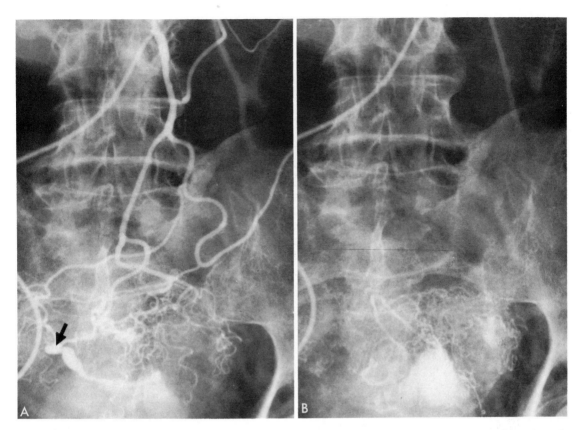

Figure 6–20. Bleeding rectal carcinoma. Inferior mesenteric angiogram in a 90 year old man with massive rectal bleeding.

A. Arterial phase. There is massive extravasation of contrast medium from a branch of the superior hemorrhoidal artery (➡). The extravasated contrast medium runs across the rectum toward the left. Infiltrated vasa recta can be seen in the region of the extravasation.

B. Parenchymal phase. The contrast medium has collected on the left side of the rectum, well away from the site of extravasation. Some superior hemorrhoidal branches empty slowly because of invasion by the tumor.

When contrast medium extravasates into a slowly bleeding diverticulum, the diverticulum appears identical to an aneurysm.

Chronic, Recurrent Gastrointestinal Bleeding

Gastrointestinal bleeding may be chronic and recurrent rather than acute. The patient has an iron deficiency anemia and guaiac or Hematest positive stools. The stools may or may not be blood tinged or melenic. Occasionally, the patient has recurrent but brief massive hemorrhage. The first diagnostic study in such a patient should be repeated, careful barium examinations of the entire gastrointestinal tract. These generally reveal a right colonic carcinoma or other bowel tumor, such as a leiomyoma. If more than one complete, careful barium examination has been normal, then angiography can be used. Prior to the advent of angiography, these patients generally underwent exploratory surgery, and empirical resections of segments of small bowel or colon were performed, often without relief of symptoms. Many patients remain undiagnosed, even after angiography. In a large series of patients with chronic, recurrent gastrointestinal bleeding, Sheedy et al. (1975) found the cause of bleeding in only 40 per cent of those studied.

Angiodysplasia

Frequently, particularly in the older age groups, an area of angiodysplasia is present in the right colon. Angiodysplasia is a gen-

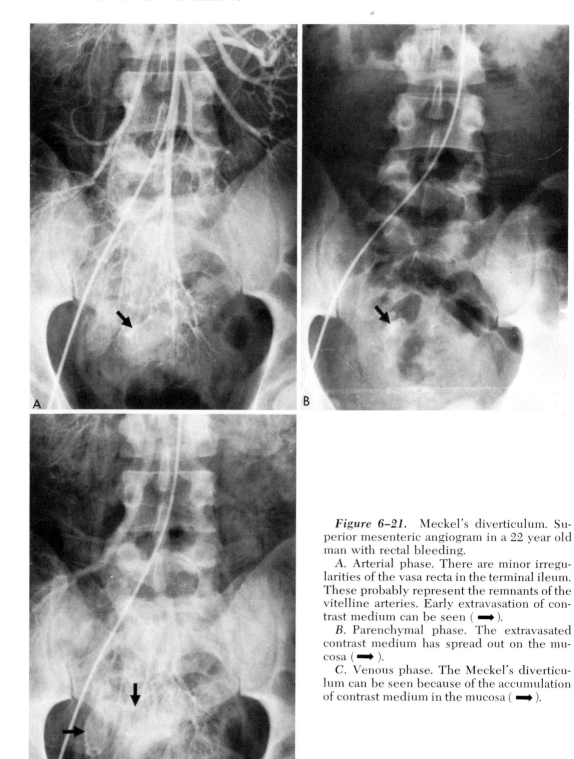

Figure 6–21. Meckel's diverticulum. Superior mesenteric angiogram in a 22 year old man with rectal bleeding.

A. Arterial phase. There are minor irregularities of the vasa recta in the terminal ileum. These probably represent the remnants of the vitelline arteries. Early extravasation of contrast medium can be seen (➡).

B. Parenchymal phase. The extravasated contrast medium has spread out on the mucosa (➡).

C. Venous phase. The Meckel's diverticulum can be seen because of the accumulation of contrast medium in the mucosa (➡).

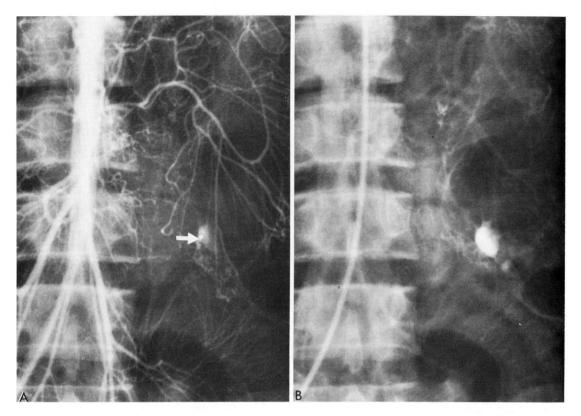

Figure 6–22. Massive lower gastrointestinal bleeding. Superior mesenteric angiogram in a 15 year old girl with massive hemorrhage from uremic ulcerations in the distal transverse colon. Prior to the angiogram she had received 100 units of blood replacement.

A. Arterial phase. Transverse colonic branches to the middle colic artery are stretched over the distended bowel. The actively bleeding artery (⟹) is well visualized, and contrast medium collects around it in the bowel.

B. Venous phase. The extravasated contrast medium collects near the bleeding site. The radiographic density of the extravasated contrast medium is the same as that in the arteries. (From Reuter, S. R., and Bookstein, J. J.: Angiographic localization of gastrointestinal bleeding. Gastroenterology 54:879, 1968.)

eral term used to describe the various vascular malformations that occur in the bowel. Although the reason for their development is uncertain, the malformations are most frequently found in the region of the cecum; more generalized forms may extend to the hepatic flexure and, uncommonly, they are found in the small bowel. The angiographic abnormalities depend on the extent of the lesions. In small, localized lesions, the angiogram reveals only a slightly dilated feeding artery with early drainage of contrast medium from the area through a slightly dilated vein (Fig. 6–24). Larger malformations may be seen as a small tangle of vessels (Fig. 6–25). In its extreme form, angiodysplasia may involve large sements of bowel (Figs. 6–26 and 6–

27). In all instances, the contrast medium in the veins draining the lesion is dense and appears in the arterial phase, the sine qua non of an arteriovenous fistula. In order to evaluate this important finding, the contrast medium must be injected in 3 seconds or less. If longer injections of contrast medium are made, the veins begin to fill normally before the arteries have emptied. Early venous drainage is best detected by evaluating the angiogram in reverse order, starting with the venous phase and moving toward the arterial phase. If the densest vein in the venous phase is traced back, the exact moment it begins to opacify can be detected. If this occurs while the arteries to the surrounding bowel remain filled, then arteriovenous shunting is present. When

Text continued on page 244

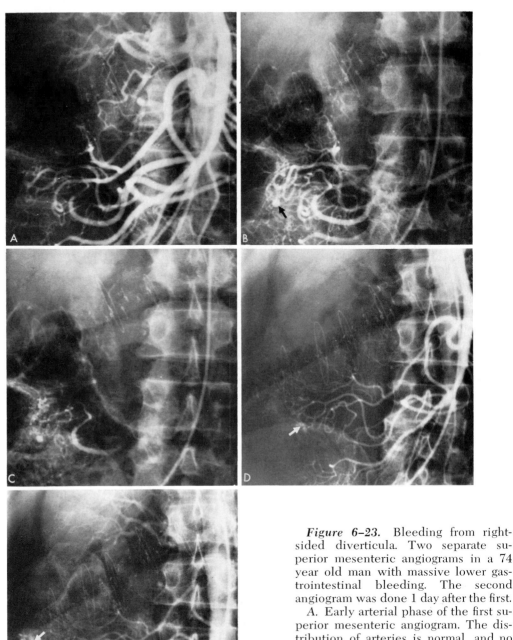

Figure 6–23. Bleeding from right-sided diverticula. Two separate superior mesenteric angiograms in a 74 year old man with massive lower gastrointestinal bleeding. The second angiogram was done 1 day after the first.

A. Early arterial phase of the first superior mesenteric angiogram. The distribution of arteries is normal, and no extravasation of contrast medium is yet seen.

B. Late arterial phase. A 3 mm in diameter collection of contrast medium (➡) resembling an aneurysm is seen on one of the terminal ileocolic artery branches.

C. Venous phase. The contrast medium remains in the diverticulum as the arteries in the area clear.

D. Arterial phase of the second superior mesenteric angiogram 1 day following the first. Extravasation of contrast medium is present at the same location as that in the previous examination (⇨).

E. Late arterial phase. Two separate areas of extravasation of contrast medium are present (⇨). Neither has the appearance of an aneurysm at this time, and the diagnosis is far more likely to be bleeding diverticula than two separate bleeding aneurysms. Bleeding was controlled, and the patient was not explored.

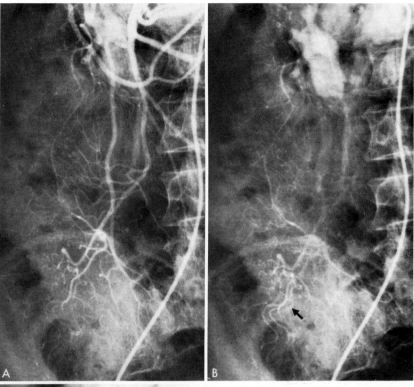

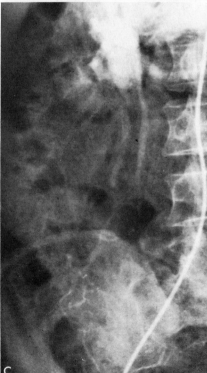

Figure 6-24. Subtle arteriovenous fistula in the cecum. Superior mesenteric angiogram in a 56 year old woman with anemia from chronic, recurrent gastrointestinal bleeding.

A. Arterial phase. The distribution of the branches of the superior mesenteric and ileocolic arteries is normal.

B. Late arterial phase. Subtle but definite early venous drainage (➡) is seen from a branch of the ileocolic artery.

C. Venous phase. The concentration of the contrast medium in the veins draining the arteriovenous fistula is much denser than that in the surrounding veins. This patient demonstrates the usefulness of finding the densest veins in the venous phase and then tracking them back into the arterial phase. (From Frey, C. F., Reuter, S. R., and Bookstein, J. J.: Localization of gastrointestinal hemorrhage by selective angiography. Surgery 67:553, 1970.)

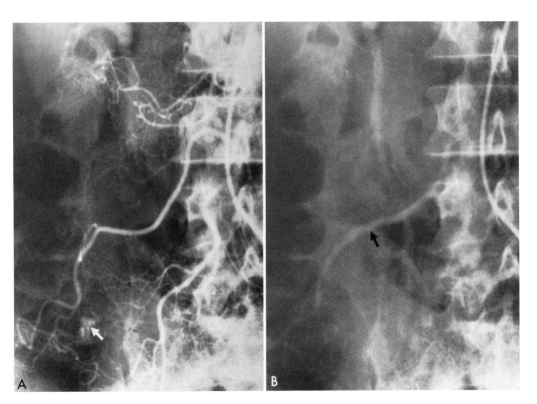

Figure 6–25. Cecal arteriovenous malformation. Superior mesenteric angiogram in a 78 year old man with chronic gastrointestinal blood loss.

A. Arterial phase. A branch of the ileocolic artery terminates in a tangle of small vessels (⟹) in the cecum.

B. Venous phase. The venous drainage (➡) from the malformation is early and dense.

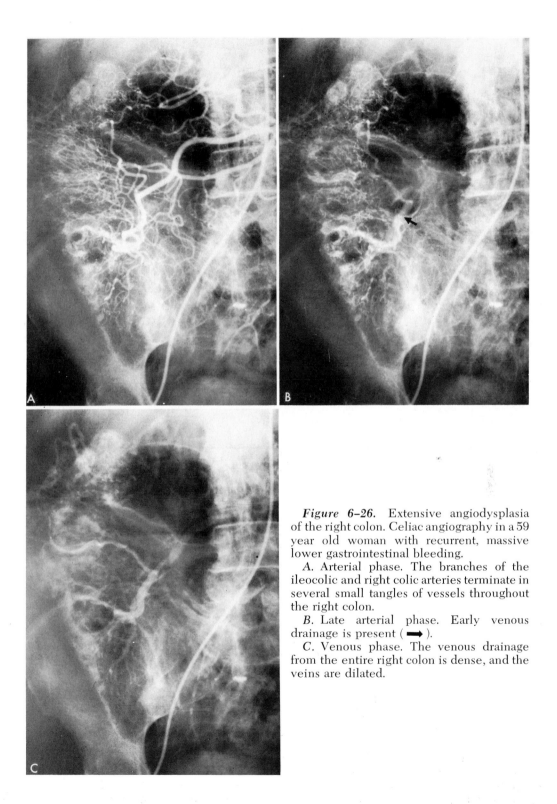

Figure 6–26. Extensive angiodysplasia of the right colon. Celiac angiography in a 59 year old woman with recurrent, massive lower gastrointestinal bleeding.

A. Arterial phase. The branches of the ileocolic and right colic arteries terminate in several small tangles of vessels throughout the right colon.

B. Late arterial phase. Early venous drainage is present (➡).

C. Venous phase. The venous drainage from the entire right colon is dense, and the veins are dilated.

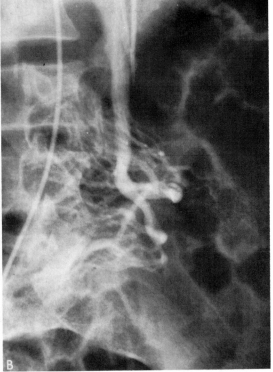

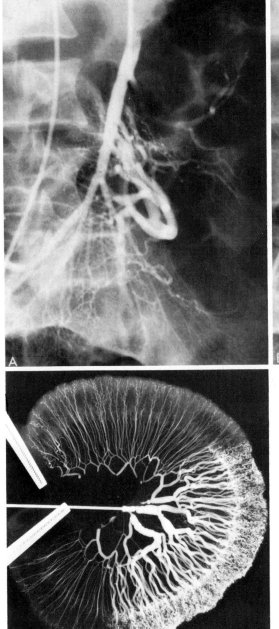

Figure 6–27. Large jejunal–ileal arteriovenous malformation. Superior mesenteric angiogram in a 45 year old man with recurrent gastrointestinal bleeding.

A. Early arterial phase. The distal jejunal and proximal ileal arteries are markedly dilated. They are also slightly angulated because the malformation has rotated the bowel toward the midline.

B. Venous phase. Dilated veins filled with dense contrast medium drain the malformation to the superior mesenteric vein.

C. Operative specimen. Normal arcades and vasa recta can be seen on either side of the segment of angiodysplasia. The arterial branches to the abnormal segment are markedly dilated and terminate in irregular tangles of mucosal arteries. The abnormal bowel is shortened and thickened.

the artery and the vein are both filled with contrast medium, two parallel vessels resembling "railroad tracks" are seen (Fig. 6–28). Even if an area of angiodysplasia is found, a careful search of the remaining angiogram should be made to exclude any other lesion, such as a small bowel carcinoma, which may be the cause of the gastrointestinal bleeding. Angiodysplasia is not uncommon in elderly patients and may

be only an incidental finding. The arterial branch that supplies the angiodysplasia should be identified in order to determine its exact location in the bowel. If necessary, a second oblique projection should be made in order to differentiate confusing, overlying arterial branches.

When an area of angiodysplasia is detected in a patient with recurrent occult bleeding, the involved segment of bowel

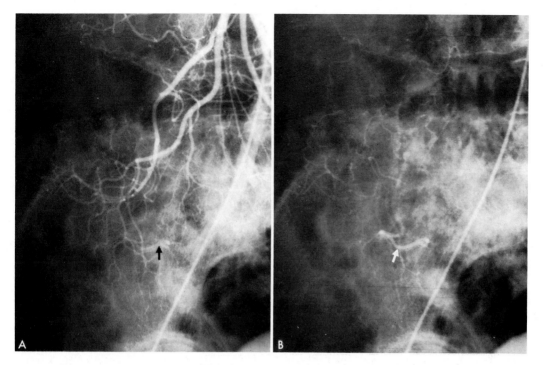

Figure 6–28. Demonstration of difficulty in exactly localizing ileocolic bleeding sites. Superior mesenteric angiography in a 48 year old woman with chronic, recurrent lower gastrointestinal bleeding.

A. Early arterial phase. Because of malposition of the ileum, the positions of the terminal portions of the superior mesenteric artery and the ileocolic artery are reversed and their branches overlap. Although early venous drainage can be demonstrated from one of the branches (➡), it cannot be determined exactly from which branch this is coming.

B. Late arterial phase. The venous drainage (⇒) from this area is dense.

should be removed. On opening the bowel, the surgeon usually sees and feels no abnormalities. Angiodysplasia is a soft, submucosal lesion. The mucosa generally appears normal, although it may be slightly reddened over the lesion, or the surgeon may palpate a small nodule. Even when he finds nothing abnormal, the surgeon must resect the suspicious area indicated by the angiogram. The pathologist will then find a tangle of dilated submucosal vessels. He can be aided in his search by a cast-clearing technique described by Baum et al. (1977). These investigators have injected Microfil (Canton Biomedical Labs) into the artery supplying the resected specimen. The specimen is then cleared in glycerin, which does not affect the histologic appearance at subsequent microscopic examinations, and the angiodysplasia is easily seen beneath the mucosa.

Patients with Osler-Weber-Rendu syndrome have many telangiectasias throughout the body. In the gastrointestinal tract the lesions are mucosal and submucosal and are a form of angiodysplasia. They are generally multiple and occur predominantly in the small bowel, although they also occur in the colon and stomach. The angiographic pattern varies from slightly nodular-appearing vasa recta (Fig. 6–29) to moderate sized areas of tangled vessels and arteriovenous shunting (Fig. 6–30). Gastrointestinal bleeding may be a chronic problem. Since it may also be the initial symptom, the angiographer may be the first to make the diagnosis. However, the actual bleeding is rarely seen. The liver is also frequently involved and has a typical "bloody" appearance (Fig. 6–31). The hepatic artery and its branches are dilated, and the blood flow is so rapid that the hepatic angiogram appears to be of poor quality.

Text continued on page 249

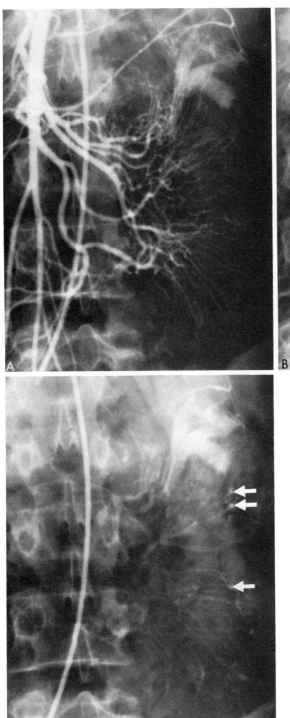

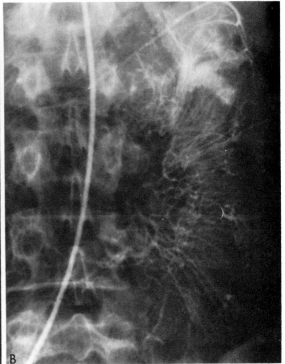

Figure 6–29. Osler-Weber-Rendu syndrome. Superior mesenteric angiogram in a 50 year old woman with recurrent melena.

A. Midarterial phase. The superior mesenteric artery and its branches appear normal.

B. Late arterial phase. Several small dilatations are present on the antimesenteric side of the vasa recta to the jejunum and ileum.

C. Venous phase. The small areas of dilatation are better visualized (⟹). They communicate with slightly dilated veins filled with contrast medium of increased density. The dilated vascular structures represent telangiectasias in the bowel mucosa, and the dense venous drainage occurs because of arteriovenous shunting.

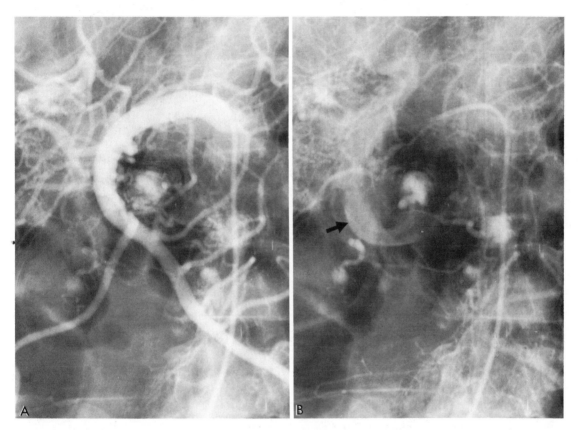

Figure 6–30. Advanced Osler-Weber-Rendu syndrome. Superior mesenteric angiogram in a 65 year old man with repeated episodes of epistaxis and melena.

A. Midarterial phase. Several tangles of dilated vessels are supplied by branches of the superior mesenteric artery.

B. Late arterial phase. Dense veins drain from the telangiectasias, and there is early filling of the portal vein with contrast medium (➡), indicating arteriovenous shunting.

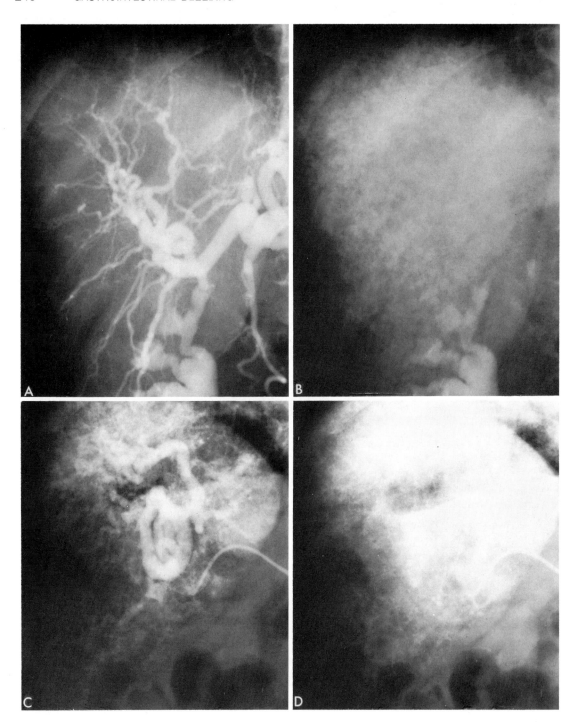

Figure 6–31. Hepatic vascularity in patients with Osler-Weber-Rendu syndrome.

A. Arterial phase of a celiac angiogram in the patient shown in Figure 6–29. The hepatic artery branches are moderately dilated.

B. Parenchymal phase. There is a markedly irregular hepatogram with dilated groups of sinusoids throughout the liver. The appearance is similar to that described for peliosis hepatis.

C. Arterial phase of a hepatic angiogram in the patient shown in Figure 6–30. The hepatic artery branches are markedly dilated, and the contrast medium is diluted by the marked increase in hepatic artery blood flow, resulting in a poor quality angiogram.

D. Parenchymal phase. There is a marked, irregular increase in the density of the hepatogram phase.

ANGIOGRAPHIC CONTROL OF MASSIVE GASTROINTESTINAL BLEEDING

The treatment of patients with massive arterial bleeding into the gastrointestinal tract has been the cornerstone of the rapidly developing field of therapeutic angiography. Since the initial reports in 1971 by Rösch et al. and Baum and Nusbaum that massive gastrointestinal bleeding can be controlled by selective infusion of vasoconstrictive drugs into the bleeding arteries, much experience has accumulated utilizing this method. More recently, several authors have reported that massive arterial bleeding can also be controlled by the selective embolization of the bleeding artery. Although not as much experience has accumulated with embolization as with infusion, the initial observations suggest that the two methods may be complementary. The best results with embolization have been obtained in those patients in whom infusion has been least effective and vice versa.

Infusion Therapy for Arterial Bleeding

Although both epinephrine and vasopressin (Pitressin) were initially used to control arterial bleeding, most angiographers now use only vasopressin. Vasopressin is an aqueous solution of the pressor principle obtained from the posterior pituitary gland and is reasonably free from the oxytocic principle. It has vasoconstrictive and antidiuretic actions and causes generalized smooth muscle contractility. In the vascular bed, it causes generalized vasoconstriction by direct action on the smooth muscle in the vascular walls, particularly in the terminal arterioles, capillaries and venules. The drug is not blocked by adrenergic blocking agents. When vasopressin is infused selectively into the celiac or superior mesenteric artery or one of their branches, the blood flow decreases rapidly, remains low during the infusion and when the infusion is terminated, gradually returns to normal over a few hours.

Side Effects

The side effects of vasopressin are arrhythmias, particularly bradycardia, and fluid retention. Vasopressin has a strong constrictive effect on the coronary arteries, and the drug should be used with extreme caution in patients with coronary artery disease. The problem of water retention is caused by the antidiuretic effect of vasopressin. Fluid and electrolyte balance should be carefully monitored during the infusion. Problems can be minimized by controlling the amount of fluid infused as much as possible. Decreasing urinary output responds to intravenous furosemide (Athanasoulis et al., 1976). More than 1 cc infusate per minute should not be used for prolonged periods of time. Because of the potentially severe side effects of vasopressin infusion, patients being infused for the control of gastrointestinal bleeding should be followed in an intensive care unit. If such a facility is not available, infusion for more than a few hours should not be undertaken.

Technique

When the bleeding site and artery have been identified on the angiogram, a catheter is placed as selectively as possible into the bleeding artery. In general, the infusion is made into the left gastric, the gastroduodenal, or the splenic artery for upper gastrointestinal bleeding or into the inferior or superior mesenteric artery for lower gastrointestinal bleeding. If superselective catheterization is not possible because of atherosclerosis or the patient's anatomy, the celiac artery can be infused.

When the artery to be infused is catheterized, the vasopressin is mixed so that the perfusate has 0.2 pressor unit per cc. This particular mixture is chosen because about 1 cc per minute of infusion is required to keep the system open, and most patients respond to an infusion of 0.2 pressor unit per minute. Infusion is best made with a rotary infusion pump (several types are commercially available). The infusion should be started in the angiography room at a rate of 0.2 pressor unit per minute. After 20 minutes the effectiveness of the infusion in controlling the bleeding should be assessed with a repeat angiogram. If the previously observed extravasation is no longer present, the infusion rate is adequate to control bleeding (Fig. 6–32; also see Fig. 6–7). If the initial infusion rate is effective, the infusion should be continued

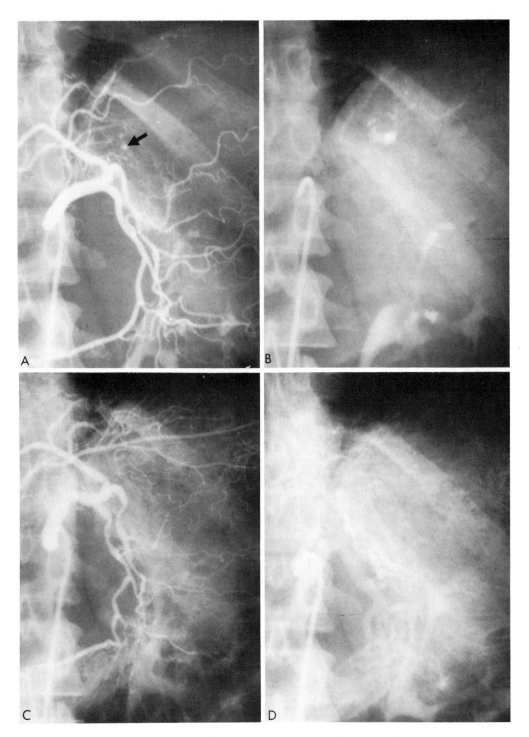

Figure 6–32. Control of gastric bleeding with vasopressin infusion. Left gastric angiogram in a 29 year old man with a Mallory-Weiss laceration at the cardioesophageal junction.

A. Arterial phase. Early extravasation of contrast medium can be seen from left gastric artery branches at the cardioesophageal junction (➡).

B. Venous phase. The extravasated contrast medium collects on the gastric mucosa.

C. Left gastric angiogram following a 20 minute infusion of vasopressin at a rate of 0.2 pressor unit per minute. Several areas of constriction are seen along the branches of the left gastric artery.

D. Venous phase. No contrast medium extravasates, indicating that this rate of infusion is adequate to control the bleeding.

for the next 12 to 24 hours at the same rate. If there is no clinical evidence of further bleeding, the dosage should then be halved, and the infusion continued at a rate of 0.1 pressor unit per minute for an additional 12 to 24 hours. Finally, 5 per cent dextrose in water should be substituted for the vasopressin and the catheter left in place several additional hours.

Different patients have different degrees of response to the same infusion rate. In some, particularly young patients, an infusion of 0.2 pressor unit per minute may cause nearly complete occlusion of the blood flow to the vascular bed being infused. In such patients the contrast medium remains in the markedly constricted and irregularly spastic branches for a long period of time, and no capillary or venous phase is seen. When this appearance is noted after the initial 20 minute infusion, the infusion rate should be decreased to 0.1 pressor unit per minute. Following 20 minutes of infusion, another angiogram should be performed. If this infusion rate controls the bleeding, it should be continued for 12 to 24 hours, then halved for an additional 12 to 24 hours if the bleeding is controlled clinically.

However, if contrast medium still extravasates at the bleeding site following the initial 20 minutes of 0.2 pressor unit per minute infusion, the dosage should be increased to 0.3 pressor unit per minute for an additional 20 minutes and the situation reassessed. If the bleeding has then stopped, the 0.3 pressor unit per minute should be maintained for about 12 hours, then cut back to 0.2 unit for the next 12 hours and then to 0.1 unit for the next 24 hours. Finally, if the bleeding has not been controlled with 0.3 pressor unit per minute, the dosage can be increased to 0.4 unit and the process repeated. If bleeding has not been controlled at 0.4 pressor unit per minute, it probably will not be controlled at higher dosages either. Such a patient should be embolized or operated on immediately. Moreover, infusion rates of more than 0.2 to 0.3 pressor unit per minute should not be maintained for periods longer than 6 to 8 hours. Investigations by Baum et al. (1974) have shown that vasopressin, when infused at a rate of 0.2 pressor unit per minute, can be cleared from the body as the infusion takes place. As the infusion rate becomes progressively higher, however, the vasopressin accumulates in the blood stream, and at rates of 0.4 to 0.6 pressor unit per minute, the amount of vasopressin per cc of blood begins to rise rapidly.

Patients should not experience pain during the infusion. If they do, the catheter tip has probably occluded a branch of the superior mesenteric artery, and its position should be checked by fluoroscopy.

Hepatic Artery Escape

Recent experiments (Barr et al., 1974) have shown that the hepatic artery reacts differently to vasopressin infusion than the other arteries of the viscera. Although the hepatic artery blood flow initially decreases following infusion of vasopressin into the celiac or superior mesenteric artery, it then reverses and rises to above preinfusion levels, remaining elevated throughout the remainder of the infusion. The phenomenon is known as hepatic artery "escape" and is attributed to a compensatory response of the hepatic artery to decreased portal blood flow. This observation is important because it means that hepatic artery branches arising from bleeding arteries may be infused without causing hepatic ischemia. The situation occurs commonly because of the large number of patients in whom accessory or replaced hepatic arteries arise from the left gastric or superior mesenteric artery.

Although this escape phenomenon allows infusion of the hepatic artery in most patients, infusion of patients with advanced cirrhosis has not yet been shown to be safe. In advanced cirrhosis, hepatic artery blood flow has already increased markedly to compensate for decreased portal blood flow and thus has already "escaped." It has not been demonstrated that the hepatic circulation in patients with advanced cirrhosis responds to vasopressin infusion in the same manner as in patients without cirrhosis. Until more information is available about the effects of vasopressin infusion on hepatic artery blood flow in advanced cirrhosis, such infusions should be undertaken with caution.

In general, vasopressin infusion has been most effective in controlling the bleeding from Mallory-Weiss lacerations, hemorrhagic gastritis, bleeding from stress ulcers and most types of bleeding from the small bowel and colon. In the latter group, vasopressin infusions have been particularly effective in controlling the bleeding from diverticula (Figs. 6–33 and 6–34). Results have been mixed in patients with bleeding gastric ulcers and poor in patients with duodenal ulcers. Usually, the larger the bleeding artery and the older the patient, the less effective vasopressin infusion is in controlling the hemorrhage.

Infusion Therapy for Variceal Bleeding

For the past few years, angiographers have treated patients with bleeding varices by infusing vasopressin into the superior mesenteric artery. The dosages used have been 0.2 pressor unit per minute for 24 hours and then 0.1 pressor unit per minute for an additional 24 hours (Athanasoulis et al., 1976). The results have been mixed. In general, the more severe the patient's cirrhosis, the less successful vasopressin infusion has been for controlling the bleeding. In a prospective study, Conn et al. (1975) controlled variceal bleeding in 71 per cent of 17 patients. However, survival was no better than in a control group.

Recently Barr et al. (1975) observed that in normal dogs an intravenous infusion of vasopressin in the same dosages as a superior mesenteric artery infusion (0.1 to 0.2 pressor unit per minute) decreases portal flow almost as much as the arterial infusion. Preliminary work by Kaufman et al. (1976) suggests that these results also pertain to cirrhotic humans, and other angiographers are now evaluating intravenous infusion. Athanasoulis et al. (1976) have reported successful control of variceal bleeding in 10 patients using an intravenous infusion rate of 0.3 pressor unit per minute of vasopressin for 12 hours, followed by 0.2 unit per minute for 24 hours and subsequently followed by 0.1 unit per minute for 24 hours.

The newly devised technique of transhepatic portal vein catheterization (Lunderquist and Vang, 1974) has led to the attempted control of variceal bleeding by selective embolization of the coronary vein. The method and its uses are described in Chapter 8.

Other Angiographic Methods for Controlling Bleeding

At present vasopressin infusion is the main angiographic method for controlling gastrointestinal hemorrhage. However, because of the side effects of the drug and the low success rate in controlling bleeding from ulcers, angiographers are continually seeking new ways to control hemorrhage. Other methods that have been investigated are balloon occlusion, intravascular coagulation and selective arterial embolization.

Balloon catheters have been moderately successful in controlling bleeding when they can be expanded close to the bleeding site. However, balloon occlusion is similar to arterial ligation, since a proximal occlusion allows collateral blood flow to develop around the occlusion. Intravascular coagulation with electrically charged guide wires placed selectively in the bleeding artery is also being evaluated. However, 30 to 40 minutes are required before thrombus begins to occlude the bleeding artery. Also, the thrombus generally develops at the catheter tip and this, like balloon occlusion and operative ligation, may be too proximal, allowing collateral blood flow to develop to the bleeding site. The most successful of the new methods has been selective arterial embolization.

Selective Arterial Embolization

Embolic material can be injected through a catheter selectively into the bleeding artery. The emboli are carried peripherally by the blood flow and occlude the branches of the artery being embolized, including the bleeding branch. Because the occlusions are peripheral, little collateral blood flow develops around the occlusion. In this sense embolization is similar to vasopressin infusion, which also primarily causes a peripheral occlusion.

The embolic materials used can be categorized as short-acting, long-acting and permanent. The only short-acting embolic material currently used is autogenous blood clot. In fact, Rösch et al. (1972), who first tried autogenous blood clot for embolization, felt that it lysed too rapidly to be useful. Therefore, subsequent investigators (Reuter and Chuang, 1974; Bookstein et al., 1974) have attempted to prolong the life of

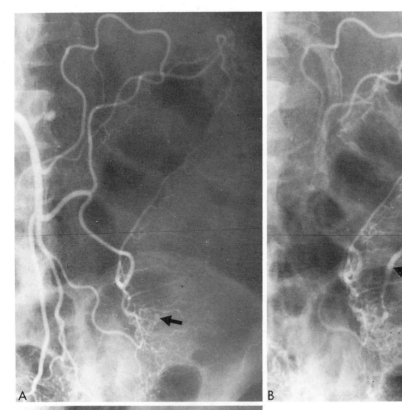

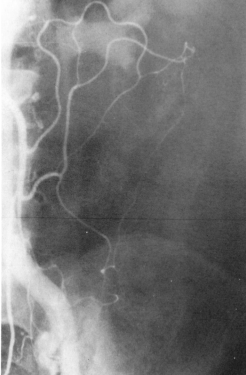

Figure 6–33. Control of colonic bleeding by vasopressin infusion. Inferior mesenteric angiogram in a 68 year old man with rectal bleeding and known diverticulosis.

A. Early arterial phase. There is faint extravasation of contrast medium into the diverticulum, which appears as an aneurysm-like structure (➡).

B. Late arterial phase. The extravasated contrast medium runs out of the diverticulum, forming a "pseudovein" (➡).

C. Inferior mesenteric angiogram following a 20 minute infusion of vasopressin at a rate of 0.2 pressor unit per minute. The branches of the inferior mesenteric artery are markedly constricted. No extravasation is seen, indicating control of the bleeding. The infusion was continued for 12 hours and terminated. No bleeding recurred.

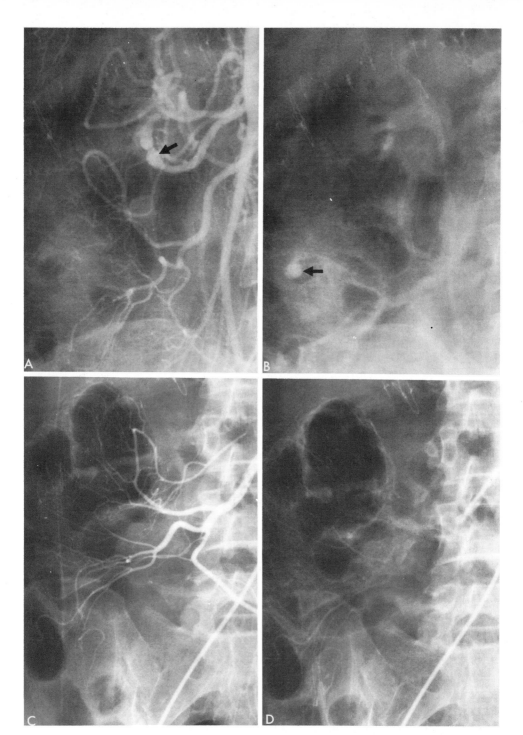

Figure 6–34. Control of colonic bleeding by vasopressin infusion. Superior mesenteric angiogram in a 53 year old woman with bleeding from right-sided diverticulosis.

A. Arterial phase. Aneurysms are present on the anterior pancreaticoduodenal arcade (➡), which is markedly dilated because of the presence of celiac stenosis. The branches to the right colon appear normal.

B. Venous phase. A rounded collection of extravasated contrast medium is present in the proximal ascending colon (➡).

C. Arterial phase of a superior mesenteric angiogram following 48 hours of vasopressin infusion. Thrombus is present around the catheter tip in the ileocolic artery. The branches of the ileocolic artery are constricted. No extravasation is seen. Initially, the bleeding in this patient was controlled only after a vasopressin infusion of 0.4 pressor unit per minute. This was continued for 12 hours, then was decreased to 0.2 pressor unit per minute for the next 12 hours and finally decreased to 0.1 pressor unit per minute for 24 hours. At the time of the angiogram the bleeding was clinically controlled, and an infusion of 5 per cent dextrose in water was substituted for the vasopressin.

D. Late arterial phase. No extravasation is seen.

the clot by mixing it with epsilon-aminocaproic acid (Amicar). Animal experiments (Chuang, et al., 1975) have shown that blood clot mixed with Amicar persists slightly longer than plain autogenous blood clot in dogs. However, a more important effect of Amicar on clot is the production of a thrombus that is firmer and easier to work with than plain autogenous clot (Fig. 6–35). Amicar clot can be squeezed between gauze sponges to express the serum and can be cut with scissors into the desired aliquots for embolization. For both reasons, therefore, most angiographers who use autogenous clot for embolization mix it with Amicar. This is done by drawing 9 cc of the patient's blood into a syringe containing 1 cc of Amicar (10 per cent mixture). The blood is drawn as soon as the catheter is placed in the aorta for the diagnostic study, before it is rinsed with heparinized saline. Only glass syringes should be used, since plastic syringes impede thrombus formation.

The clot takes about 30 minutes to form, approximately the time required to perform the diagnostic examination and place the catheter selectively into the artery to be embolized. The clot can then be taken from the syringe, and as much serum as possible is expressed with sponges. Approximately a 0.5 cc aliquot is cut from the thrombus with scissors and placed in a tuberculin syringe with about 0.5 cc of unheparinized saline. The syringe is then coupled to the catheter and the clot injected. As it passes through the stopcock and catheter, the clot becomes fragmented, resulting in embolization of several branches (Fig. 6–36, also see Figs. 6–1 and 6–5). Experience has shown that the bleeding artery is generally among the first to be occluded (Fig. 6–37). The emboli are probably directed toward the bleeding artery by the increased blood flow caused by the absence of peripheral resistance.

A repeat angiogram is then made to confirm the occlusion. If contrast medium still extravasates at the bleeding site, additional

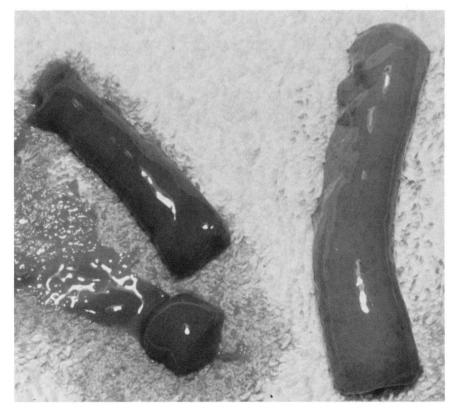

Figure 6–35. Amicar clot. The clot at the right has been prepared by mixing 9 cc of the patient's blood with 1 cc of Amicar. That on the left is the patient's clot without Amicar. As can be seen, the Amicar clot is much firmer and easier to work with than the non-Amicar clot, which tends to fall apart more easily and may be somewhat gelatinous.

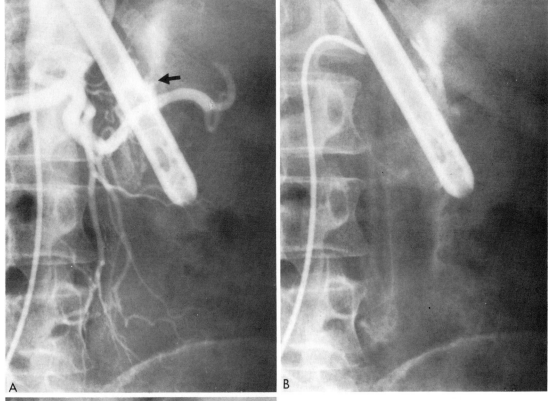

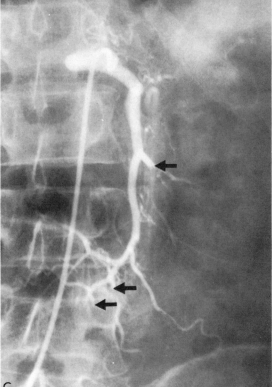

Figure 6–36. Control of gastric bleeding with Amicar-mixed blood clot. Celiac angiogram in a 48 year old man with massive hemorrhage from a gastric ulcer.

A. Arterial phase. There is early extravasation of contrast medium in the region of the fundus just to the left of the Ewald tube (➡). Note the presence of the wide bore nasogastric tube, which is important for clearing the stomach of blood clots.

B. Venous phase. The extravasated contrast medium collects on the gastric mucosa.

C. Selective left gastric angiogram following selective embolization with 1 cc autogenous clot mixed with Amicar. Most of the branches of the left gastric artery have been occluded by fragments of the blood clot (➡).

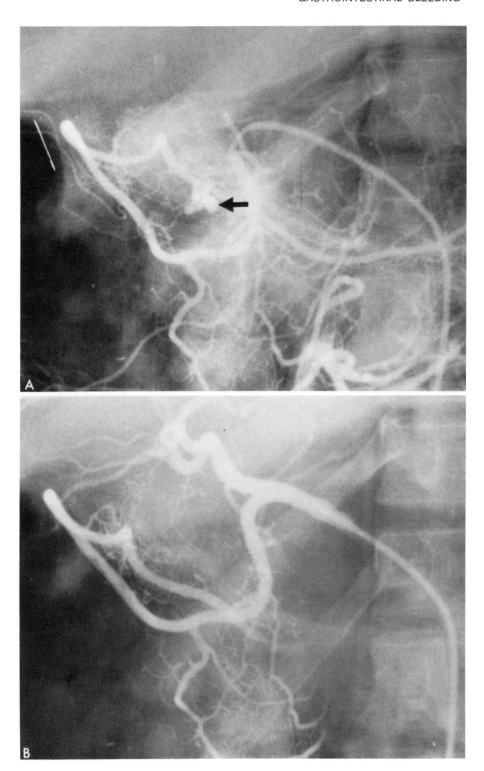

Figure 6–37. Embolic control of duodenal hemorrhage. Gastroduodenal angiogram in a 47 year old man with a bleeding duodenal ulcer.

A. Arterial phase. Extravasating contrast medium has collected in the duodenal bulb (➡).

B. Gastroduodenal angiogram following selective embolization of the gastroduodenal artery with 0.5 cc autogenous blood clot mixed with Amicar. Several of the branches in the gastroduodenal artery have been occluded by fragments of clot. No contrast medium extravasates into the duodenal bulb, indicating that the bleeding has been controlled.

0.5 cc aliquots of clot are injected until the bleeding branch is occluded. Total amounts greater than 1.5 cc should probably not be used. The effectiveness of the embolization in controlling the bleeding can also be checked by observing the return of nasogastric lavage. If the embolization is effective, the lavage rather rapidly turns pink and then clear. The catheter is left in place for approximately 6 hours in case the clot lyses and bleeding recurs. The embolized artery infrequently bleeds again, but when it does, the repeat bleeding generally occurs at 1 to 3 hours; if no further bleeding has occurred by 6 hours, the catheter can be removed.

Most autogenous clot emboli undergo lysis, and angiography done 24 hours after embolization demonstrates that the previously occluded branches have become patent, except for the artery that was bleeding (Fig. 6–38). This phenomenon has been observed consistently with the use of autogenous blood clot, regardless of the organ or artery being embolized (Fig. 6–39). Why the clot in the bleeding branch does not also lyse is unknown. Possibly this phenomenon is related to the reversal of polarity of damaged arterial intima, as might occur at the base of an ulcer. It may also be related to the amount of plasminogen activator in damaged intima, or the bleeding artery may simply remain occluded long enough to give the body's clotting mechanisms a chance to function.

Intermediate embolic materials that have been used to control bleeding in the gastrointestinal tract are Gelfoam (Reuter and Chuang, 1974; Reuter et al., 1975) and Oxycel fiber (Bookstein et al., 1974). Animal experiments have shown that these materials cause an arterial occlusion which lasts from a few weeks to several months, and some of the embolized branches remain occluded permanently. Of the two materials, Gelfoam is more generally used because it is easier to handle. Gelfoam comes in strips which can be cut into small cubes measuring 2 to 3 mm on a side or into larger rectangular pieces measuring 2 to 3 mm on a side and 10 mm in length (Fig. 6–40). When placed in saline, Gelfoam becomes soft and pliable and can be placed in the back of a tuberculin syringe and injected along with saline through the catheter. Generally, four to five cubes are injected at a time until the bleeding is controlled (Figs. 6–41 and 6–42). No more than about 1.0 to 1.5 cc of Gelfoam should be injected. Oxycel fibers are more difficult to handle but can be mixed with the patient's blood and irregular pieces of the matted mixture are then injected through a tuberculin syringe. Unlike the autogenous blood clot emboli, Gelfoam and Oxycel emboli are not lysed at 24 hours, and the artery that has been embolized generally thromboses as far back as the next proximal major branch (Figs. 6–43 and 6–44). Repeat studies at 24 hours reveal the embolized vessel to be completely occluded. However, injection of another artery to the stomach reveals the development of a rich collateral blood supply to the distribution of the occluded artery (Fig. 6–44).

Several types of permanent occluding agents are available. However, permanent occlusion is not necessary to control gastrointestinal bleeding, and these agents

Text continued on page 262

Figure 6–38. Control of massive gastric hemorrhage from a high lesser curvature ulcer with a follow-up study at 24 hours. Left gastric angiogram in a 56 year old man.

A. Arterial phase. Contrast medium extravasates from a fundal branch of the left gastric artery (⇨).

B. The extravasating contrast medium collects on the gastric mucosa.

C. Left gastric angiogram following embolization of the left gastric artery with 0.5 cc Amicar-mixed autogenous blood clot. Fragments of emboli have occluded several of the left gastric artery branches. No contrast medium extravasates at the site of the ulcer.

D. Left gastric angiogram 24 hours following embolization. The patient has a cascade stomach, and the orientation of the left gastric arteries has changed from the previous day's study. However, most of the previously occluded left gastric artery branches are again patent. A shred of thrombus persists in one of the branches (➡).

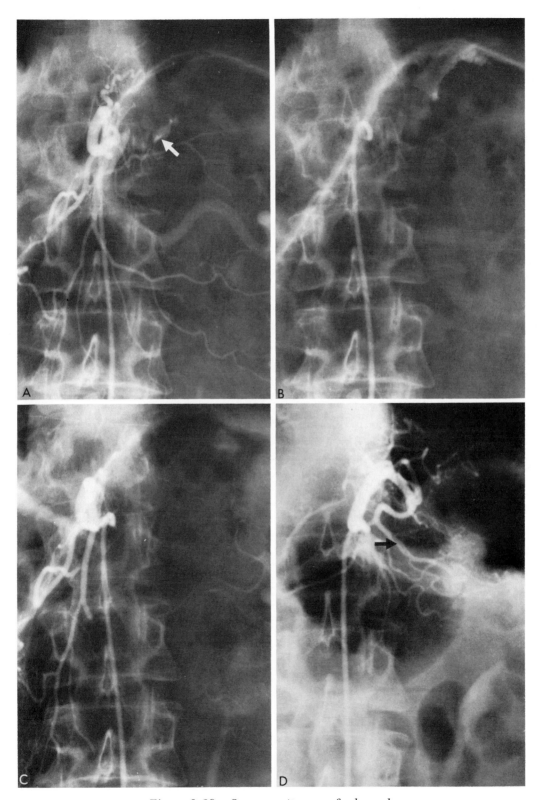

Figure 6–38. See opposite page for legend

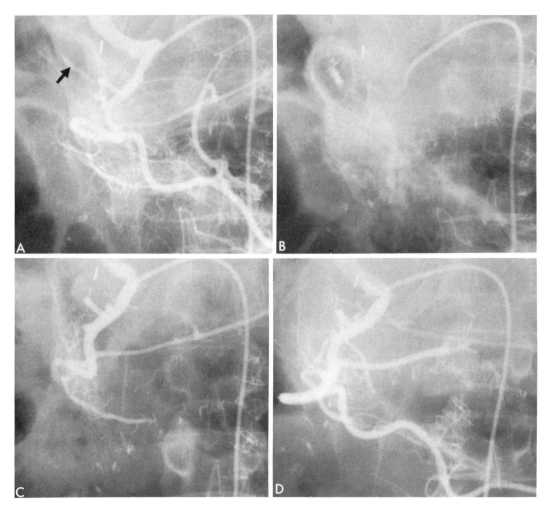

Figure 6–39. Control of duodenal hemorrhage by embolization with Amicar-mixed autogenous blood clot. Gastroduodenal angiogram in a 44 year old man with chronic alcoholic cirrhosis who was in hepatic coma because of his gastrointestinal bleeding.

A. Arterial phase. Early extravasation of contrast medium can be seen in the midportion of the duodenal bulb (➡).

B. Venous phase. The extravasated contrast medium collects in the bulb. The bulb can be identified by the increased accumulation of contrast medium in the mucosa.

C. Gastroduodenal angiogram following selective embolization of the gastroduodenal artery with 1 cc of Amicar-mixed autogenous blood clot. Several branches of the gastroduodenal artery, including the gastroepiploic artery and both pancreaticoduodenal arcades, have been occluded by fragments of clot. No contrast medium extravasates into the duodenal bulb, indicating that the bleeding has been controlled.

D. Gastroduodenal angiogram 24 hours following embolization. The previously occluded gastroduodenal artery branches are again patent, including those to the duodenal bulb. No contrast medium extravasates.

The patient came out of hepatic coma after 2 days and went home in 7 days.

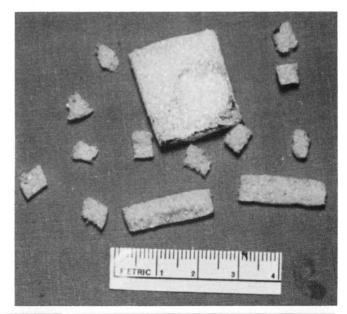

Figure 6–40. Gelfoam emboli. Small cubes of emboli are cut from the strip of Gelfoam shown in the center of the illustration. These measure 3 to 4 mm on a side. Longer lengths of Gelfoam (1.5 to 2.0 cm) can be used when bleeding is not controlled with the small cubes. When the Gelfoam cubes are placed in saline, they become soft and are easily injected through most catheters.

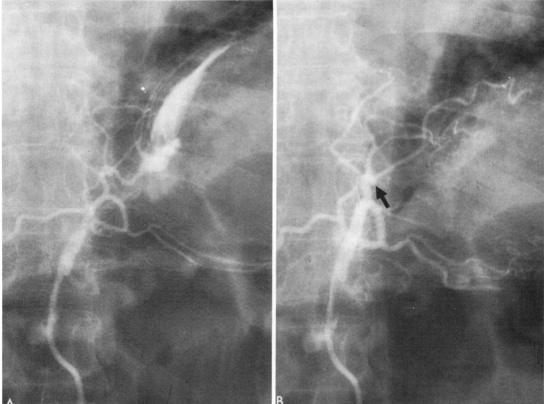

Figure 6–41. Control of gastric hemorrhage with Gelfoam emboli. Left gastric angiogram in a 57 year old man with a large fundal ulcer.

A. Arterial phase. There is massive extravasation of contrast medium from a fundal branch of the left gastric artery.

B. Following selective embolization of the left gastric artery with 4 small Gelfoam cubes, the bleeding artery is occluded (➡). The remaining gastric arteries are dilated as compared with the pre-embolization study. The changes resulting from shock, including visceral vasoconstriction and depressed blood pressure, frequently reverse rapidly when the bleeding is controlled, even before the blood volume reexpands. (Courtesy of Dr. Joseph J. Bookstein.)

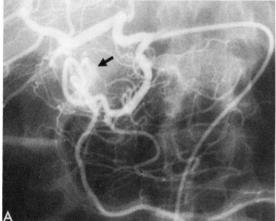
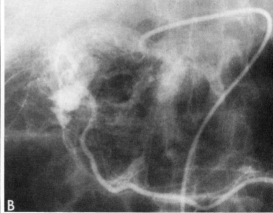
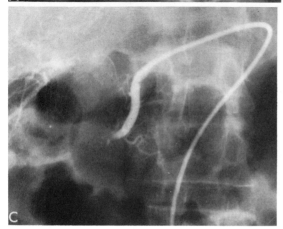

Figure 6-42. Control of duodenal hemorrhage by Gelfoam embolization. Gastroduodenal angiogram in a 68 year old man with known duodenal ulcer disease.

A. Arterial phase. Early extravasation of contrast medium is seen from the duodenal branches of the pancreaticoduodenal arcades (➡).

B. Late arterial phase. The extravasated contrast medium collects in the duodenal bulb.

C. Gastroduodenal angiogram following the injection of 10 small cubes of Gelfoam. The gastroduodenal artery and most of its branches are occluded by the emboli. No contrast medium extravasates. The patient's clinical condition improved rapidly, and he was placed on an aggressive ulcer regimen.

should not be used to treat arterial bleeding in the gastrointestinal tract. They should be reserved for use in the treatment of arteriovenous malformations, in the transhepatic, transportal embolization of the coronary vein and in other applications for which a permanent occlusion is desired.

Only temporary control is needed in the treatment of gastrointestinal bleeding. Therefore, Amicar-mixed autogenous blood clot should be the embolic material of choice. Occasionally, however, the patient's blood will not clot following several transfusions or because of depleted platelets or clotting factors. In such a patient either the clot is gelatinous and mushy, or no clot forms at all. Mixing the blood with a small amount of thrombin may cause a clot to form, but the resulting clot is soft and does not produce good emboli. When clot does not form, Gelfoam should be used for the embolization. In other patients, a good clot forms, but when it is injected into the

bleeding artery, the clot passes through the artery into the lumen of the stomach or duodenum. The injection of additional clot only blocks off normal arteries without affecting the bleeding artery. Gelfoam should be used in these patients, beginning with small 2 to 3 mm cubes. In rare instances, these also pass through the bleeding artery, and longer lengths of Gelfoam emboli should be used (Fig. 6-43).

A potential complication of embolization is infarction. Although gastric infarction following gastric embolization has been reported (Prochaska, 1973), the patient studied also had approximately 50 hours of vasopressin infusion along with the embolization. It is unlikely that infarction will occur in an intact stomach following embolization alone, since the stomach has such a rich blood supply from several individual arteries. The duodenum also has a dual blood supply, and to date infarction has not been reported with the embolization for

Text continued on page 266

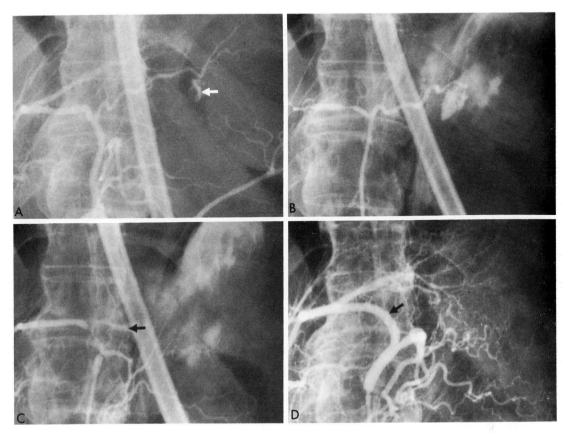

Figure 6–43. Control of gastric hemorrhage by Gelfoam embolization in a 58 year old man with a gastric ulcer following initial failure of autogenous blood clot embolization.

A. Arterial phase of a celiac angiogram. The bleeding (⟹) comes from a branch of the left gastric artery to the fundus, arising just proximal to the left hepatic artery. In order to avoid embolization of the liver, the catheter was advanced through the left gastric artery into the bleeding branch.

B. Selective angiogram of the bleeding left gastric artery branch. Massive extravasation of contrast medium occurs when the injection is made. A total of 1.5 cc of Amicar-mixed autogenous blood clot was injected into the artery without occluding it. The clot went through the bleeding artery into the lumen of the stomach. This was followed by the embolization of the artery with 10 small cubes of Gelfoam. These also passed through into the stomach. Finally, a 1.5 cm length of Gelfoam was injected. This occluded the artery. The catheter was then drawn back into the distal left gastric artery.

C. Distal left gastric angiogram. A great deal of catheter spasm is present in the distal left gastric artery and in the proximal left hepatic artery. The main left gastric artery branch can be seen, but the embolized branch (➡) does not fill with contrast medium.

D. Left gastric angiogram 24 hours following the embolization. The left gastric and hepatic arteries and their branches are now dilated as compared with the previous examinations because the patient is out of shock. The left gastric artery branch that was embolized has thrombosed as far back as its origin (➡) and is not seen.

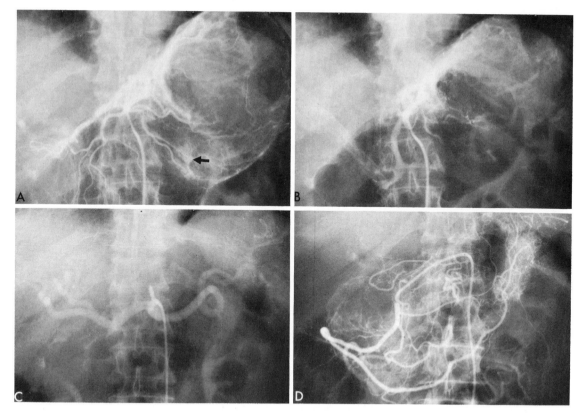

Figure 6–44. Control of gastric hemorrhage by Gelfoam embolization. Left gastric angiogram in a 62 year old man with melena.

A. Arterial phase. The branches of the left gastric artery are slightly dilated, and there is a diffuse increase in mucosal accumulation of contrast medium, demonstrating the typical appearance of gastritis. In addition, localized extravasation of contrast medium is present in the body of the stomach (➡).

B. Left gastric angiogram following embolization of the left gastric artery with 12 small cubes of Gelfoam. Most of the left gastric artery branches are occluded. The extreme tortuosity of the small branches in the body and the fundus of the stomach is typical of gastritis. No contrast medium extravasates.

C. Left gastric angiogram 24 hours after Gelfoam embolization. The left gastric artery has thrombosed backward toward its origin. The catheter tip had entered soft thrombus at the origin, and all of the injected contrast medium refluxes back into the splenic and hepatic arteries.

D. Gastroduodenal angiogram 24 hours after embolization. A rich collateral blood supply to the fundus of the stomach has developed over the gastroepiploic artery. On injection of the splenic artery, the development of the short gastric artery collaterals was similar.

Figure 6–45. Control of right colon hemorrhage by Gelfoam embolization. Superior mesenteric angiogram in a 74 year old man in whom a right-sided abdominal abscess had eroded into the right colic artery. At the time of the angiogram, blood was pouring out through the abscess drains. Embolization was elected as therapy because the patient could not tolerate an exploratory operation.

A. Superior mesenteric angiogram. Contrast medium extravasates from a branch of the right colic artery (➡). The catheter was advanced down the superior mesenteric artery and introduced selectively into the right colic artery.

B. Right colic angiogram. The bleeding site is well demonstrated. Following this angiogram, small Gelfoam cubes were injected into the right colic artery but passed through the bleeding branch into the abscess cavity. The cubes were followed by 1 cm lengths of Gelfoam plug. These also passed through the bleeding branch. Finally, a 3 cm length of Gelfoam was injected. This controlled the extravasation.

C. Right colic angiogram following control of the bleeding. The branches of the right colic artery are occluded (➡), as is the ileocolic artery (▶).

D. Superior mesenteric angiogram 24 hours after embolization. The right colic artery is thrombosed as far back as its origin (➡), and the ileocolic artery (▶) remains occluded.

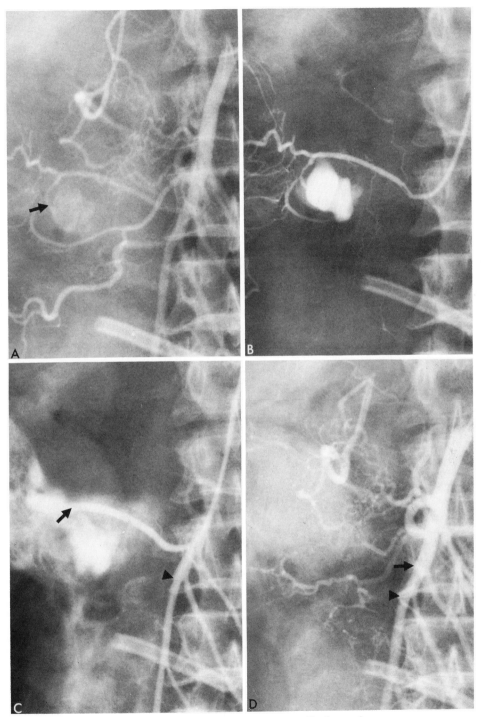

Figure 6–45. *See opposite page for legend*

duodenal bleeding. However, embolization should not be used in patients following gastric or duodenal surgery, since infarction is a potential problem when arteries have been ligated. Little experience has accumulated with embolization for small bowel or colonic bleeding as yet, and because of the nature of the blood supply to the bowel, an occasional infarction might be anticipated. A few patients with bowel bleeding who were poor operative risks have been successfully embolized with Amicar-mixed blood clot and Gelfoam without any apparent infarction (Fig. 6–45). Until greater experience has accumulated, however, small bowel or colonic embolization should be reserved only for patients who have failed to respond to vasopressin infusion and who are not candidates for operative control of the bleeding. As with the stomach and duodenum, embolization of the small bowel or colon should not be used postoperatively.

BIBLIOGRAPHY

Abu-Dalu, J., Urca, I., and Garti, I.: Selective angiography as a diagnostic aid in acute massive gastrointestinal bleeding. Arch. Surg. 106:17, 1973.

Athanasoulis, C. A.: Angiographic methods for the control of gastric hemorrhage. Amer. J. Digest. Dis. 21:174, 1976.

Athanasoulis, C. A., Baum, S., Waltman, A. C., et al.: Control of acute gastric mucosal hemorrhage: Intra-arterial infusion of posterior pituitary extract. New Eng. J. Med. 290:597, 1974.

Athanasoulis, C. A., Waltman, A. C., Novelline, R. A., et al.: Angiography: Its contribution to the emergency management of gastrointestinal hemorrhage. Radiol. Clin. N. Amer. 14:265, 1976.

Athanasoulis, C. A., Waltman, A. C., Ring, E. J., et al.: Angiographic management of postoperative bleeding. Radiology 113:37, 1974.

Baer, J. W., and Ryan, S.: Analysis of cecal vasculature in the search for vascular malformations. Amer. J. Roentgenol. 126:394, 1976.

Barr, J. W., Larkin, R. C., and Rösch, J.: Vasopressin and hepatic artery: Effect of selective celiac infusion of vasopressin on the hepatic artery blood flow. Invest. Radiol. 10:200, 1974.

Barr, J. W., Larkin, R. C., and Rösch, J.: Similarity of arterial and intravenous vasopressin on portal and systemic hemodynamics. Gastroenterology, 69:13, 1975.

Baum, S., Athanasoulis, C. A., Galdabrini, J., et al.: Angiodysplasia of the right colon: A cause of gastrointestinal bleeding. In Amer. J. Roentgenol. (in press).

Baum, S., Coggins, C., Misch, A. B., et al.: Vasopressin blood levels in patients undergoing selective arterial mesenteric infusion for control of gastrointestinal bleeding (abstract). Invest. Radiol. 9:327, 1974.

Baum, S., and Nusbaum, M.: The control of gastrointestinal hemorrhage by selective mesenteric arterial infusion of vasopressin. Radiology 98:497, 1971.

Baum, S., Nusbaum, M., Blakemore, W. S., et al.: The preoperative radiographic demonstration of intra-abdominal bleeding from undetermined sites by percutaneous selective celiac and superior mesenteric arteriography. Surgery 58:797, 1965.

Baum, S., Rösch, J., Dotter, C. T., et al.: Selective mesenteric arterial infusions in the management of massive diverticular hemorrhage. New Eng. J. Med. 288:1269, 1973.

Boijsen, E., and Reuter, S. R.: Angiography in diagnosis of chronic unexplained melena. Radiology 89:413, 1967.

Boijsen, E., Göthlin, J., Hallböök, T., et al.: Preoperative angiographic diagnosis of bleeding aneurysms of abdominal visceral arteries. Radiology 93:781, 1969.

Bookstein, J. J., Chlosta, E., Foley, D., et al.: Transcatheter hemostasis of gastrointestinal bleeding using modified autogenous clot. Radiology 113:277, 1974.

Brant, B., and Rösch, J.: Experiences with angiography in diagnosis and treatment of acute gastrointestinal bleeding of various etiologies: Preliminary report. Ann. Surg. 176:419, 1972.

Carey, L. S., and Grace, D. M.: The brisk bleed: control by arterial catheterization and Gelfoam plus. J. Can. Assoc. Radiol. 25:113, 1974.

Casarella, W. J., Galloway, S. J., Taxin, R. N., et al.: "Lower" gastrointestinal tract hemorrhage: New concepts based on arteriography. Amer. J. Roentgenol. 121:357, 1974.

Cavaluzzi, J. A., Kaufman, S. L., and White, R. I., Jr.: Vasopressin control of massive hemorrhage in chronic ulcerative colitis. Amer. J. Roentgenol. 127:672, 1976.

Chuang, V. P., Reuter, S. R., Cho, K. J., et al.: Alterations in gastric physiology caused by selective embolization and vasopressin infusion of the left gastric artery. Radiology 120:533, 1976.

Chuang, V. P., Reuter, S. R., and Schmidt, R. W.: Control of experimental traumatic renal hemorrhage by embolization with autogenous blood clot. Radiology 117:55, 1975.

Conn, H. O., Ramsby, G. R., Storer, E. H., et al.: Intra-arterial vasopressin in the treatment of upper gastrointestinal hemorrhage: A prospective, controlled clinical trial. Gastroenterology 68:211, 1975.

Cooley, R. N.: The diagnostic accuracy of upper gastrointestinal radiologic studies. Amer. J. Med. Sci. 242:628, 1961.

Cooley, R. N.: The diagnostic accuracy of radiologic studies of the biliary tract, small intestine and colon. Amer. J. Med. Sci. 246:610, 1963.

Davis, G. B., Bookstein, J. J., and Coel, M. N.: Advantage of intraarterial over intravenous vasopressin infusion in gastrointestinal hemorrhage. Amer. J. Roentgenol. 128:733, 1977.

Davis, G. B., Bookstein, J. J., and Hagan, P. L.: The relative effects of selective intra-arterial and intravenous vasopressin infusion. Radiology 12:537, 1976.

Finley, J. W., and Paulson, P. S.: Selective arteriography and infusion in diagnosis and treatment of acute gastrointestinal bleeding. Amer. Surg. 39:448, 1973.

Frey, C. F., Reuter, S. R., and Bookstein, J. J.: Localization of gastrointestinal hemorrhage by selective angiography. Surgery 67:548, 1970.

Galloway, S. J., Casarella, W. J., and Shimkin, P. M.: Vascular malformations of the right colon as a cause of bleeding in patients with aortic stenosis. Radiology 113:11, 1974.

Goldberger, L. E., and Bookstein, J. J.: Transcatheter embolization for treatment of diverticular hemorrhage. Radiology 122:613, 1977.

Goldman, M. L., Land, W. C., Jr., Bradley, E. L., et al.: Transcatheter therapeutic embolization in the management of massive upper gastrointestinal bleeding. Radiology 120:513, 1976.

Gray, R. K., and Grollman, J. H.: Acute lower gastrointestinal bleeding secondary to varices of the superior mesenteric venous system: Angiographic demonstration. Radiology 111:559, 1974.

Halpern, M., Turner, A. F., and Citron, B. P.: Hereditary hemorrhagic telangiectasia. Radiology 90:1143, 1968.

Harris, R. D., Anderson, J. E., and Coel, M. N.: Aneurysms of the small pancreatic arteries: A cause of upper abdominal pain and gastrointestinal bleeding. Radiology 115:17, 1975.

Kanter, I. E., Schwartz, A. J., and Fleming, R. J.: Localization of bleeding point in chronic and acute gastrointestinal hemorrhage by means of selective visceral arteriography. Amer. J. Roentgenol. 103:386, 1968.

Katzen, B. T., Rossi, P., Passariella, R., et al.: Transcatheter therapeutic arterial embolization. Radiology 120:523, 1976.

Kaufman, S. L., Harrington, D. P., Barth, K. H., et al.: Control of variceal bleeding by superior mesenteric artery vasopressin infusion. Amer. J. Roentgenol. 128:567, 1977.

Kaufman, S. L., Maddrey, W. C., Harrington, D. P., et al.: Hemodynamic effect of intra-arterial and intravenous vasopressin infusion in patients with portal hypertension. (Abstract). Invest. Radiol. 11:368, 1976.

Koehler, P. R.: New approaches to the radiological diagnosis of Mallory-Weiss syndrome. Brit. J. Radiol. 42:354, 1969.

Koehler, P. R., Nelson, J. A., and Berenson, M. M.: Massive extra-enteric gastrointestinal bleeding: angiographic diagnosis. Radiology 119:41, 1976.

Koehler, P. R., and Salmon, R. B.: Angiographic localization of unknown acute gastrointestinal bleeding sites. Radiology 89:244, 1967.

Koehler, P. R., Nelson, J. A., and Berenson, M. M.: Massive extraenteric gastrointestinal bleeding. Angiographic diagnosis. Radiology 119:41, 1976.

Lande, A., Bedford, A., and Schechter, L. S.: The spectrum of arteriographic findings in Osler-Weber-Rendu disease. Angiology 27:223, 1976.

Lande, A., and Meyers, M. M.: Iatrogenic embolization of the superior mesenteric artery: arteriographic observations and clinical implications. Amer. J. Roentgenol. 126:822, 1976.

Lipp, W. F., and Lipsitz, M. H.: The clinical significance of the coexistence of peptic ulcer and portal cirrhosis, with special reference to the problem of massive hemorrhage. Gastroenterology 22:181, 1952.

Lopata, H. I., and Berlin, L.: Colon varices: A rare cause of lower gastrointestinal bleeding. Radiology 87:1048, 1966.

Lunderquist, A., and Vang, J.: Trahshepatic catheterization and obliteration of the coronary vein in patients with portal hypertension and esophageal varices. New Eng. J. Med. 291:646, 1974.

Margulis, A. R., Heinbecker, P., and Bernard, H. R.: Operative mesenteric arteriography in the search for the site of bleeding in unexplained gastrointestinal hemorrhage. Surgery 48:534, 1960.

McCray, R. S., Martin, F., Amir-Ahmadi, H., et al.: Erroneous diagnosis of hemorrhage from esophageal varices. Amer. J. Dig. Dis. 14:755, 1969.

Merino-deVillasante, J., Alvarez-Rodriguez, R. E., and Hernandez-Ortiz, J.: Management of post-biopsy hemobilia with selective arterial embolization. Amer. J. Roentgenol. 128:668, 1977.

Meyers, M. A., Alonso, D. R., and Baer, J. W.: Pathogenesis of massively bleeding colonic diverticulosis: new observations. Amer. J. Roentgenol. 127:901, 1976.

Meyers, M. A., Volberg, F., Katzen, B., et al.: Angioarchitecture of colonic diverticula: Significance in bleeding diverticulosis. Radiology 108:249, 1973.

Nordentoft, E. L., and Larsen, E. A.: Rupture of a jejunal intramural aneurysm causing massive intestinal bleeding. Acta Chir. Scand. 133:256, 1967.

Nusbaum, M., and Baum, S.: Radiographic demonstration of unknown sites of gastrointestinal bleeding. Surg. Forum 14:374, 1963.

Perchik, L., and Max, T. C.: Massive hemorrhage from varices of the duodenal loop in a cirrhotic patient. Radiology 80:641, 1963.

Perlberger, R. R.: Control of hemobilia by angiographic embolization. Amer. J. Roentgenol. 128:672, 1977.

Pessel, J. F., Beairsto, E. B., Wise, J. S., et al.: Unusual causes of gastrointestinal hemorrhage. Gastroenterology 31:538, 1956.

Prochaska, J. M., Flye, M. W., and Johnsrude, I. S.: Left gastric artery embolization for control of gastric bleeding: Complications. Radiology 107:521, 1973.

Rastelli, G. C., Magnani, L., and Bocchialini, C.: L'impiego dell' arteriografia nella deiagnostica dele emorragie del tubo digerente. Minerva Chir. 14:1188, 1959.

Reuter, S. R., and Bookstein, J. J.: Angiographic localization of gastrointestinal bleeding. Gastroenterology 54:876, 1968.

Reuter, S. R., Fry, W. J., and Bookstein, J. J.: Mesenteric artery branch aneurysms. Arch. Surg. 97:497, 1968.

Reuter, S. R., and Chuang, V. P.: Control of abdominal bleeding with autogenous embolized material. Radiologe 14:86, 1974.

Reuter, S. R., Chuang, V. P., and Bree, R. L.: Selective arterial embolization for control of massive upper gastrointestinal bleeding. Amer. J. Roentgenol. 125:119, 1975.

Richardson, J. D., McInnis, W. D., Ramos, R., et al.: Occult gastrointestinal bleeding: An evaluation of available diagnosis methods. Arch. Surg. 110:661, 1975.

Ring, E. J., Athanasoulis, C. A., Waltman, A. C., et al.:

Pseudovein: An angiographic appearance of arterial hemorrhage. J. Can. Assoc. Radiol. 24:242, 1973.

Ring, E. J., Baum, S., Athanasoulis, C. A., et al.: Angiography in the diagnosis and treatment of nonvariceal bleeding in patients with portal hypertension. Surg. Gynec. Obstet. 139:205, 1974.

Roberts, C., and Maddison, F. E.: Partial mesenteric arterial occlusion with subsequent ischemic bowel damage due to pitressin infusion. Amer. J. Roentgenol. 126:829, 1976.

Rösch, J., Dotter, C. T., and Antonvic, R.: Selective vasoconstrictor infusion in the management of arterio-capillary gastrointestinal hemorrhage. Amer. J. Roentgenol. 116:279, 1972.

Rösch, J., Dotter, C. T., and Brown, M. J.: Selective arterial embolization: New method for control of acute gastrointestinal bleeding. Radiology 102:303, 1972.

Rösch, J., Dotter, C. T., and Rose, R. W.: Selective arterial infusions of vasoconstrictors in acute gastrointestinal bleeding. Radiology 99:27, 1971.

Schoenbaum, S. W., Sprayregen, S., Kron, E. S., et al.: Angiographic demonstration of bleeding gastric leiomyomas. Amer. J. Roentgenol. 119:277, 1973.

Sheedy, P. F., II, Fulton, R. E., and Atwell, D. T.: Angiographic evaluation of patients with chronic gastrointestinal bleeding. Amer. J. Roentgenol. 123:338, 1975.

Tadavarthy, S. M., Knight, L., Ovitt, T. W., et al.: Therapeutic transcatheter arterial embolization. Radiology 112:13, 1974.

Tegtmeyer, C. J., Smith, T. H., Shaw, A., et al.: Renal infarction: a complication of Gelfoam emboliza-

tion of a hemangioendothelioma of the liver. Amer. J. Roentgenol. 128:305, 1977.

Thompson, W. M., Pizzo, S. V., Jackson, D. C., et al.: Transcatheter electrocoagulation: a therapeutic angiographic technique for vessel occlusion. Invest. Radiol. 12:146, 1977.

Wagner, M., Kiselow, M. C., Keats, W. L.: Varices of the colon. Arch. Surg. 100:718, 1970.

20. Walter, J. F., Passo, B. T., and Cannon, W. B.: Successful transcatheter embolic control of massive hematobilia secondary to liver biopsy. Amer. J. Roentgenol. 127:847, 1976.

Weinstein, E. C., Moertel, C. G., and Waugh, J. M.: Intussuscepting hemangiomas of the gastro-intestinal tract: Report of a case and review of the literature. Ann. Surg. 157:265, 1963.

Wenz, W., and Krebs, H.: Angiographic demonstration of a bleeding neurinoma of the small intestine. Germ. Med. Mth. 13:77, 1968.

White, R. I., Girargiana, F. A., Jr., and Bell, W.: Bleeding duodenal ulcer control: Selective arterial embolization with autogenous blood clot. J.A.M.A. 229:546, 1974.

White, R. I., Jr., Harrington, D. P., Novak, G., et al.: Pharmacologic control of hemorrhagic gastritis: Clinical and experimental results. Radiology 111:549, 1974.

Whitehouse, G. H.: Solitary angiodysplastic lesions in the ileocaecal region diagnosed by angiography. Gut 14:977, 1973.

Wittenberg, J., Athanasoulis, C. A., Shapiro, J. H., et al.: A radiological approach to the patient with acute, extensive bowel ischemia. Radiology 106:13, 1973.

INFLAMMATORY DISEASE

The use of angiography is rarely indicated in the evaluation of patients with inflammatory disease of the gastrointestinal tract. The angiographic abnormalities caused by inflammatory disease must be known and recognized, however, because they are encountered when angiography is performed for other reasons.

Two generalizations can be made about the angiographic abnormalities caused by inflammation. The first is that a wide range of findings may be present in a given disease process. This variation is caused by the degree of acute inflammation present at the time of the examination as well as the overall duration of the inflammatory process. In acute, active bacterial inflammation, the main findings are hypervascularity of the diseased area with dilatation of the supplying arteries, increased accumulation of contrast medium in the involved parenchyma and dense, early venous drainage. Abscesses are seen as avascular or bubbly mass lesions, displacing the adjacent arteries. As the inflammatory process regresses, the angiogram may return to normal. If fibrosis follows, the vascularity may actually be decreased. The second generalization is that the angiographic findings most typical of inflammatory disease may also resemble those of neoplasm, athero-

sclerosis, trauma and some of the less common vascular diseases, making inflammatory disease a great imitator. In most patients, however, some clinical factor suggests that inflammatory disease should be strongly considered in the differential diagnosis. These common denominators of inflammation must be kept in mind as the angiographic abnormalities caused by inflammatory diseases of specific gastrointestinal organs are discussed.

BENIGN GASTRIC AND DUODENAL ULCERS

Angiography should not be used in the evaluation of patients with peptic ulcers of the stomach or duodenum, since endoscopy and barium examinations are easy to perform, safe and reliable. Moreover, the angiographic abnormalities caused by ulcers are neither specific nor consistent. Since gastric and duodenal ulcers may be encountered during angiography for gastrointestinal bleeding or other reasons, we have included a short description of our experience in evaluating these lesions. When the ulcer has not penetrated the gastric or duodenal wall, angiographic abnormalities are minimal. Fine, irregular vessels may be

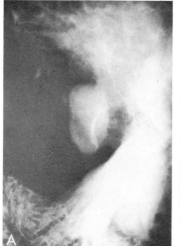
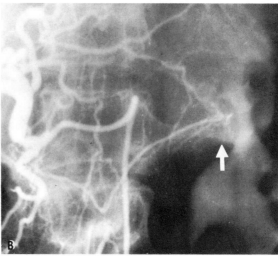

Figure 7–1. Gastric ulcer with fine, irregular vessels at the ulcer base.

A. Upper gastrointestinal series in a 52 year old woman reveals a large lesser curvature penetrating ulcer.

B. Common hepatic angiogram. The right gastric artery supplies the region of the ulcer. There are multiple indistinct abnormal arteries (⇨) which resemble tumor vessels at the base of the ulcer. The surgical specimen showed a benign ulcer.

present in the region immediately adjacent to the ulcer (Fig. 7–1), and a localized area of increased contrast medium accumulation may be seen during the parenchymal phase. The venous phase is generally normal; rarely, venous drainage may be early and dense. However, when the ulcer is large and penetrating, major vessels around the lesion may be involved, resulting in deformity of the left gastric or gastroduodenal artery similar to that caused by carcinoma (Fig. 7–2). If the ulcer is actively bleeding

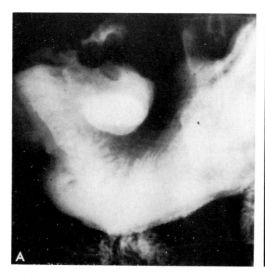
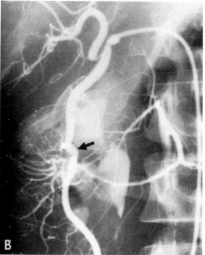

Figure 7–2. Benign penetrating duodenal ulcer simulating neoplastic encasement in a 44 year old woman.

A. Upper gastrointestinal series. A large penetrating ulcer is demonstrated.

B. Gastroduodenal angiogram. Arterial phase. The gastroduodenal artery is irregularly narrowed and altered in course (➡). Some fine, irregular arteries are seen in the same region. (From Reuter, S. R., Redman, H. C., and Bookstein, J. J.: Differential problems in angiographic diagnosis of carcinoma of the pancreas. Radiol. *96:*96, 1970.)

at the time of angiography, contrast medium may extravasate into the gastric or duodenal lumen.

ENTERITIS AND COLITIS

The typical angiographic findings associated with inflammatory disease of the bowel are increased vascularity and arteriovenous shunting. The arteries supplying the diseased areas are dilated, blood flow is rapid, the bowel wall shows markedly increased contrast medium accumulation during the parenchymal phase and the venous drainage is early and dense. These changes are proportional to the severity of inflammation and are relatively independent of the cause of the inflammatory process. When the inflammation decreases and the bowel wall returns to normal, these changes regress, and the arteries and veins in the diseased segment have a normal appearance; if fibrosis ensues, the vascularity may actually be decreased. Thus, the early angiographic changes of regional enteritis, ulcerative colitis, diverticulitis, acute bacterial enterocolitis and ischemic colitis are similar and depend primarily upon the degree of bacterial inflammation present. Particularly in the early stages, angiography is not a reliable method for differentiating these conditions and has little use in their diagnosis.

Regional Enteritis

The angiographic findings of regional enteritis are related to both the activity and duration of the disease. The early findings are those of acute inflammation and are nonspecific. During periods of activity, prominent hypervascularity is accompanied by dilated arteries and early, dense venous filling (Fig. 7–3). Increased parenchymal contrast medium accumulation may reveal a thickened bowel wall. When the inflammation becomes quiescent, the vascular abnormalities usually return to normal.

In the later stages of progressive and recurrent disease, fibrosis may cause irregularities of the vasa recta, some of which

may be occluded. The arterial branches in the mesentery may show areas of narrowing (Fig. 7–4), and the vasa recta tend to arise at right angles from the mesenteric branches instead of at the usual acute angle. A severely diseased and fibrosed segment of bowel may have a decrease in the number of vasa recta. In the authors' experience, these angiographic abnormalities which accompany long-standing regional enteritis are specific. They have not been encountered in other inflammatory diseases of the bowel.

Ulcerative Colitis

The angiographic appearance of ulcerative colitis also varies with the severity of the inflammatory process and tends to return to normal with remissions of the disease. During exacerbations, arterial blood flow to the involved portion of the colon increases, with prominent parenchymal accumulation of contrast medium and early, dense venous drainage. The vasa recta do not taper normally and remain dilated across the entire bowel (Fig. 7–5). This is not a specific change and is seen in other colonic inflammations. The vasa recta may terminate before reaching the antimesenteric border of the colon. When this happens, some fine, irregular collateral arteries may be present on the antimesenteric border. Late in the course of ulcerative colitis, when the colon has become fibrotic and shortened, the angiogram may be normal or the vascularity in the colon may be slightly decreased, with fewer vasa recta. Ulcerative colitis does not cause thickening of the mesentery, and the irregularities of the mesenteric arteries seen in regional enteritis have not been observed.

The increased incidence of carcinoma of the colon in patients with long-standing ulcerative colitis is well known. These tumors may be multiple and are difficult to detect by barium enema in colons with many pseudopolyps. Therefore, angiography may be used to reveal neoplastic degeneration in one or more areas. The angiographic abnormalities in such patients are the same as those of colonic carcinoma, primarily, encasement of colonic vessels and tumor neovascularity. Insufflation of

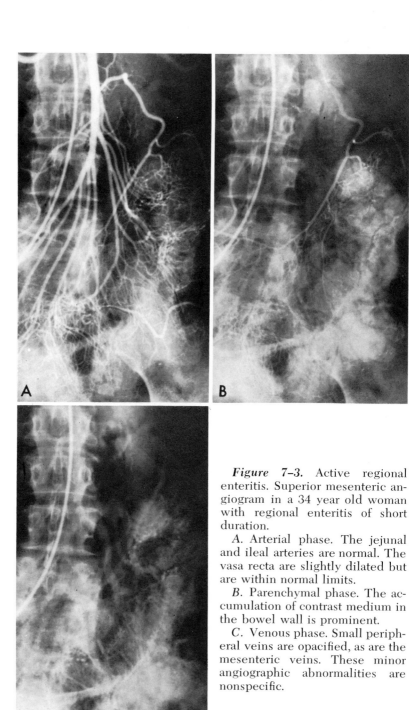

Figure 7–3. Active regional enteritis. Superior mesenteric angiogram in a 34 year old woman with regional enteritis of short duration.

A. Arterial phase. The jejunal and ileal arteries are normal. The vasa recta are slightly dilated but are within normal limits.

B. Parenchymal phase. The accumulation of contrast medium in the bowel wall is prominent.

C. Venous phase. Small peripheral veins are opacified, as are the mesenteric veins. These minor angiographic abnormalities are nonspecific.

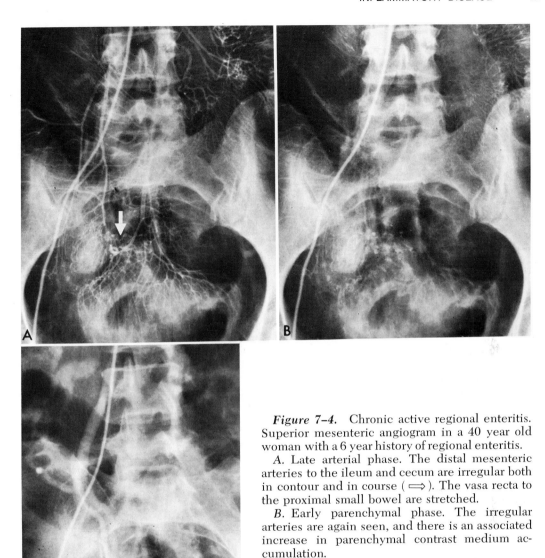

Figure 7-4. Chronic active regional enteritis. Superior mesenteric angiogram in a 40 year old woman with a 6 year history of regional enteritis.

A. Late arterial phase. The distal mesenteric arteries to the ileum and cecum are irregular both in contour and in course (⇒). The vasa recta to the proximal small bowel are stretched.

B. Early parenchymal phase. The irregular arteries are again seen, and there is an associated increase in parenchymal contrast medium accumulation.

C. Venous phase. Dense venous drainage is present.

the colon with air via a rectal tube helps in the detection of small carcinomas but should be avoided if toxic megacolon is present.

Diverticulitis

Angiography has little application in the evaluation of patients with diverticulitis since the disease is diagnosed easily by clinical history and barium enema. However, angiography can be used in an attempt to differentiate an atypical colonic carcinoma from an atypical diverticulitis. Although most patients with diverticulitis who have been reported in the literature have had inactive inflammatory disease at the time of examination, a few have had active inflammation. The latter have the typical changes of inflammatory disease of the

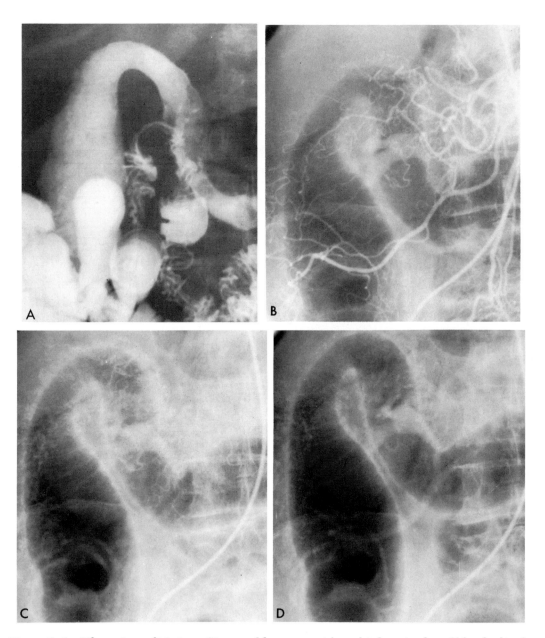

Figure 7-5. Ulcerative colitis in an 81 year old woman with multiple episodes of bloody diarrhea. The disease was diagnosed by proctoscopy.

A. Barium enema. The hepatic flexure has multiple fine ulcerations and loss of haustrations.

B. Superior mesenteric angiography. Arterial phase. The vasa recta show little tapering, and the bowel wall appears thickened, especially laterally.

C. Late arterial phase. The number of vessels in the bowel wall and parenchymal accumulation of contrast medium are increased.

D. Venous phase. Venous drainage is fairly prominent but is neither early nor dense. All these findings are nonspecific changes seen in inflammatory bowel disease. (Courtesy of Dr. Philip A. Hoskins).

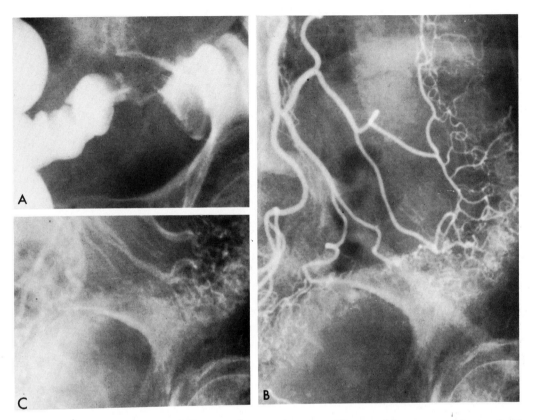

Figure 7-6. Sigmoid stricture following diverticulitis in a 79 year old woman with constipation.

A. Barium enema demonstrates a sigmoid stricture about 2 cm in length. There are no overhanging edges and no clear-cut mass. Normal mucosa does appear to go through the lesion.

B. Inferior mesenteric angiogram, arterial phase. The vasa recta in the area of the stricture are decreased both in number and in length. The marginal artery is discontinuous, but there is no neoplastic encasement.

C. Venous phase reveals diminished venous return from the region of the stricture.

bowel, with increased blood flow to the involved segments of colon, moderately dense accumulation of contrast medium in the parenchymal phase and prominent, early venous drainage. The vasa recta may be normal or dilated and tortuous. Associated pericolonic abscesses may result in displacement of mesenteric arterial branches, and contrast accumulation may be seen adjacent to the inflammatory mass. In long-standing or inactive disease, the primary finding is interruption of the marginal artery, perhaps related to fibrosis from recurrent abscess formation on the mesenteric side of the bowel wall (Fig. 7–6). The vasa recta may be completely normal or diminished in number in an area of fibrosis.

Ischemic Colitis

Ischemic colitis is an inflammatory disease of the colon caused by decreased arterial perfusion leading to mucosal devitalization and a secondary inflammation. Two mechanisms may cause this disease process. The most common is a low perfusion state caused by decreased cardiac output, often seen in patients with heart disease or in prolonged shock of any etiology. The second mechanism is actual occlusive vascular disease in which the collateral circulation is not adequate to maintain complete bowel wall integrity. Regardless of the mechanism, the disease follows the same course. The decreased blood flow causes mucosal devitalization. The resultant sloughing permits bacterial invasion and an inflammatory response with formation of granulation tissue. Mucosal edema and hemorrhage, which may be prominent, are seen as "thumbprinting" at barium enema. If the arterial blood flow is restored before the muscular layers are damaged, the bowel wall generally heals completely; however, with more severe damage, fibrosis and stricture occur. If blood flow is not restored, necrosis, perforation and death ensue.

The angiographic appearance of ischemic colitis is not specific. Immediately after the onset of symptoms, the angiogram is usually normal unless a vascular occlusion is present. As the inflammatory process progresses, dilated arteries, prominent parenchymal contrast medium accumulation and dense, early venous drainage appear (Fig. 7–7). With healing, the angiogram returns to normal unless fibrosis has been significant, in which case the vascularity to the involved segment may be diminished.

The nonspecificity of the angiographic changes in ischemic colitis does not allow differentiation of this disease from ulcerative colitis, which it may also resemble both clinically and histologically.

Differential Diagnosis of Inflammatory Lesions of the Bowel

The nonspecific nature of the hypervascularity accompanying bowel inflammation has been stressed in each of the previous sections. In the early stages of these diseases, differentiation by angiography is not possible. Only regional enteritis has specific findings in the late stages when fibrosis and mesenteric thickening occur. Therefore, angiography has little place in the primary evaluation of inflammatory disease of the bowel.

Moreover, normal variations can mimic the changes in inflammatory disease. Food passing through the small bowel increases the vascularity to the segment containing the bolus of food at the time of angiography. We have seen this appearance in patients studied under emergency conditions who have been eating or drinking

---

Figure 7–7. Reversible mesenteric ischemia in a 63 year old woman with sudden onset of bloody diarrhea.

A. Barium enema. Thumbprinting of the splenic flexure indicates that there has been submucosal hemorrhage.

B. Inferior mesenteric angiogram. Early arterial phase. No occluded vessels and little evidence of atherosclerosis are seen. A small nonoccluding embolus is present at the origin of a sigmoid branch; however, the bowel is hyperemic at the splenic flexure.

Legend continued on opposite page

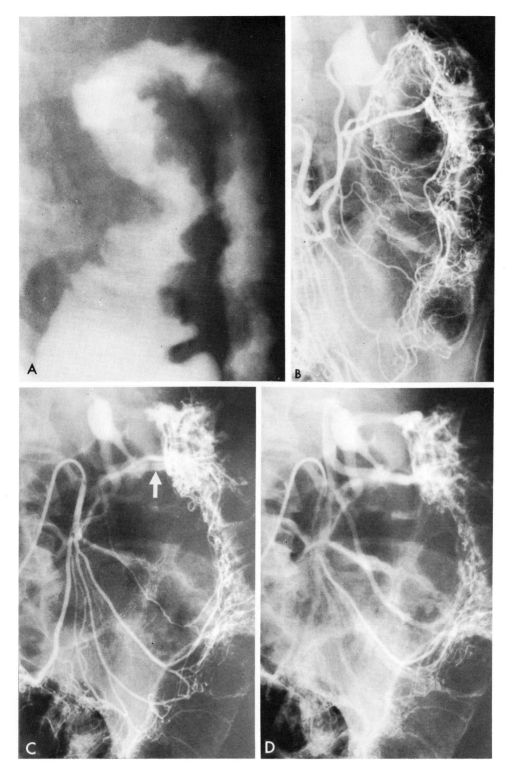

Figure 7–7 Continued. *C.* Late arterial phase. Early dense venous drainage occurs from the splenic flexure (⟹), while arteries are still filled with contrast medium.

D. Venous phase. The venous drainage from the diseased bowel has greater contrast medium density than that from the remainder of the colon. (From Reuter, S. R., Kanter, I. E., and Redman, H. C.: Angiography in reversible colonic ischemia. Radiology 97:371, 1970.)

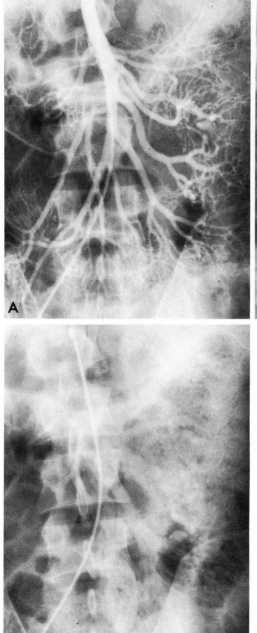

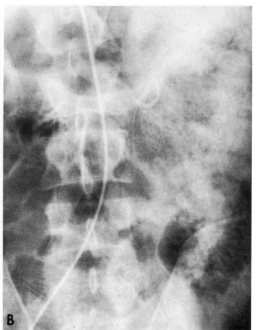

Figure 7-8. Postprandial increase in vascularity in the small bowel. Superior mesenteric angiogram in a 24 year old man who had drunk beer and eaten during the 2 hours before angiography. The angiogram was performed because of blunt abdominal trauma, and paracentesis was positive for blood.

A. Arterial phase. The jejunal and ileal arteries including the vasa recta are dilated.

B. Parenchymal phase. The contrast medium accumulation in the jejunum especially is dense.

C. Venous phase. The veins appear early and are well opacified.

prior to angiography (Fig. 7-8). Also, the jejunum is occasionally hypervascular and has dense venous drainage in patients who have had Billroth II gastrojejunostomies.

Therefore, the few indications for the occasional use of angiography in inflammatory diseases of the bowel are: (1) to determine the degree and extent of the inflammatory process when not possible by barium studies, (2) to help in the evaluation of indeterminate or bizarre small bowel series and barium enema examinations, (3) to try to differentiate between atypical diverticulitis and atypical colonic carcinoma and (4) to detect carcinomatous degeneration of ulcerative colitis.

INFLAMMATORY DISEASE OF THE BILIARY TRACT

Angiography is rarely used in the diagnosis of biliary tract disease unless carcinoma is suspected clinically. However, the cystic arteries are demonstrated on most celiac angiograms, and inflammatory changes of the biliary tract are sometimes seen.

Cholecystitis

Cholecystitis has a spectrum of angiographic findings related to the stage and activity of the disease. In chronic cholecystitis, the arterial blood supply to the gallbladder is generally diminished. The branches of the cystic artery are diminutive or absent, and no contrast medium accumulates in the gallbladder wall.

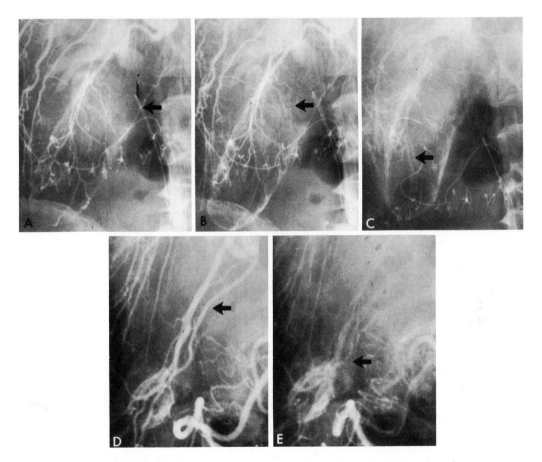

Figure 7–9.   Subacute cholecystitis.

A. Hepatic angiogram in a 43 year old man with recurrent abdominal pain. A gallbladder series showed nonvisualization. The surgical specimen revealed chronic acalculus cholecystitis. Early arterial phase. The deep cystic artery (➡) is quite small, but branches from the superficial artery are prominent and supply the gallbladder.

B. Late arterial phase. Some of the finer branches are tortuous and irregular (➡). Accumulation of contrast medium in the gallbladder wall is moderate.

C. Venous phase. Prominent veins are present (➡). The gallbladder wall is still opacified and is slightly thickened.

D. Celiac angiogram in a 52 year old woman with recurrent cholecystitis. Arterial phase. The cystic artery (➡) supplies fine tortuous arteries to a small hypervascular gallbladder.

E. Parenchymal phase. Part of the gallbladder wall has dense accumulation of contrast medium; the remainder is faintly opacified (➡).

Subacute cholecystitis, however, often shows an increased blood supply to the gallbladder with dilatation of the cystic artery and its branches. Parenchymal accumulation of contrast medium may occur early and be prominent, demonstrating a thickened gallbladder wall (Fig. 7–9). Gallbladder veins, which are seldom seen normally, are sometimes visualized in patients with subacute cholecystitis.

Patients with acute cholecystitis are rarely studied by angiography. Marked hypervascularity with dilatation of the cystic artery and its branches may be present, as well as an additional arterial supply from hepatic artery branches. Contrast medium accumulation may be increased in the gallbladder and in any associated inflammatory mass (Rösch et al., 1969).

Empyema may occur in patients with cholecystitis or with relatively healthy gallbladders. In the first situation, the gallbladder is often too fibrotic to dilate, and the angiographic appearance may be that of subacute cholecystitis (Fig. 7–10). Empyema in patients with less chronically diseased gallbladders usually causes dilatation and stretching and straightening of the major cystic arterial branches. Accumulation of contrast medium in the gallbladder wall reveals that the wall is not thickened. Perivesical inflammatory response may be marked, with some fine arteries in the area of inflammation. Rarely, veins draining the gallbladder may be seen in an empyema. The mesentery and omentum may adhere to the gallbladder fossa, and the anterior and posterior epiploic arteries may dilate.

Cholelithiasis

Cholelithiasis in an otherwise normal gallbladder causes no angiographic ab-

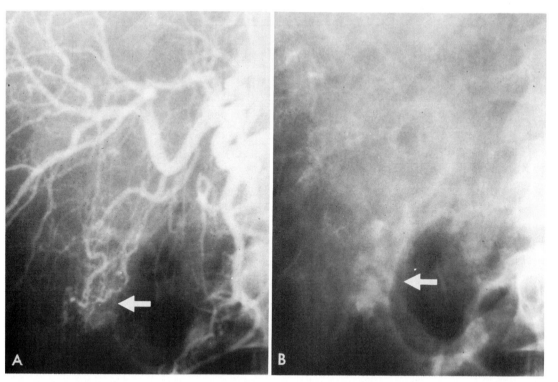

Figure 7–10. Gallbladder empyema. Hepatic angiogram in a 74 year old man. At autopsy an empyema of the gallbladder was found with evidence of long-standing cholecystitis.

A. Arterial phase. Many small, irregular branches (⟹) arise from the cystic artery. The gallbladder is not enlarged.

B. Parenchymal phase. Contrast medium accumulation (⟹) in the gallbladder is irregular. No veins are clearly identified.

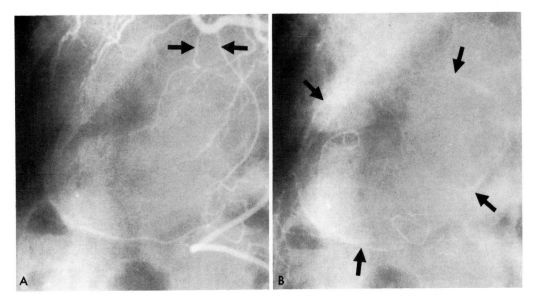

Figure 7–11. Impacted common bile duct stone. Celiac angiogram in 54 year old man with obstructive jaundice.

A. Arterial phase. The deep and superficial cystic arteries (➡) originate separately from the right hepatic artery. The deep branch appears stretched.

B. Parenchymal phase. The gallbladder contour is rounded and tense (➡), and the gallbladder wall is thin.

abnormality. Hydrops of the gallbladder secondary to a stone gives the angiographic appearance of gallbladder dilatation with stretching of the deep and superficial cystic arteries (Fig. 7–11). The fine branches tend to arise at right angles and are stretched and straightened. If parenchymal accumulation of contrast medium is present, the gallbladder contour appears rounded and tense.

Cholangitis

Cholangitis of all varieties is relatively uncommon and is not studied intentionally with angiography. However, some patients have unexplained right upper quadrant pain with intermittent jaundice, and angiography is requested to evaluate these symptoms. We have studied two patients with chronic cholangitis secondary to stenosis of the ampulla of Vater; both had mildly abnormal hepatic angiograms. The major hepatic arteries were normal in size and distribution, though the peripheral branches were tortuous. The major abnormality was many fine, tortuous hepatic ar-

tery branches throughout the liver, which emptied slowly. The portal vein was normal. The moderate fine vessel hypervascularity may represent hepatic inflammatory response. These patients did not have cirrhosis or persistent obstructive jaundice.

INFLAMMATORY DISEASE OF THE LIVER

Hepatic Abscesses

Abscesses in and around the liver develop from hematogenous spread of bacterial pathogens, from hepatic trauma or surgery and from indolent pathogens such as *Entamoeba* or *Echinococcus*. Abscesses around the liver also develop as complications of surgery, following perforation of an abdominal viscus or are secondary to other abdominal and pelvic inflammatory diseases. Bacterial pathogens are generally responsible for these perihepatic abscesses.

A spectrum of angiographic abnormalities similar to that in other inflammatory processes occurs in hepatic abscesses. The angiographic abnormalities may be only those of an avascular mass lesion (Fig. 7–12), with displacement of normal arteries and veins and a decreased accumulation of contrast medium in the hepatogram phase (Fig. 7–13). The abscess cavity is generally avascular but may have a bubbly appearance in the parenchymal phase (see Fig. 5–12). A halo of compressed normal parenchyma may surround the lesion. This constellation is more common with indolent pathogens but is also seen with acute pathogens and may be very difficult to distinguish from avascular metastases or cysts, especially when the abscesses are multiple.

Hepatic abscesses may also cause increased vascularity both in and around the lesion (Fig. 7–14). The hepatic arteries to the lesion may be slightly dilated, and many fine, irregular arteries may surround the abscess. The hepatogram around the abscess may have increased density and may be quite irregular. Rarely, arteriovenous shunting occurs, and some hepatic veins are demonstrated.

The clinical history is important in the interpretation of the angiographic abnormalities. Abscesses in hepatic subcapsular hematomas or contusions often have no features to distinguish the abscess from the initial traumatic lesion. Also, diffuse hematogenous seeding of abscesses throughout the liver closely simulates liver metastases at angiography. A clinical history of an infecting source and febrile course helps to distinguish between these lesions in many patients.

Indolent abscesses of the liver caused by *Echinococcus* and *Entamoeba* are not commonly encountered in the United States. The angiographic appearance of hydatid cysts is not specific for hydatid disease since they are primarily abnormalities of any mass lesion. Hepatic arteries and portal veins are displaced by the cyst or cysts, and radiolucent defects are present in the hepatogram phase. Compressed hepatic parenchyma often forms a thin halo around the cyst (Fig. 7–15), which some authors consider to be specific for hydatid disease. Since the inflammatory process is low grade, neovascularity, hypervascularity and prominent venous drainage are usually not present. Angiography can be used to localize the hydatid cysts before surgery. Ultrasound, computed tomography and isotopic liver scans have generally replaced angiography for the diagnosis and localization of hydatid cysts.

Text continued on page 286

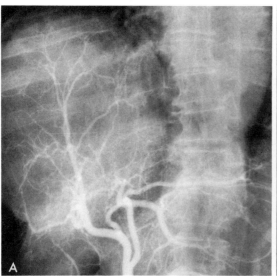 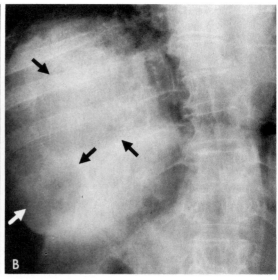

Figure 7–12. Intrahepatic abscesses. Hepatic angiogram in a 67 year old woman with fever.

A. Arterial phase. Both right and left hepatic artery branches are moderately stretched. No abnormal arteries are seen.

B. Parenchymal phase. Two rounded areas of decreased contrast accumulation ($\rightrightarrows$) are present in the right lobe of the liver. The abscess in the left lobe is not as well visualized.

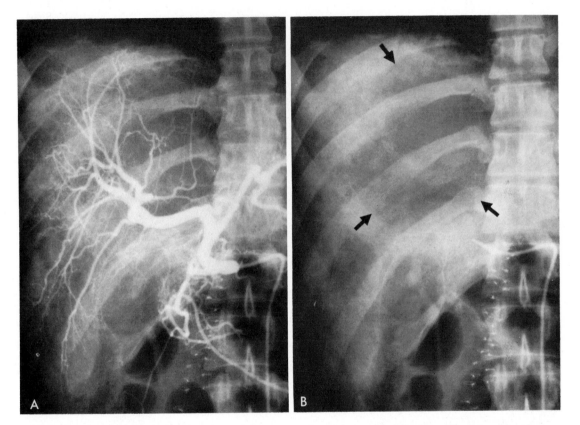

Figure 7–13. Hepatic abscess. Hepatic angiogram in a 35 year old man with fever of unknown origin.

A. Arterial phase. The hepatic artery branches in the region of the quadrate lobe are displaced around a large, avascular-appearing mass.

B. The abscess stands out against the normal hepatogram phase as an area of decreased contrast accumulation (➡). The compressed normal hepatic parenchyma around the abscess cavity appears dense. A second, smaller abscess can be seen in the lower portion of the right lobe of the liver.

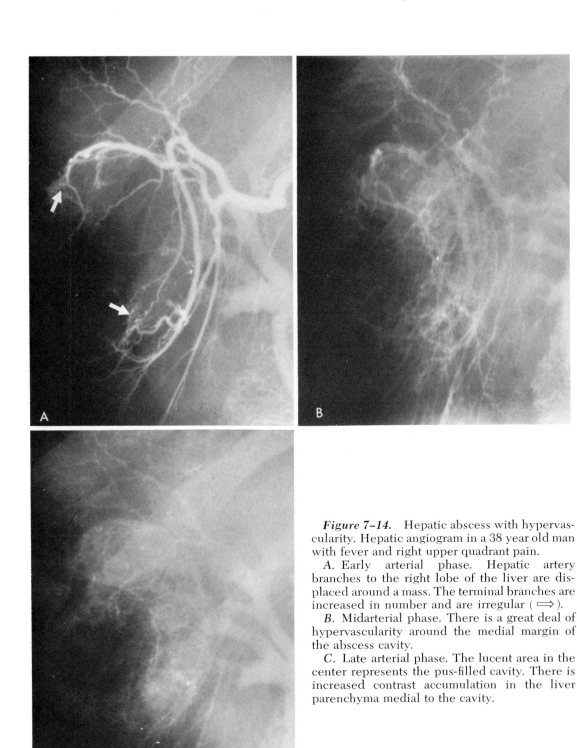

Figure 7–14. Hepatic abscess with hypervascularity. Hepatic angiogram in a 38 year old man with fever and right upper quadrant pain.

A. Early arterial phase. Hepatic artery branches to the right lobe of the liver are displaced around a mass. The terminal branches are increased in number and are irregular (⟹).

B. Midarterial phase. There is a great deal of hypervascularity around the medial margin of the abscess cavity.

C. Late arterial phase. The lucent area in the center represents the pus-filled cavity. There is increased contrast accumulation in the liver parenchyma medial to the cavity.

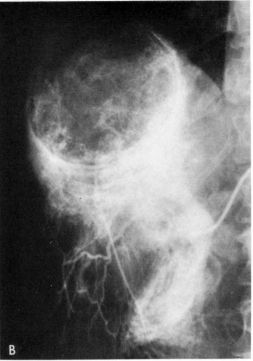

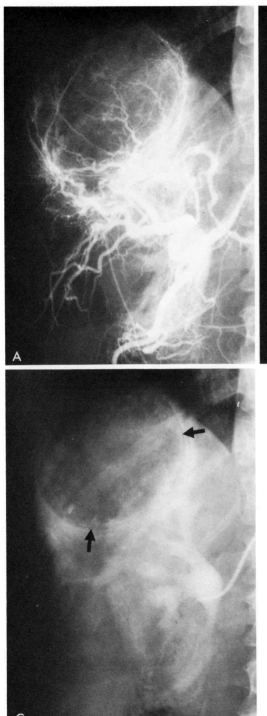

Figure 7–15. Hepatic echinococcal cyst. Hepatic angiogram in a 60 year old woman who had had an echinococcal cyst removed from the right lobe of her liver 2 years previously.

A. Early arterial phase. The hepatic artery branches to the upper lateral portion of the right lobe of the liver are dilated and tortuous and are stretched around a mass.

B. Late arterial phase. A great deal of hypervascularity is present around the rim of the cyst cavity. The terminal arterial branches are tortuous and irregular and have a fuzzy appearance typical of inflammatory vessels.

C. A halo (➡), caused by the wall of the cyst, surrounds the lesion.

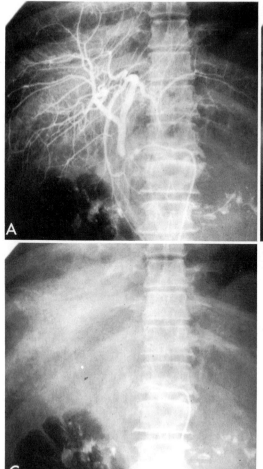

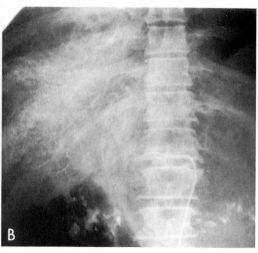

Figure 7-16. Amebic abscesses in the liver. Hepatic angiogram in a 27 year old Mexican farm worker. At operation, amebic abscesses were found in both lobes of the liver.

A. Arterial phase. The intrahepatic arteries are stretched by masses, and the number of small arteries is increased. The left hepatic artery branches are especially displaced.

B. Early hepatogram phase. Contrast medium accumulation and arterial emptying are irregular.

C. Late hepatogram phase. Areas of both decreased and increased contrast medium accumulation are present.

Amebic abscesses of the liver are also low-grade inflammatory processes, which generally cause mass defects at angiography (Fig. 7–16). Arteries and veins are displaced, and a rim of compressed parenchyma surrounds a lucency in the hepatogram phase.

Abscesses in the subphrenic and subhepatic spaces and in contiguous organs can cause angiographic abnormalities in the liver (Fig. 7–17). Adjacent inflammation may cause increased vascularity in the liver with an irregular hepatogram and arteriovenous shunting. Most commonly, however, only a nonspecific increase in fine arterial branches is demonstrated.

Subphrenic abscesses can impress the liver parenchyma, displacing the intrahepatic arteries in a fashion similar to that of a subcapsular hematoma. While such abscesses can be localized by angiography, it is often impossible to tell whether the ab-

scesses are intrahepatic or not. More commonly, subphrenic abscesses cause no hepatic abnormality or only a slight increase in fine arterial branches (Fig. 7–18). Hepatic capsular and inferior phrenic artery branches may dilate and may supply some irregular arteries to the abscess. Angiography can help differentiate a subphrenic abscess from pulmonary or pleural empyema if the abscess lies below the inferior phrenic artery branches in more than one projection. Ultrasound and computed tomography have replaced angiography in the evaluation of most perihepatic abscesses.

Serum and Infectious Hepatitis

Reports of the use of angiography in hepatitis are few. We have examined one patient for right upper quadrant pain fol-

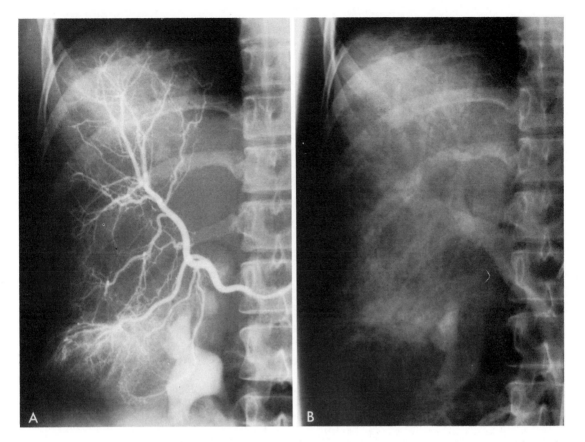

Figure 7-17. Infrahepatic abscess. Right hepatic arteriogram in a 29 year old woman with a right upper quadrant mass and right lower quadrant pain.

A. Arterial phase. There is a great deal of hypervascularity in the inferior portion of the right lobe of the liver and the bed of the gallbladder. The arteries have the tortuous, fuzzy appearance of inflammatory vessels.

B. Venous phase. There is a diffuse, fine, irregularly increased contrast accumulation in the region of the hypervascularity.

At operation an abscess was found that involved the bed of the gallbladder, the inferior portion of the right lobe of the liver and the hepatic flexure of the colon.

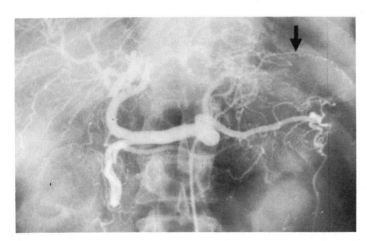

Figure 7-18. Subphrenic abscess. Celiac angiogram in a 45 year old man who developed a left subphrenic abscess 3 weeks after a splenectomy was performed for trauma. Two days after the angiogram, more than 1000 cc of pus was drained from the left subphrenic space. The splenic artery is small. The left inferior phrenic artery (➡) gives off a few irregular, fine branches. Some fine, irregular arteries are present in the left upper quadrant, and the left gastric artery branches are displaced.

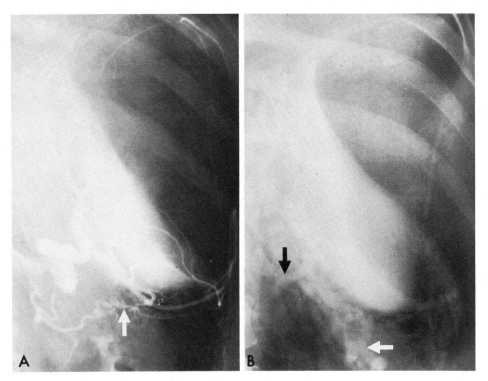

Figure 7–19. Splenic abscess. Splenic angiogram in a 32 year old man.

A. Arterial phase. The splenic artery is compressed to the right, and the capsular branches surround an avascular mass. The splenic parenchyma is compressed medially. Some distorted, tortuous arteries (⇨) are seen at the lower pole of the spleen.

B. Venous phase. The splenic vein (➡) is markedly narrowed, and collateral veins (⇨) are present along the medial border of the spleen. The abnormal arteries and venous compromise do not occur in subcapsular hematoma, which this case closely resembles.

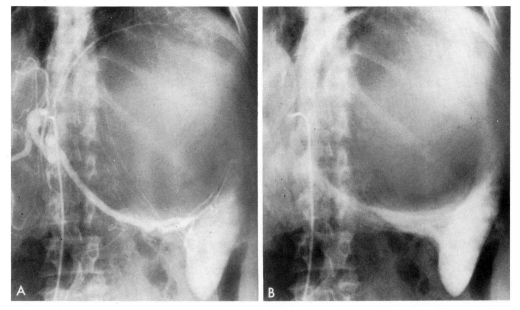

Figure 7–20. Echinococcal cyst of the spleen. Celiac angiogram in a 21 year old man with a left upper quadrant mass.

A. Arterial phase. The splenic artery is bowed caudally, and the left gastric artery is displaced cephalad by an avascular mass which displaces the spleen inferiorly.

B. Parenchymal phase. The splenic parenchyma is somewhat distorted by the large mass, which has a moderately dense wall of compressed parenchyma in some areas. A hydatid cyst was found at surgery. (Courtesy of Dr. Ghassan Rizk. From Rizk, G. K., Tayyarah, K. A., and Ghandur-Mnaymneh, L.: The angiographic changes in hydatid cysts of the liver and spleen. Radiology 99:303, 1971.)

lowing an automobile accident who developed classical infectious hepatitis 2 days later. The angiogram was normal in all respects. A second patient studied during the acute stage of hepatitis had a hypervascular liver with slowed arterial emptying and a very dense, irregular parenchymal phase. Evans (1964) reports stretching of intrahepatic arteries in hepatitis with attenuation of the peripheral arterial branches. Angiography in a patient with chronic active hepatitis revealed diffuse increased vascularity, especially of fine vessels, with some tortuosity of the peripheral arteries.

SPLENIC ABSCESSES

Splenic abscesses may occur secondary to hematogenous spread of acute bacterial pathogens, following trauma or secondary to indolent pathogens such as *Entamoeba*. Abscesses from all these causes have a similar angiographic appearance. An avascular mass with little or no arterial supply displaces and compresses the splenic parenchyma, often with an appearance similar to that seen in subcapsular hematoma (Fig. 7–19). The spleen is generally enlarged. Evidence of inflammation with increased arterial supply and some irregular arteries may

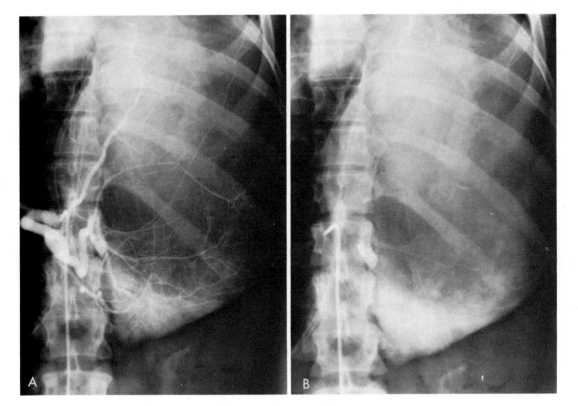

Figure 7–21. Splenic abscess. Celiac angiogram in a 26 year old heroin addict with a left upper quadrant mass and fever.

A. Arterial phase. The area of the spleen is markedly enlarged, the main splenic artery is displaced medially and the intrasplenic arterial branches are displaced around an avascular mass.

B. Parenchymal phase. The residual normal splenic parenchyma can be seen inferiorly. The large intrasplenic mass is relatively avascular. This appearance is difficult to differentiate from that caused by a cyst.

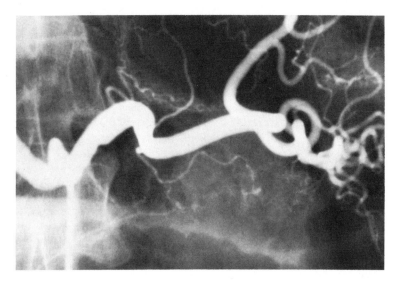

Figure 7–22. Celiac angiogram in a 37 year old woman with chronic pancreatitis. The pancreatica magna artery is mildly irregular, as are its branches through the tail of the pancreas. This nonspecific irregularity of the intrapancreatic arteries is frequently seen in patients with chronic pancreatitis. (From Reuter, S. R., Redman, H. C., and Joseph, R. R.: Angiographic findings in pancreatitis. Amer. J. Roentgenol. *107*:56, 1969.)

be present adjacent to the spleen. The splenic vein may be narrowed, occluded or have an irregular caliber. The omentum may migrate to the left upper quadrant, and the epiploic arteries may dilate. Splenic abscesses may also be intrasplenic, displacing splenic arteries and parenchyma (Figs. 7–20 and 7–21). Ultrasound, computed tomography and isotopic scans have generally replaced angiography in the evaluation of patients with suspected splenic abscesses.

INFLAMMATORY DISEASE OF THE PANCREAS

Pancreatitis

Pancreatitis is usually an easy clinical diagnosis, and angiography is rarely used as a primary diagnostic procedure. Angiography has a central role in the diagnosis of pancreatic carcinoma, however, and the changes of pancreatitis must be known and recognized so that pancreatitis and carcinoma can be differentiated.

Angiographic abnormalities in pancreatitis are related to the duration and severity of the disease. Abnormal findings are generally minimal and nonspecific in patients who have had the disease less than 2 years. The initial attack of acute pancreatitis usually has no specific abnormal angiographic findings. If the pancreas is edematous and swollen, the area covered by the pancreatic branches may appear increased. Occasionally, the pancreaticoduodenal arcades are widened or appear slightly stretched. In general, however, evaluation of changes in shape and size of the pancreas is difficult unless there is associated hypervascularity. The increased parenchymal accumulation of contrast medium accompanying hypervascularity makes evaluation of size easier. Patients with hemorrhagic pancreatitis and pancreatic necrosis can have an entirely normal angiogram.

If the disease becomes recurrent, the early angiographic abnormalities are nonspecific, minor arterial irregularities of the intrapancreatic branches (Fig. 7–22). These irregularities suggest atherosclerosis. Prominent hypervascularity also occurs, manifested by both an increased number of arterial branches in part or all of the pancreas (Fig. 7–23) and an increased parenchymal accumulation of contrast medium in the capillary phase. Arteriovenous shunting sometimes accompanies this hypervascularity.

If the disease has been present for a long time, the angiographic changes of chronic pancreatitis ensue. A specific change in the major intrapancreatic arteries and their branches is a beaded appearance, with short, dilated segments alternating with normal or narrowed segments (Fig. 7–24). The range in severity of this abnormality is wide; however, in our experience it is specific for pancreatitis. The irregular arterial contour may be due to repeated attacks on the vascular wall by pancreatic enzymes,

which weaken the vessel, or to perivascular fibrosis. The recurrent release of pancreatic enzymes may also account for the increased incidence of aneurysms on arteries around the pancreas (Fig. 7–25; also see Fig. 3–24) (Boijsen, 1969).

The major vessels around the pancreas may be involved by long-standing pancreatitis. The splenic artery is particularly susceptible to pancreatitis, and a sleevelike narrowing of the splenic artery may occur (Fig. 7–26). The sleeving or cuffing may appear similar to that seen in atherosclerosis; however, in pancreatitis the splenic artery is straight and narrowed, while in atherosclerosis it is generally tortuous and irregularly narrowed. Encasement by carcinoma may also cause a similar sleeving-type deformity, but usually only a short segment is involved. Therefore, a long, smooth narrowing of the splenic artery in the presence of other signs of pancreatitis is supportive evidence for this diagnosis.

Differentiation of a typical, beaded configuration of pancreatic arteries in chronic pancreatitis from arterial changes caused by carcinoma of the pancreas is important (see Fig. 4–1). The major differentiating factors follow. First, the courses of the involved arteries remain relatively unchanged in pancreatitis. Most pancreatic arteries have a gently undulating course through the pancreas, and this is unaltered by pancreatitis. In contrast, carcinoma of the pancreas usually changes the arterial course, causing abrupt angulations and distortions. However, fibrosis accompanying long-standing pancreatitis rarely results in abrupt angulation of pancreatic arteries, and these changes appear very similar to carcinoma (Fig. 7–27). Second, the changes in arterial caliber in chronic pancreatitis are smooth and even, while those in carcinoma tend to be irregular and jagged. Third, the characteristic arterial changes in pancreatitis tend to be accompanied by an increased number of arterial branches, while in carcinoma the overall vascularity tends to be decreased. Finally, the angiographic abnormalities in pancreatitis are more generalized, while the changes in carcinoma tend to occur in localized areas of the pancreas. Using these criteria one can generally differentiate between pancreatitis and carcinoma.

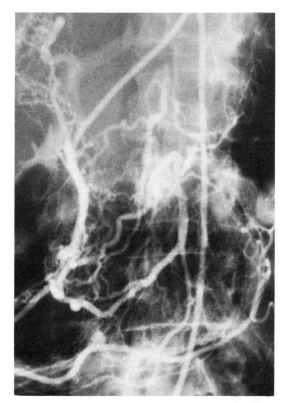

Figure 7–23. Hypervascularity in pancreatitis. Gastroduodenal angiogram in a 47 year old woman with chronic pancreatitis. The pancreaticoduodenal arcades and their branches are dilated, and the number of arterial branches through the head of the pancreas is increased.

Text continued on page 295

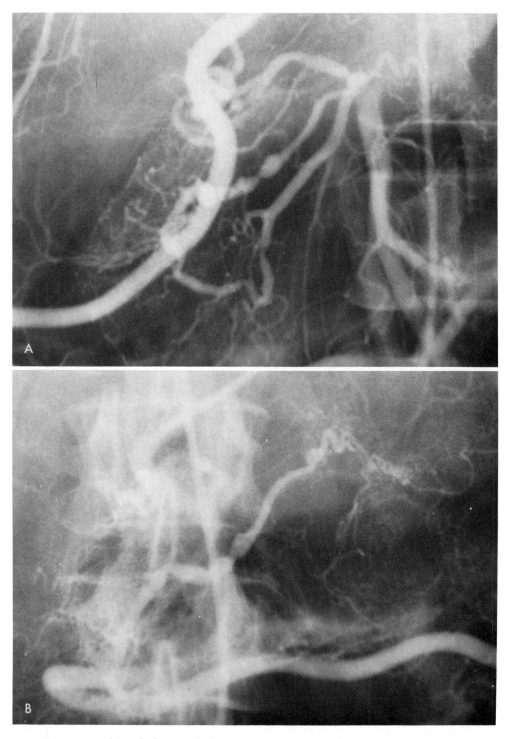

Figure 7-24. Typical beaded arterial changes of pancreatitis. Gastroduodenal angiogram in a 49 year old man with chronic, relapsing pancreatitis.

A. Early arterial phase. The pancreaticoduodenal arcades are markedly dilated and beaded. Aneurysmal dilatations are present along the course of these vessels.

B. Late arterial phase. The transverse pancreatic artery is filled with contrast medium, revealing similar aneurysmal dilatations.

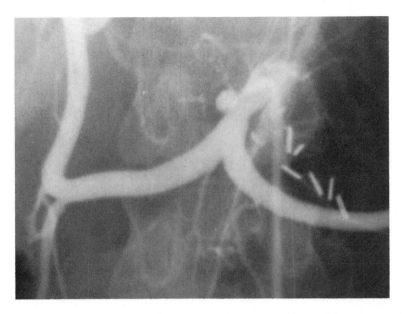

Figure 7–25. Celiac artery aneurysm. Celiac angiogram in a 40 year old woman with chronic pancreatitis. A saccular aneurysm 3 mm in diameter arises from the proximal celiac artery.

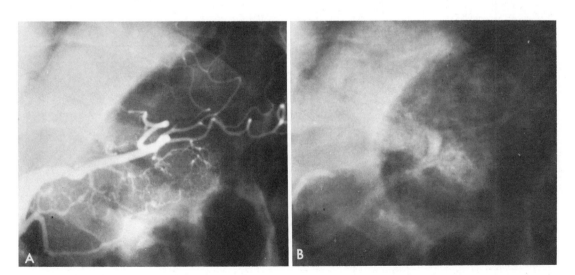

Figure 7–26. Chronic pancreatitis with typical arterial changes. Splenic angiogram in a 40 year old man with long-standing pancreatitis and alcoholism.

A. Arterial phase. The splenic artery is smoothly narrowed shortly after its origin, a finding which has been called cuffing or sleeving. This is nonspecific and may also be caused by atherosclerosis or neoplasm. The arteries to the tail of the pancreas show several smooth constrictions and dilatations without distortion of their course. This change is characteristic of chronic pancreatitis but is present in less than 50 per cent of cases.

B. Venous phase. The splenic vein is moderately narrowed. (From Reuter, S. R., Redman, H. C., and Joseph, R. R.: Angiographic findings in pancreatitis. Amer. J. Roentgenol. *107*:56, 1969; and reprinted from CRC Critical Reviews in Radiological Sciences, *1*, pg. 304, 1970, with permission.)

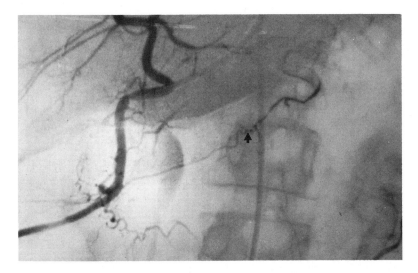

Figure 7–27. Chronic pancreatitis simulating neoplastic encasement. Gastroduodenal angiogram in a 50 year old woman with chronic pancreatitis. An anastomotic branch from the anterior pancreaticoduodenal arcade to the dorsal pancreatic artery is abruptly angulated at its midportion (➡), and is associated with alterations in caliber. These findings mimic those caused by carcinoma of the pancreas. (From Reuter, S. R., Redman, H. C., and Bookstein, J. J.: Differential problems in the angiographic diagnosis of carcinoma of the pancreas. Radiology 96:93, 1970.)

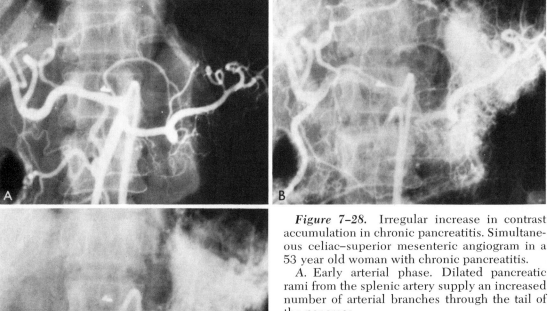

Figure 7–28. Irregular increase in contrast accumulation in chronic pancreatitis. Simultaneous celiac–superior mesenteric angiogram in a 53 year old woman with chronic pancreatitis.

A. Early arterial phase. Dilated pancreatic rami from the splenic artery supply an increased number of arterial branches through the tail of the pancreas.

B. Late arterial phase. Contrast accumulation throughout the tail of the pancreas is increased and has a mottled, irregular appearance.

C. Venous phase. The mottled, irregularly increased contrast accumulation can be better visualized. The splenic vein appears slightly stretched.

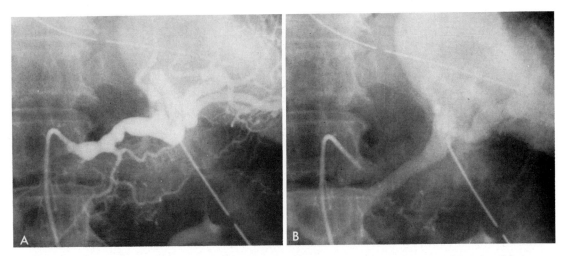

Figure 7–29. Splenic vein narrowing in pancreatitis. Splenic angiogram in a 68 year old man.

A. Arterial phase. The narrowings in the proximal splenic artery are caused by catheter spasm. The dorsal pancreatic artery is slightly dilated and supplies dilated branches through the tail of the pancreas.

B. Venous phase. The splenic vein is slightly narrowed as it passes over the tail of the pancreas.

In long-standing pancreatitis, the patchy fibrosis which occurs throughout the pancreas results in an unhomogeneous accumulation of contrast medium (Fig. 7–28). If the fibrosis is diffuse enough, both the number of pancreatic arteries and the parenchymal accumulation of contrast medium are decreased.

The splenic and superior mesenteric veins may be narrowed or may have luminal irregularities in long-standing pancreatitis (Fig. 7–29). The splenic vein is not infrequently occluded, and epiploic collateral veins from the spleen bypass the occlusion (Fig. 7–30). Demonstration of these veins can be enhanced by vasodilatory pharmacoangiography and the subtraction technique.

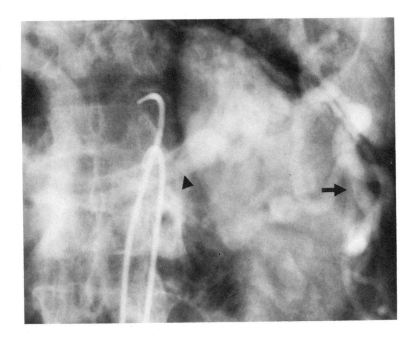

Figure 7–30. Splenic vein occlusion in chronic pancreatitis. Venous phase of a simultaneous celiac-superior mesenteric angiogram in a 76 year old woman with long-standing chronic pancreatitis. The splenic vein is occluded in the splenic hilus. Collateral veins run caudally (➡) to the systemic venous system in the abdominal wall and also run medially (▶) to the gastroepiploic vein, which flows directly into the portal vein. Some smaller collateral veins run superiorly and enter the portal system through the left gastric vein.

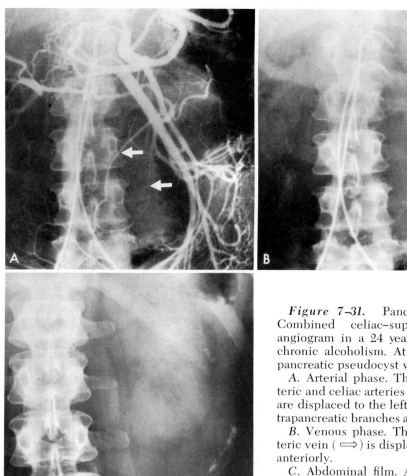

Figure 7–31. Pancreatic pseudocyst. Combined celiac–superior mesenteric angiogram in a 24 year old woman with chronic alcoholism. At operation a large pancreatic pseudocyst was found.

A. Arterial phase. The superior mesenteric and celiac arteries and their branches are displaced to the left and anteriorly. Intrapancreatic branches are stretched (⟹).

B. Venous phase. The superior mesenteric vein (⟹) is displaced to the left and anteriorly.

C. Abdominal film. A left upper quadrant mass with calcification is present.

Pancreatic Pseudocyst

Pancreatic pseudocysts can develop in patients with pancreatitis or may be secondary to abdominal trauma. The angiographic appearances in these two instances are similar. The primary angiographic abnormality in a pseudocyst is stretching of the arteries around the lesion (Fig. 7–31). A significant degree of stretching of an intrapancreatic artery is fairly specific for cyst formation and is rarely seen in carcinoma or pancreatitis without a cyst. Which vessels are stretched depend upon the size and position of the cyst. Small cysts displace only the intrapancreatic branches (Fig. 7–32; also see Fig. 5–28), but large cysts may displace the splenic, hepatic, gastroduodenal and mesenteric arteries. The angiogram may be normal, even in patients with moderate-sized cysts, if the cyst is anterior and exophytic. The splenic artery in particular is frequently spared (Fig. 7–33). In the capillary phase, contrast accumulation in the cyst is absent, causing a filling defect in the pancreaticogram. Large cysts in the body and tail of the pancreas can occlude the splenic vein, and collateral venous channels are then demonstrated. Extra care should be taken to demonstrate the splenic vein when pseudocysts are suspected. Cysts rarely erode into arteries within the pancreas and fill with blood, simulating aneurysms (Figs. 7–34 and 7–35). Massive hemorrhage may occur when larger cysts erode arteries (Fig. 7–36). The angiographic changes of chronic pancreatitis frequently accompany pancreatic pseudocysts. The primary differential problem in the angiographic diagnosis of pancreatic pseudocyst is an atypical, avascular cystadenoma, which rarely may mimic a pseudocyst.

The primary diagnostic methods in patients with suspected pancreatic pseudocysts should be ultrasound or computed tomography, not only because they are noninvasive but also because angiograms are normal in a significant number of patients with pseudocysts.

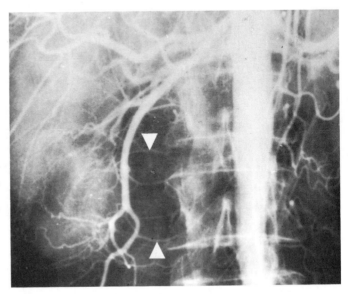

Figure 7–32. Small pancreatic pseudocyst. Celiac angiogram in a 54 year old woman with gastric outlet obstruction. Gastroduodenal arterial branches to the duodenum are prominent, owing to inflammatory response. The posterior and anterior pancreaticoduodenal arcades and all their branches (▷) are stretched and bowed around an avascular mass in the head of the pancreas. At autopsy, an 8 cm pancreatic pseudocyst was found.

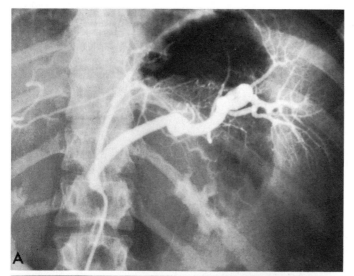

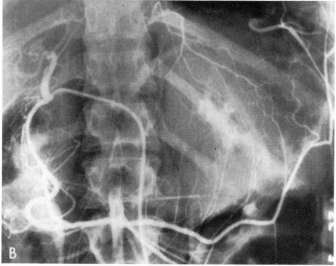

Figure 7–33. Pancreatic pseudocyst. Angiography in a 22 year old woman with alcoholism who complained of abdominal swelling. A pancreatic pseudocyst containing more than 1500 cc of fluid was found at exploration.

A. Arterial phase of a splenic angiogram. The splenic artery shows no definite abnormality, but the left gastric artery is elevated and bowed. The splenic vein was normal.

B. Arterial phase of a gastroduodenal angiogram. The gastroduodenal artery is displaced to the right, and the branches of the right gastroepiploic artery to the stomach are stretched. No angiographic abnormality is present in the few intrapancreatic arteries filled with contrast medium.

Figure 7–34. Small pancreatic pseudocysts communicating with intrapancreatic arteries. Combined celiac–superior mesenteric angiogram in a 33 year old man with chronic pancreatitis. Small, round collections of contrast medium ($\Longrightarrow$) are seen in the tail of the pancreas. The operative specimen contained many small cysts, some in communication with arteries and others in communication with the duct of Wirsung. (From Reuter, S. R., Redman, H. C., and Joseph, R. R.: Angiographic findings in pancreatitis. Amer. J. Roentgenol. 97:56, 1969.)

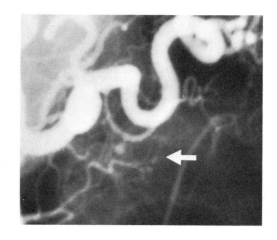

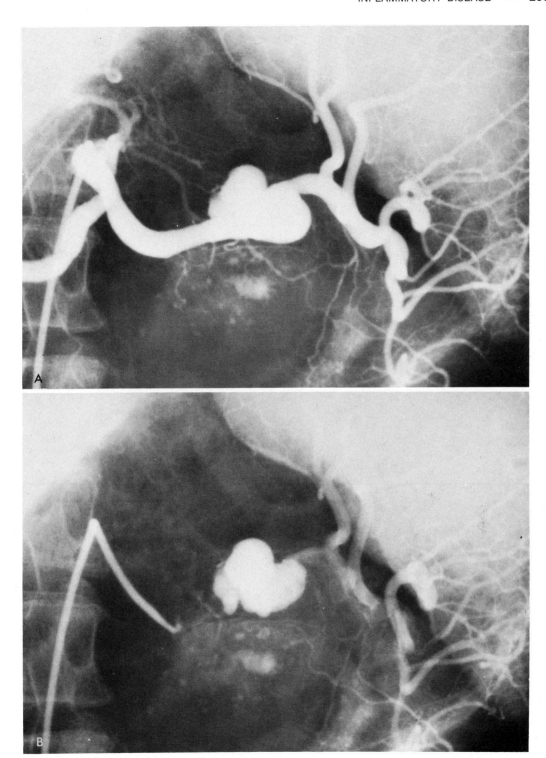

Figure 7-35. Bleeding into a pseudocyst in chronic pancreatitis. Celiac angiogram in a 59 year old man.

A. Early arterial phase. A pseudoaneurysm representing the pseudocyst fills with contrast medium from the midsplenic artery. The pancreatic rami through the tail of the pancreas have the nonspecific arterial irregularities seen in pancreatitis. Some calcifications are present.

B. Late arterial phase. The pseudocyst retains the contrast medium as the splenic artery empties. The findings were confirmed at operation.

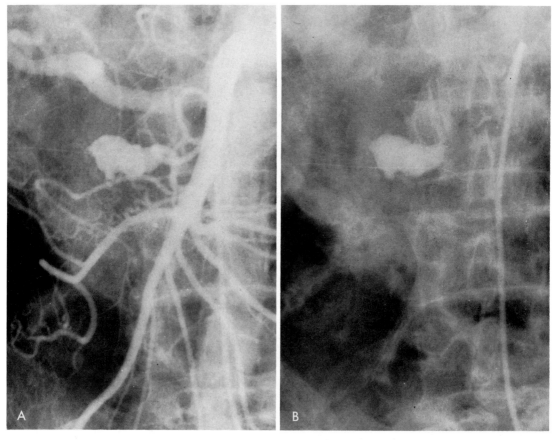

Figure 7–36. Pancreatic pseudocyst causing massive upper gastrointestinal bleeding. Superior mesenteric angiogram in a 68 year old man with chronic pancreatitis and upper gastrointestinal bleeding.

A. Arterial phase. Contrast medium fills a pseudocyst from a branch of the inferior pancreaticoduodenal artery.

B. Parenchymal phase. The contrast medium remains in the pseudocyst. At operation, the pseudocyst was found in the region of the uncinate process. The cyst did not communicate directly with the duodenum; however, the blood reached the duodenum through the duct of Wirsung.

INTRAPERITONEAL ABSCESSES

Abscesses may occur anywhere within the peritoneal cavity. These occur following bowel perforation, secondary to pelvic or other abscesses, following trauma and as complications of surgery. Hematogenous spread generally involves solid organs, such as the liver and the spleen. The majority of intraperitoneal abscesses are caused by acute pathogens; however, abscesses can be due to *Mycobacterium tuberculosis, Entamoeba, Echinococcus* or other indolent pathogens.

A wide range of angiographic abnormalities similar to changes seen with other in-flammatory processes occur with these abscesses. The simplest changes are those of an avascular mass (Fig. 7–37). While a 2 to 3 cm in diameter abscess in a solid organ may displace arteries and cause a defect in the parenchymal phase, avascular abscesses in the mesentery, omentum, subphrenic space or lesser sac must be larger to cause enough arterial displacement to be recognized. Clinical history may help to distinguish an avascular abscess from cysts or metastatic neoplasm.

When an abscess has a more prominent inflammatory component, vascularity is often increased. Arterial supply to the region may be dilated, and omental arteries

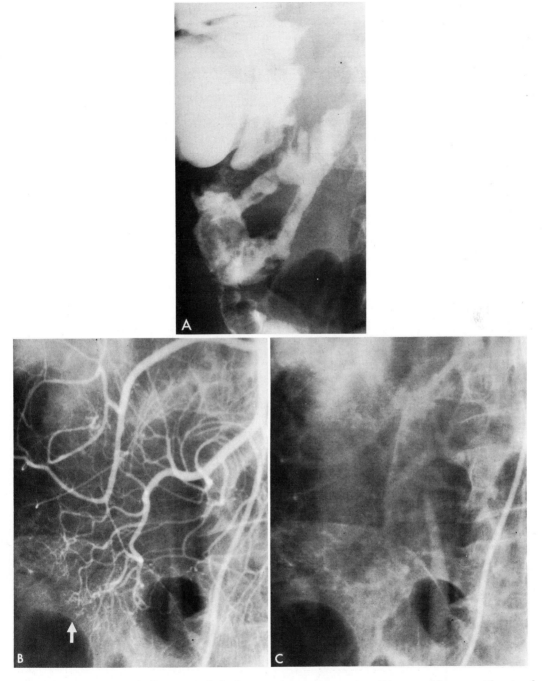

Figure 7–37. Pericecal abscess with little vascular response in a 74 year old man with a tender right lower quadrant mass. At operation a small pericecal abscess with many adhesions and adherent omentum was found.

A. Barium enema demonstrates a distorted and irritable medial cecal wall with reflux into abnormal small bowel.

B. Superior mesenteric angiogram. A few, fine, irregular arteries (⟹) are present in the cecum. Some of the ileal branches of the ileocolic artery have an unusual course, suggesting adhesions.

C. Venous phase. No early or dense veins or increase in contrast medium accumulation is seen near the lesion.

supply the abscess (Fig. 7–38). Small, irregular arteries may be present around the periphery of the abscess. With the increased arterial supply, a parenchymal accumulation of contrast medium often surrounds the abscess. Early, dense venous drainage can also accompany increased vascularity. When vascular response is prominent, differentiation from vascular metastases may be difficult.

Abscesses in the omentum and mesentery are especially hard to demonstrate by angiography. Displacement of arteries is hard to detect since the positions of these vessels are variable normally. A minimal increase in arterial supply with fixed, distorted arteries and minimal inflammatory response is frequently all that is present. Omentum may migrate to the area, taking along the epiploic arteries, which may be dilated.

Intraperitoneal adhesions can sometimes be detected by angiography (Fig. 7–39). The mesenteric branches to the small bowel and colon may be distorted and fixed in position, and the vasa recta may be markedly angled in an abnormal or unusual position. Parenchymal contrast medium accumulation and venous drainage are usually normal. The vasa recta to the obstructed bowel are stretched and distended. An uncommon disease, chronic sclerosing fibrinous peritonitis, causes thickening and shortening of the mesentery. At angiography, the mesenteric vessels are markedly tortuous and shortened (Fig. 7–40). While the vascularity appears to be increased overall, this appearance is caused by contraction of the mesenteric arterial branches, and no true neovascularity occurs. The vasa recta are normal unless fibrosis has led to small bowel obstruction. The angiographic appearance of chronic sclerosing fibrinous peritonitis is similar to that of a carcinoid tumor or pancreatic carcinoma invading the mesentery.

As has been noted frequently throughout this chapter, noninvasive methods have replaced angiography for evaluation of patients with suspected abscesses. Ultrasound and computed tomography should be the primary, and generally the only, special procedures to be used. The angiographic findings in inflammatory diseases are important primarily because of problems they cause in the differential diagnosis of carcinomas.

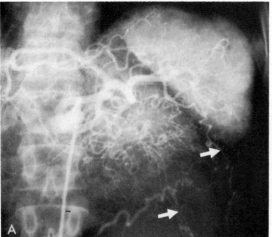 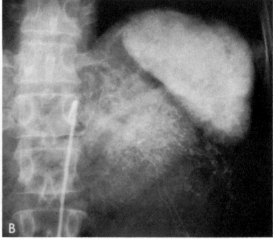

Figure 7–38. Omental abscess. Celiac angiogram in a 42 year old woman with fever and a left upper quadrant mass. At operation a clostridial omental abscess was found.

A. Midarterial phase. Dilated, irregular, tortuous anterior epiploic and omental arteries (⟹) from both the right and left gastroepiploic arteries supply the left upper quadrant mass.

B. Late arterial phase. Contrast accumulation in the mass is not particularly increased, and no early venous drainage is seen.

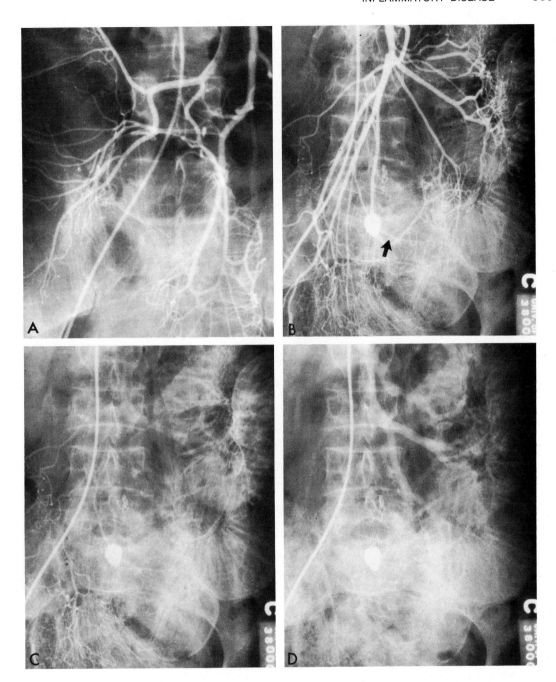

Figure 7–39. Adhesions.

A. Superior mesenteric angiogram in a 43 year old man with small bowel obstruction from adhesions. The patient had had two operations for lysis of adhesions following appendectomy for a ruptured appendix. Arterial phase. The distal ileal arteries are angled and displaced to the patient's left. The vasa recta are stretched and distorted.

B. Superior mesenteric angiogram in a 52 year old woman with diffuse abdominal pain and suspected mesenteric infarction. Abdominal films showed no abnormalities. At operation, adhesions obstructing the ileum were found. Arterial phase. The ileal arteries are displaced to the right and the vasa recta to the jejunum are stretched and spread. A distal ileal branch is abruptly angulated cephalad (➡). Beyond the angulation, the bowel is not distended.

C. Late arterial phase. The jejunal loops are dilated, accumulation of contrast medium in the bowel wall is increased and there is early venous drainage.

D. Venous phase. Venous drainage from the jejunum is prominent.

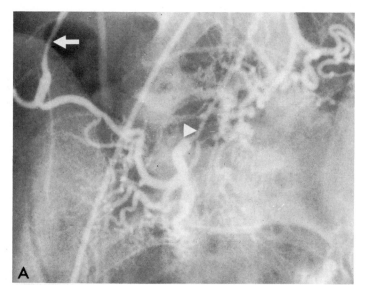

Figure 7–40. Chronic sclerosing fibrinous peritonitis. Superselective distal superior mesenteric angiogram in a 52 year old man admitted for evaluation of progressive bowel obstruction. The patient had had peritonitis and wound dehiscence following a partial gastrectomy. At operation, the bowel was encased in a thick, fibrinous material.

A. The mesenteric branches form an accordion pattern, but the vasa recta are normal. Catheter spasm (▷) has narrowed one artery, but another (⇒) was narrowed by the fibrotic process.

B. Small bowel series. A mass impression is present against the cecum. There are several nodular defects impressing the small bowel.

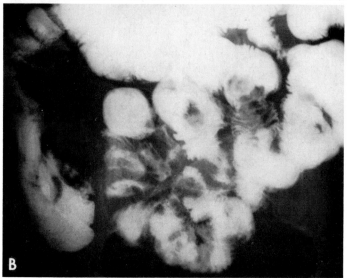

BIBLIOGRAPHY

Aakhus, T., Hofsli, M., and Vestad, E.: Angiography in acute pancreatitis. Acta Radiol., 8:119, 1969.

Alfidi, R. J., Rastogi, H., Buonocore, E., et al.: Hepatic arteriography. Radiology, 90:1136, 1968.

Baltaxe, H. A., and Fleming, R. J.: The angiographic appearance of hydatid disease. Radiology 97:599, 1970.

Boijsen, E.: Angiographic diagnosis of pancreatic disease. T. Gastroent. 12:219, 1969.

Boijsen, E., and Olin, T.: Zöliakographie und Angiographie der Arteria Mesenterica superior. Ergebn. Med. Strahlenforsch. 1:112, 1964.

Boijsen, E., and Reuter, S. R.: Mesenteric angiography in the evaluation of inflammatory and neoplastic disease of the intestine. Radiology 87:1028, 1966.

Boijsen, E., and Tylén, U.: Vascular changes in chronic pancreatitis. Acta Radiol. 12:34, 1972.

Boijsen, E., Göthlin, J., Hallböök, T., et al.: Preoperative angiographic diagnosis of bleeding aneurysms of abdominal visceral arteries. Radiology 93:781, 1969.

Bosniak, M. A., and Phanthumachinda, P.: Value of arteriography in the study of hepatic disease. Amer. J. Surg. 112:348, 1966.

Bradley, E. L., and Clements, J. L.: Implications of diagnostic ultrasound in the surgical management of pancreatic pseudocysts. Amer. J. Surg. 127:163, 1974.

Brahme, F.: Mesenteric angiography in regional enterocolitis. Radiology 87:1037, 1966.

Brahme, F., and Hildell, J.: Angiography in Crohn's disease revisited. Amer. J. Roentgenol. 126:941, 1976.

Busson, A., and Hernandez, C.: L'artériographie sélective mésentérique dans la rectocolite hémorragique et la colite ulcéreuse d'emblée. Arch. Mal. Appar. Dig. 54:441, 1965.

Chermet, J., Bigot, J. M., and Monnier, J. P.: Gastrointestinal hemorrhage from arterial erosion in pancreatitis. Preoperative diagnosis by emergency arteriography. J. Radiol. Electrol. Med. Nucl. 35:117, 1974.

Cho, K. J., and Reuter, S. R.: Angiographic assessment of pancreatic pseudocyst: a reappraisal. J. Can. Ass. Radiol. 27:193, 1976.

Dencker, H., Holmdahl, K. H. S., Lunderquist, A., et al.: Mesenteric angiography in patients with radiation injury of the bowel after pelvic irradiation. Amer. J. Roentgenol. 114:476, 1972.

Deutsch, V.: Cholecysto-angiography. Amer. J. Roentgenol. 101:608, 1967.

Deutsch, V., Adar, R., and Mozes, M.: Angiography in the diagnosis of subphrenic abscess. Clin. Radiol. 25:133, 1974.

Dombrowski, H., and Korb, G.: Das Gefässbild bei Enteritis regionalis (Morbus Crohn) und sein diagnostische Bedeutung. Radiologe 10:17, 1970.

Ekelund, L., Lunderquist, A., Dencker, H., et al.: Hepatic angiography in ulcerative colitis and Crohn's disease. Amer. J. Roentgenol. 126:952, 1976.

Evans, J. A.: Specialized roentgen diagnostic technics in the investigation of abdominal disease. Radiology 82:579, 1964.

Friday, R. O., Barriga, P., and Crummy, A. B.: Detection and localization of intra-abdominal abscesses by diagnostic ultrasound. Arch. Surg. 110:335, 1975.

Fu, W.-R., and Stanton, L. W.: Angiographic study of pseudocysts of the pancreas. J. Canad. Ass. Radiol. 20:176, 1969.

Glickman, M. G., and Itzchak, Y.: Angiographic diagnosis of intrinsic duodenal inflammatory disease. Radiology 123:297, 1977.

Hernandez, C.: L'angiographie de l'ileite terminale de Crohn. Actualités Hépatogastroentérol. 4:77, 1968.

Jacobs, J. B., Hammond, W. G., and Doppman, J. L.: Arteriographic localization of suprahepatic abscesses. Radiology 93:1299, 1969.

Jacobs, R. P., Shanser, J. D., Lawson, D. L., et al.: Angiography of splenic abscesses. Amer. J. Roentgenol. 122:419, 1974.

Kadell, B. M., and Riley, J. M.: Major arterial involvement by pancreatic pseudocysts. Amer. J. Roentgenol. 99:632, 1967.

Kuiper, D. H., Papp, J. P., and Thompson, N. W.: Solitary splenic abscess. Mich. Med. 69:293, 1970.

Lomba Viana, R.: Selective arteriography in the diagnosis and evaluation of amebic abscess of the liver. Amer. J. Dig. Dis. 20:632, 1975.

Longstreth, G. F., Newcomer, A. D., and Green, P. A.: Extrahepatic portal hypertension caused by chronic pancreatitis. Ann. Intern. Med. 75:903, 1971.

Lunderquist, A., and Lunderquist, A.: Angiography in ulcerative colitis. Amer. J. Roentgenol. 99:18, 1967.

Lunderquist, A., Lunderquist, A., and Knutsson, H.: Angiography in Crohn's disease of the small bowel and colon. Amer. J. Roentgenol. 101:338, 1967.

McNulty, J. G.: Angiographic manifestations of hydatid disease of the liver. Amer. J. Roentgenol. 102:380, 1968.

Meyers, M. A.: Griffiths' point: Critical anastomosis at the splenic flexure. Significance in ischemia of the colon. Amer. J. Roentgenol. 126:77, 1976.

Nebesar, R. A., and Pollard, J. J.: A critical evaluation of selective celiac and superior mesenteric angiography in the diagnosis of pancreatic diseases, particularly malignant tumor: Facts and "artefacts." Radiology 89:1017, 1967.

Nebesar, R. A., Tefft, M., Bawter, J. F., et al.: Angiography in radiation "hepatitis." Brit. J. Radiol. 47:588, 1974.

Nebesar, R. A., Tefft, M., and Colodny, A. H.: Angiography of liver abscess in granulomatous disease of childhood. Amer. J. Roentgenol. 108:628, 1970.

Phillips, J. F., Cockrill, H., Jorge, E., et al.: Radiographic evlauation of patients with schistosomiasis. Radiology 114:31, 1975.

Pinchuk, L., Debray, C., and Hernandez, C.: La angiografia total en el diagnóstico y tratamiento del quiste hidatidíco de hígado. Pren. Méd. Argent. 54:2085, 1967.

Pollard, J. J., and Nebesar, R. A.: Abdominal angiography. New Eng. J. Med. 279:1093, 1968.

Pollard, J. J., Nebesar, R. A., and Mattoso, L. F.: Angiographic diagnosis of benign diseases of the liver. Radiology 86:276, 1966.

Reuter, S. R., Kanter, I. E., and Redman, H. C.: Angiography in reversible colonic ischemia. Radiology 97:371, 1970.

Reuter, S. R., and Redman, H. C.: Pancreatic angiography. CRC Crit. Rev. Radiol. Sci. 1:287, 1970.

Reuter, S. R., Redman, H. C., and Joseph, R. R.: Angiographic findings in pancreatitis. Amer. J. Roentgenol. 107:56, 1969.

Rizk, G. K., Tayyarah, K. A., and Ghandur-Mnaymneh, L.: The angiographic changes in hydatid cysts of the liver and spleen. Radiology 99:303, 1971.

Roe, M., and Greenough, W. G.: Marked hypervascularity and arteriovenous shunting in acute pancreatitis. Radiology, 113:47, 1974.

Rösch, J., Grollman, J. H., Jr., and Steckel, R. J.: Arteriography in the diagnosis of gallbladder disease. Radiology 92:1485, 1969.

Sato, T., Watanabe, K., Saitoh, Y., et al.: Selective arteriography for gallbladder disease. Arch. Surg. 99:598, 1969.

Smith, S. L., Tutton, R. H., and Ochsner, S. F.: Roentgenographic aspects of intestinal ischemia. Radiology 107:239, 1973.

Tylén, U.: Angiographic differentiation between inflammatory disease and carcinoma of the pancreas. Acta Radiol. (Diagn.) (Stockh.) 14:257, 1973.

Tylén, U., and Arnesjö, B.: Angiographic diagnosis of inflammatory disease of the pancreas. Acta Radiol. (Diagn.) (Stockh.) 14:215, 1973.

Tylén, U., and Dencker, H.: Roentgenologic diagnosis of pancreatitic abscess. Acta Radiol. (Diagn.) (Stockh.) 14:9, 1973.

Viana, R. L.: Selective arteriography in the diagnosis and evaluation of amebic abscess of the liver. Amer. J. Dig. Dis. 20:632, 1975.

Westcott, J. L.: Angiographic demonstration of arterial occlusion in ischemic colitis. Gastroenterology 63:486, 1972.

White, A. F., Baum, S., and Buranasiri, S.: Aneurysms secondary to pancreatitis. Amer. J. Roentgenol. 127:393, 1976.

CIRRHOSIS AND PORTAL HYPERTENSION

The term cirrhosis is applied to diffuse hepatic fibrosis. In this disease, hepatic cellular death, fibrosis and hepatic regeneration occur simultaneously. Several factors may be responsible for the fibrosis. Alcoholism and malnutrition result in diffuse nodular or Laennec's cirrhosis, bile duct obstruction in biliary cirrhosis, schistosomiasis in parasitic cirrhosis, prolonged congestive heart failure in congestive cirrhosis and hepatitis in postnecrotic cirrhosis. From a hemodynamic point of view, the common denominator in all types of cirrhosis is a progressive increase in resistance to portal vein blood flow, resulting in portal hypertension. In turn, the portal hypertension leads to the development of portal–systemic collateral veins and usually to the development of esophageal varices and gastrointestinal hemorrhage. The patient comes to angiography because of hemorrhage, either for elucidation of the cause or for evaluation of the patient's blood flow patterns prior to portacaval shunt surgery. Portal and hepatic vein obstruction also lead to portal hypertension and are, therefore, included in this chapter.

Until recently, the angiographic litera-

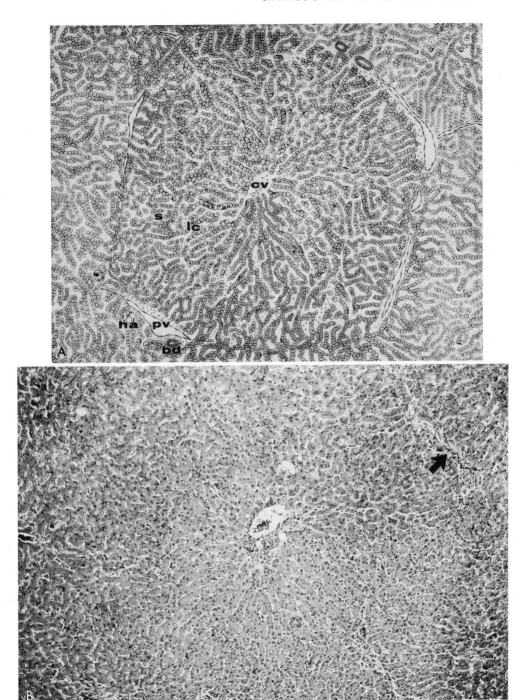

Figure 8–1. Normal hepatic lobule.

A. Line drawing. Sinusoidal spaces (s) and cords of hepatic cells (lc) radiate from the central vein (cv) to the periphery of the hexahedral-shaped lobule. Portal spaces containing a hepatic artery (ha), portal vein (pv), bile ducts (bd) and lymphatics are evenly interspersed around the periphery of the lobule.

B. Histologic appearance of a normal lobule. The central vein can be seen in the center of the picture. Cords of liver cells and sinusoids radiate toward the periphery. A portal space can be recognized in the upper right hand corner (➡).

ture concerning cirrhosis and portal hypertension has been confusing and contradictory. The main problem has been the lack of correlation between the angiographic findings, the hepatic histology and the portal blood flow dynamics. Moreover, several different types of angiographic examinations have been available for evaluation of patients with cirrhosis and portal hypertension. Generally, only one method was used in a given patient, and this has led to a lack of correlation between the findings of the different studies. Only a few investigators, most notably Warren et al. (1967) and Viamonte et al. (1970), have made correlations between the angiographic findings and portal blood flow dynamics and between different types of angiographic examinations in the same patient. Their work has provided a basis for understanding the angiographic abnormalities found in cirrhosis.

HISTOLOGY AND BLOOD FLOW IN THE NORMAL LIVER

The primary functional unit of the liver is the hepatic lobule (Fig. 8–1). The lobule resembles a rough hexahedron. In the middle, the central or intralobular vein drains to the tributaries of the hepatic veins. Cores of cells and hepatic sinusoids are arranged in a radial pattern around the central vein and extend to the periphery of the lobule. Around the periphery at regular intervals are four to five portal spaces, containing a portal vein, hepatic artery, hepatic bile duct and lymphatics. The terminal arterioles of the hepatic artery and the terminal radicles of the portal vein empty into the sinusoids; the mixed hepatic arterial and portal venous blood flows through the sinusoids, past the liver cells, to the central vein. This common drainage of arterial and venous blood into the same space is unique in the body and, as will be discussed later, results in some of the angiographic findings that occur in the cirrhotic patient.

In the normal person, 75 to 80 per cent of the total hepatic blood flow comes from the portal vein; the remainder comes from the hepatic artery (Fig. 8–2A). The supply from these two sources is reciprocal; any reduction in one normally results in an immediate, compensatory increase in the other. Thus, if the portal vein is ligated, hepatic arterial blood flow increases immediately and markedly. The response of portal venous blood flow to a decrease in hepatic arterial blood flow is immediate but much less pronounced. Although the mechanism for this reciprocal relationship is not known, it helps explain the angiographic appearance of dilated hepatic arteries in patients with advanced cirrhosis and decreased portal blood flow.

PATHOLOGIC CHANGES IN CIRRHOSIS AND RESULTING ALTERATIONS IN HEPATIC BLOOD FLOW

Cirrhosis is generally classified as postsinusoidal or presinusoidal, depending on where the primary block to blood flow lies. Laennec's, congestive and postnecrotic cirrhosis cause postsinusoidal blocks. Presinusoidal cirrhosis is caused by schistosomiasis and occasionally by reticuloendothelial tumors, viral hepatitis and chronic biliary tract obstruction. From an angiographic point of view, portal vein thrombosis can also be considered a presinusoidal, and hepatic vein thrombosis, a postsinusoidal block. This division is convenient for explaining the different hemodynamic and angiographic findings in the two types of block. It should be remembered, however, that the massive fibrosis, cellular death and regenerating liver cells in end stage cirrhosis cause severe aberrations in all the hepatic blood vessels.

Postsinusoidal Cirrhosis

Another look at Figure 8–1 reveals the precarious position of the sinusoids and central veins, surrounded as they are by liver cells. As hepatic cells die in patients with cirrhosis, they are replaced by fibrosis, fat and irregularly arranged regenerating cells. The fibrotic process occurs early and relatively equally in lobules, portal spaces and central veins, but the first of the hepatic vessels to be affected are the vulnerable sinusoids (Fig. 8–3). Fibrotic replacement of sinusoids and distortion of

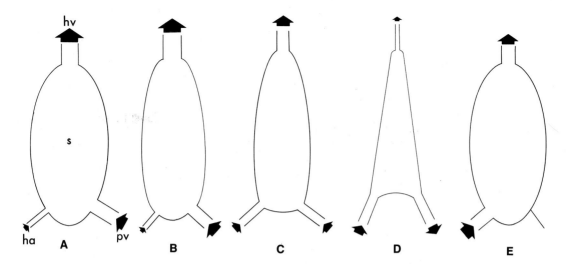

Figure 8-2. Hemodynamic changes accompanying cirrhosis.

A. Normal liver. Seventy-five to 80 per cent of the blood in the sinusoids (**s**) comes from the portal vein (**pv**); the remainder comes from the hepatic artery (**ha**). Blood in the sinusoids bathes the hepatic cells and leaves the liver via the central veins to the hepatic veins (**hv**).

B. Early cirrhosis (Stage I). Sinusoidal volume is restricted by fibrosis, and the central veins become distorted. The portal pressure elevates, and portal blood flow is maintained. The ratio of portal vein to hepatic artery blood flow is not yet altered.

C. Moderate to severe cirrhosis (Stage II). Further fibrosis leads to further restriction of sinusoidal volume and results in obliteration of central veins and hepatic venules. Resistance to the flow of portal vein blood through the liver becomes greater than resistance through portal-systemic collateral veins, and blood is diverted from the portal system. As portal flow through the liver decreases, hepatic artery flow increases.

D. Advanced cirrhosis (Stage III). Fibrosis has obliterated many central veins and hepatic venules; regenerating nodules have distorted larger hepatic venules. Resistance to flow through these veins is so great that the hepatic artery blood entering the markedly restricted sinusoids exits via the portal vein radicles. The liver becomes totally dependent on arterial blood supply.

E. Portal vein thrombosis. Portal blood flow ceases without a decrease in sinusoidal volume or increased resistance to hepatic venous drainage. The hepatic artery dilates markedly as it takes over the complete hepatic blood flow.

central veins cause an increased resistance to blood flow through the liver. In the early stages of cirrhosis, when the fibrosis is not yet severe, an increased portal pressure overcomes the increased resistance to outflow, and portal venous flow through the liver is maintained (Fig. 8–2B). Progressive fibrosis and increasing resistance for hepatic venous flow are compensated for by increasing portal venous pressure. At some stage along this progressive course, however, the resistance to flow through the several small communicating channels between the portal system and the systemic veins becomes equal to resistance through the liver. At this point, portal–systemic collateral veins begin to develop, and portal venous blood is diverted from the liver.

Once portal venous blood is diverted through the portal–systemic collateral veins, the portal pressure no longer correlates with the degree of hepatic fibrosis but is dependent upon the effectiveness of the collateral veins in decompressing the portal system.

Until the development of portal–systemic collateral veins (or "hepatofugal" collaterals, since they take flow away from the liver), arterial perfusion of the liver continues essentially unchanged. Once portal venous blood is diverted from the liver, the hepatic arterial blood flow increases compensatively (Fig. 8–2C). However, it never compensates completely for the decrease in portal venous flow, and total hepatic blood flow is decreased.

Although fibrosis of the portal spaces occurs early in cirrhosis, portal vein radicles and hepatic arteries are relatively protected from compression compared with the sinusoids and central veins. In advanced stages of the cirrhotic process, however, fibrotic distortion of the distal portal vein radicles accentuates the resistance to portal blood flow through the liver, and even more blood is diverted through the portal–systemic collateral veins. Finally, even the hepatic arteries are distorted by portal fibrosis.

In the end stages of cirrhosis, resistance to drainage of hepatic blood flow through the distorted, fibrosed sinusoids and hepatic veins becomes so great that the hepatic arterial flow to the liver is drained by the valveless portal vein. Thus, the portal vein is converted to an outflow tract (Fig. 8–2D). This progression is gradual, and, for a time, blood flow in the portal vein is to and fro; however, eventually it reverses, and both the portal venous flow and the hepatic arterial flow drain through the portal–systemic collateral veins. When this occurs, the portal pressure still depends upon the effectiveness of the portal–systemic collateral veins in decompressing the system, but the pressure is generally very high.

The reversal of blood flow in the portal vein signals the onset of very advanced cirrhosis. In this stage, the continued functioning of the liver is dependent entirely upon hepatic arterial blood flow. Unfortunately, this is one of the remaining unclear areas in the pathogenesis of hepatic cirrhosis. As mentioned earlier, hepatic arterial blood flow increases reciprocally when portal flow decreases, and all patients with advanced cirrhosis have some degree of increased arterial blood flow. Some patients have a marked increase and others a moderate increase. The degree of increase probably depends in part on the extent of fibrosis around the terminal arterioles and in

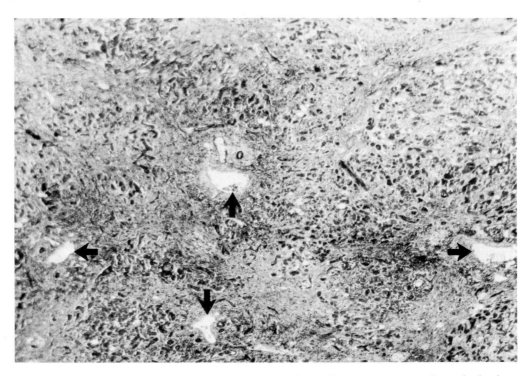

Figure 8–3. Histologic appearance of cirrhosis. Wide cords of fibrosis run through the liver, replacing sinusoids and hepatic cells. The fibrosis has divided lobules into pseudolobules and small groups of cells. Four portal spaces are seen (➡), but no central veins can be recognized. This photomicrograph demonstrates that although portal spaces are involved early in the fibrotic process, they are much more resistant to the ravages of fibrosis than the sinusoidal spaces or central veins.

part on how many functioning liver cells remain. Although the mechanisms are not understood, it is generally recognized that patients with advanced cirrhosis who do not develop a markedly increased hepatic arterial blood flow have a poor prognosis.

Presinusoidal Cirrhosis

In schistosomiasis and portal vein thrombosis, the obstruction to portal blood flow occurs in the portal vein radicles themselves. There is little change in the hepatic lobules. The sinusoids and hepatic veins remain patent, so that portal blood flow to the liver is decreased without a compromise in hepatic venous outflow (Fig. 8–2E). In this situation, the decreased portal vein blood flow is immediately compensated for by a marked increase in hepatic arterial blood flow. Only late in the course of schistosomiasis does the portal fibrosis extend to involve the lobules.

As with patients who have a postsinusoidal block, portal–systemic collateral veins develop to divert the portal venous flow from the liver. The degree of portal hypertension depends upon the effectiveness of these collateral veins in decompressing the portal system.

The liver is frequently small in patients with portal vein thrombosis, and the triad of a small liver, a marked increase in hepatic artery blood flow and a normal liver biopsy establishes the diagnosis even without angiographic demonstration of the venous thrombosis. In general, when portal venous blood flow to the liver ceases, the liver shrinks. A small liver, therefore, is a frequent angiographic feature in patients with portal vein thrombosis, in patients with severe alcoholic cirrhosis and reversal of flow in the portal vein and in patients following portacaval decompressive shunts.

PORTAL VENOUS ANATOMY

The portal venous system drains the small bowel, colon, spleen, stomach, pancreas and omentum. As with the arterial supply to the viscera, portal venous anatomy is variable, and a thorough analysis of the variations was given by Douglass et al. (1950). The most common branching pattern is shown in Figure 8–4. Several

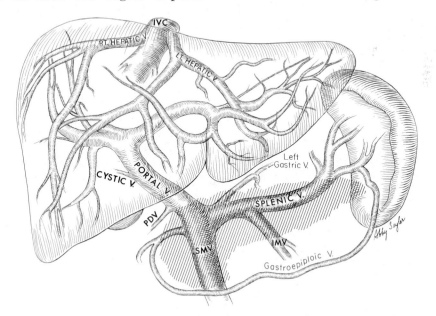

Figure 8–4. Portal vein anatomy in a normal person. The splenic vein, arising from its splenic tributaries, receives the short gastric and left gastroepiploic veins. It then passes craniodorsal to the tail of the pancreas, generally receiving the left gastric (coronary) and inferior mesenteric veins (IMV). The confluence of splenic and superior mesenteric veins (SMV) forms the portal vein. Pancreaticoduodenal (PDV) and cystic veins join the portal vein before it bifurcates into right and left portal radicles. Portal vein radicles and hepatic veins cross each other at approximately right angles.

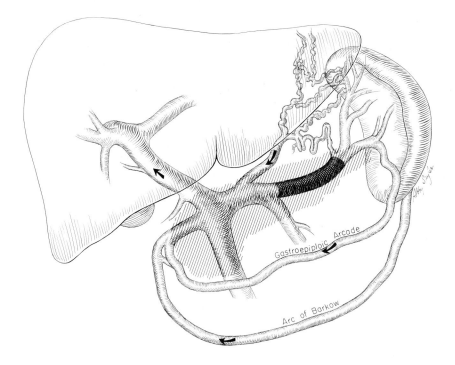

Figure 8-5. Development of portal–portal collateral veins in splenic vein thrombosis. The major collateral pathways develop over gastric (splenic → short gastric → coronary → portal veins) and omental (splenic → gastroepiploic or arc of Barkow → superior mesenteric → portal veins) veins. In patients with portal vein thrombosis, small collaterals in the head of the pancreas and gallbladder communicate with pancreaticoduodenal or cystic veins.

splenic vein tributaries join together to form the splenic vein, which passes with the splenic artery across the dorsal aspect of the tail and body of the pancreas. In the region of the body of the pancreas, the splenic vein generally receives the inferior mesenteric vein just before joining the superior mesenteric vein to form the portal vein. The inferior mesenteric vein may also join the superior mesenteric vein or the portal vein at the confluence of the splenic and superior mesenteric veins. On its superior surface, just before its junction with the superior mesenteric vein, the splenic vein receives the left gastric (coronary) vein from the lesser curvature of the stomach. In addition, the inferior mesenteric, superior mesenteric and portal veins have several smaller tributaries shown in Figure 8-4.

As with the arterial blood supply to the viscera, many anastomotic arcades exist in the portal system. Also, the veins of the portal venous system have important communications with the systemic veins.

Portal Venous Arcades

The potential arcades that exist in the portal system are shown in Figure 8-5. These arcades are most important in patients with splenic or portal vein occlusions. The splenic vein is most commonly occluded in patients with pancreatitis or carcinoma of the pancreas or stomach. The portal vein may also be occluded by these diseases, but, more commonly, portal vein thrombosis is idiopathic. The portal venous arcades function as portal–portal collateral veins (or "hepatopetal" collateral veins, since blood continues flowing toward the liver).

In splenic vein occlusion, the most important portal–portal collateral pathways develop through omental veins (see Figs. 4-6 and 4-67). In addition to the direct pathway through the left gastroepiploic to the right gastroepiploic vein along the greater curvature of the stomach, there is a large potential collateral vein, the arc of Barkow, along the free edge of the greater omentum. This connects the left gastroepiploic vein with the right gastroepiploic vein. There is no gastroduodenal vein to correspond with the gastroduodenal artery. Another venous collateral pathway in splenic vein occlusion is from the short gastric veins to the left gastric vein (see Fig. 3–45). Although this collateral route may be adequate to prevent the development of esophageal varices, gastric varices may be prominent and may bleed.

In patients with portal vein occlusion,

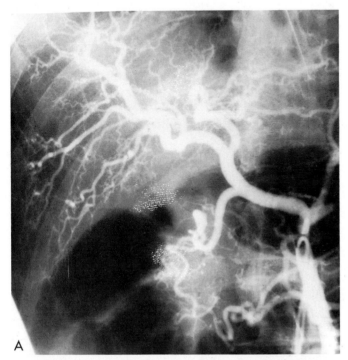

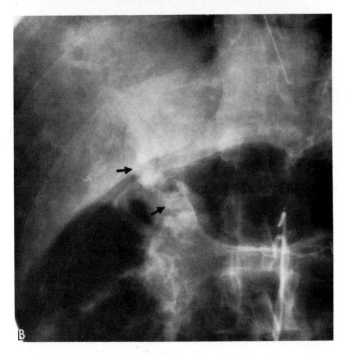

Figure 8-6. Appearance of cavernomatous transformation of the portal vein. Combined celiac–superior mesenteric angiogram in a 56 year old man with portal vein occlusion secondary to chronic pancreatitis.

A. Arterial phase. Branches of the pancreaticoduodenal arcades are dilated and mildly irregular. Some hypervascularity is present in the head of the pancreas.

B. Venous phase. Veins over the head of the pancreas drain into many tortuous, wormlike veins (➡) extending along the portal vein to portal vein radicles in the liver. No main portal vein is demonstrated.

these collateral pathways have no importance. Instead, numerous small veins along the common bile duct and gallbladder bring venous blood flow to the cystic and pyloric veins, as do small unnamed veins in the hilum of the liver from the pancreaticoduodenal and gastroepiploic veins. On angiograms these veins are seen as tangles of tortuous, dilated venous channels which represent the typical angiographic appearance of portal venous occlusion (Figs. 8–6 and 8–33.

Although these portal–portal collateral veins reestablish blood flow around occluded splenic or portal veins, they are usually not completely effective in decompressing the portal system, and most of these patients have persistent portal hypertension and develop portal–systemic collateral veins as well.

Portal–Systemic Collateral Veins

In most patients with progressive liver disease, a stage is reached at which resistance to blood flow through the liver is equal to or greater than that through collateral veins to the systemic circulation (Fig. 8–7). The most significant portal–systemic collateral veins in patients with cirrhosis and portal hypertension develop from the left gastric and short gastric veins via the esophageal veins to the azygos system. It is these collaterals that are responsible for bleeding esophageal varices, the major cause of death in patients with portal hypertension. The inferior mesenteric vein has communications through the superior hemorrhoidal veins to the inferior hemorrhoidal veins and the internal iliac veins. The splenic veins in the hilum of the spleen have communications with retroperitoneal veins and these, in turn, communicate with veins on the abdominal wall and with the inferior phrenic and renal veins. The latter communication is the general pathway of the well known "spontaneous splenorenal shunt." Another significant portal–systemic collateral pathway is the reopening of the umbilical vein, passing from the left portal vein to the umbilicus and thence to systemic veins on the anterior abdominal wall.

The final significant group of portal–systemic collaterals is rarely demonstrated on angiograms. These are numerous small por-

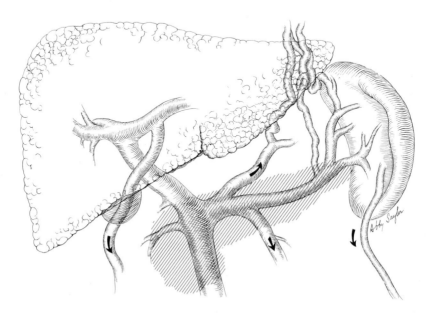

Figure 8–7. Major portal–systemic collateral veins in portal hypertension. In Stage II and III cirrhosis, blood flows to the systemic veins through the umbilical vein, left gastric vein, inferior mesenteric vein and an unnamed vein from the hilum of the spleen (arrows, left to right). The blood flow in these veins reverses from its normal direction. Since the superior mesenteric vein has no communication with systemic veins, blood flow in this vessel continues in its normal direction.

tal tributaries along the bowel wall and in the mesentery that connect with small retroperitoneal veins draining to the inferior vena cava. These collateral veins produce a characteristic coloration of the peritoneum in patients with portal hypertension and account for most of the blood loss during dissection of the inferior vena cava and portal vein in a portacaval shunt operation.

In addition, the middle colic and other colic veins may communicate with the inferior mesenteric vein over the marginal vein accompanying the marginal artery of Drummond. This is uncommon and may account for the occasional colonic varices in patients with portal hypertension (see Fig. 6–15).

Although these collateral channels develop most commonly to decompress the portal venous system, they may also be seen in patients with inferior vena cava obstruction (Hipona and Gabriele, 1967). In this instance, the blood flow in them is reversed, and systemic venous flow is shunted through the portal system to bypass the caval obstruction.

ANGIOGRAPHIC EVALUATION OF PATIENTS WITH CIRRHOSIS AND PORTAL HYPERTENSION

Angiography is frequently used as part of the evaluation of three groups of patients with cirrhosis and portal hypertension.

1. The patient with known cirrhosis and portal hypertension in whom a portal–systemic shunt operation is planned.

2. The patient without a history of chronic alcoholism or hepatitis who bleeds from esophageal varices.

3. The patient who has had a portal–systemic shunt and has complications suggesting thrombosis of the shunt.

The Patient with Known Cirrhosis and Portal Hypertension in Whom a Portal–Systemic Shunt Operation is Planned

The most frequent use of angiography in the evaluation of patients with cirrhosis and portal hypertension is prior to a portal–systemic shunt operation. The patients fall into two groups: those who are examined at the time of massive upper gastrointestinal bleeding prior to an emergency portacaval shunt and those who have ceased to bleed and are evaluated prior to an elective shunt operation. The two groups are considered together in this discussion because the hemodynamic alterations and the angiographic appearances are essentially the same. In these patients, angiography permits an exact measurement of portal pressure, demonstrates the presence of portal–systemic collateral veins (particularly esophageal varices), gives important information about the dynamics of portal blood flow and, if performed at the time of hematemesis, excludes arterial sources as the cause of bleeding.

A review of the angiographic abnormalities in patients with cirrhosis and portal hypertension requires some correlation between the angiogram and the stage of the patient's disease. Since the progression of hemodynamic alterations roughly parallels the severity of the histologic changes in the liver, one reasonable correlation is between the angiographic findings and the changes in hepatic blood flow. Based upon the previous description of the hemodynamic changes that accompany postsinusoidal cirrhosis, three stages of severity can be identified. Stage I extends from the onset of the disease to the development of portal–systemic collateral pathways (early or mild cirrhosis). In this stage, portal pressure is mildly to moderately elevated, and portal venous blood flow to the liver is maintained at approximately its normal level. Stage II extends from the development of portal–systemic collateral veins up to, but not including, the reversal of blood flow in the main portal vein (moderate cirrhosis). These patients have significant elevations of portal pressure. Portal vein blood flow to the liver is decreased, and the hepatic arterial flow is compensatively increased. Total hepatic blood flow is decreased. Stage III extends from the reversal of portal vein blood flow to death (advanced or decompensated cirrhosis). The liver in these patients is perfused entirely by arterial blood flow. The arterial inflow leaves the liver, in part, by retrograde flow through the portal vein, and this blood, as well as the venous drainage from the viscera, must be returned to the heart through portal–systemic collateral veins. Portal pressure depends upon the effectiveness of these collaterals, but the incidence of bleeding from varices in this group is high.

Although most patients fall into one or another of these groups, gray areas exist between the stages. Most patients coming to angiography for evaluation of cirrhosis and portal hypertension fall into Stage II. The patients in Stage I have not developed varices, and their angiograms are generally performed for unrelated reasons. Many patients in Stage III die of hepatic failure or gastrointestinal hemorrhage.

A number of angiographic methods are available by which hepatic blood flow can be evaluated. These fall into three major groups:

1. Hepatic venous (wedged hepatic venography and manometry, free hepatic venography and manometry, inferior vena cavography and manometry).

2. Arterial (celiac, superior mesenteric, hepatic, splenic and left gastric angiography and arterial portography).

3. Portal venous (splenoportography and splenic manometry, transhepatic portography and manometry, and umbilical portography and manometry). Each of these groups gives important information about hepatic and splanchnic hemodynamics in patients with cirrhosis.

Hepatic Venous Studies

Hepatic vein examinations are an important part of the angiographic evaluation of patients with cirrhosis and portal hypertension. The transmitted sinusoidal pressure can be obtained through a catheter wedged in a peripheral hepatic vein. In addition, an injection of contrast medium through the wedged hepatic vein catheter gives information about the degree of sinusoidal fibrosis, the speed of emptying of the portal vein and the direction of flow in the portal vein. An injection with the catheter free in a hepatic vein gives information about the degree of distortion of hepatic veins by fibrosis. Finally, pressures taken above and below the liver in the right atrium and inferior vena cava provide an essential baseline to which the hepatic wedge pressure must be compared. Occasionally, these pressures indicate the degree to which hepatic venous flow is obstructed by distortion of the inferior vena cava by an enlarged and nodular liver.

The hepatic veins are approached from the inferior vena cava, either from above or below. If the femoral vein approach is used, a manipulator instrument generally must be employed to reverse the direction of the catheter downward into the hepatic veins in order to wedge the catheter tip.

WEDGED HEPATIC VENOGRAPHY. When the catheter tip is wedged in a small hepatic vein, pressures can be measured either with a transducer or simply with a saline manometer. In patients with the common forms of cirrhosis, all of whom have sinusoidal or postsinusoidal obstruction, this pressure represents the pressure transmitted through a static column of blood extending from the portal vein through the sinusoids and hepatic venules to the catheter. It is the same as the splenic pulp pressure measured at splenoportography, and both measurements accurately reflect total portal pressure. Normal portal pressures measured in this manner range from 40 to 150 mm of saline. If the pressure is above 150 mm of saline, the patient has portal hypertension.

Portal hypertension has two components. The first is due to the intrahepatic obstruction of portal flow and the second to transmitted pressure from the inferior vena cava. These two components can be separated by measuring inferior vena caval pressure in addition to the wedged hepatic venous pressure. Wedged hepatic venous pressure minus inferior vena caval pressure is the corrected sinusoidal pressure, or that part of the portal pressure due to intrahepatic resistance to blood flow. Elevated corrected sinusoidal pressure is due to hepatic disease and is relatively constant. Inferior vena caval pressure may be elevated by anatomic factors, such as distortion of the inferior vena cava by an enlarged liver or, more commonly, by elevated systemic venous pressure. The concept of a corrected sinusoidal pressure is useful because it reflects the steady state of the patient's liver disease, and this is what causes the development of portal–systemic collateral veins and bleeding varices. A corrected sinusoidal pressure up to approximately 100 mm of saline is normal. When the corrected sinusoidal pressure rises above this point, the patient can be considered to have a significant increase in the intrahepatic resistance to portal blood flow. The higher the corrected sinusoidal pressure, the greater the resistance.

Although corrected sinusoidal pressure constitutes the major component of portal pressure in most patients with significant cirrhosis and is that component of portal pressure that is the major cause of the development of portal-systemic collateral veins, it must be remembered that the total pressure is the cause of hemorrhage in patients with esophageal varices. Thus, a patient with both cirrhosis and congestive heart failure may bleed from esophageal varices because of the temporarily elevated central venous pressure and may cease to bleed when the central venous pressure returns to normal. In general, patients with cirrhosis do not bleed from varices unless the portal pressure is above 200 to 250 mm of saline. In patients with massive upper gastrointestinal bleeding and a portal pressure of less than 200 mm of saline, the bleeding is almost always from a source other than the esophageal varices.

Although portal pressure correlates in a general way with the severity of liver disease, an absolute correlation should not

be expected, since the effectiveness of collateral veins in decompressing the portal system varies from patient to patient.

When the wedged hepatic venous pressure has been established, an injection of contrast medium is made with the catheter in the wedged position. The rate of this injection should be 2 cc per second or less. The quantity of contrast medium used is not critical but should not exceed 8 cc. The purpose of this injection is to flood the venules and sinusoids that drain to the hepatic vein blocked by the catheter. When this is done in a normal person, the contrast medium drains from the flooded sinusoids through other hepatic venules and veins. The angiographic appearance is that of a homogeneous blush of hundreds of sinusoids with the contrast medium draining to other hepatic veins (Fig. 8–8). Too rapid an injection results in a reflux of contrast medium into portal veins, even in normal people. As sinusoidal fibrosis and obstruction to venous outflow from the sinusoids progress in cirrhotic patients, two changes occur. First, the pattern of sinusoidal filling becomes irregular and unhomogeneous.

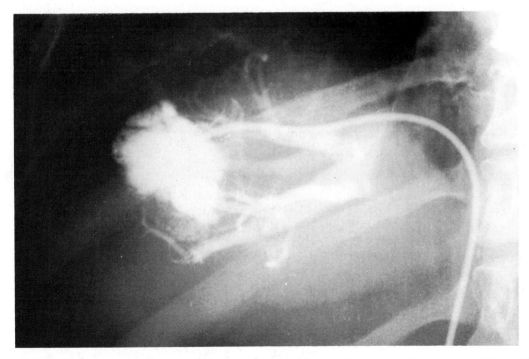

Figure 8–8. Wedged hepatic venogram in a patient without liver disease. The pattern of sinusoidal filling is homogeneous. The contrast medium passes freely to hepatic veins other than the vein injected, and these drain to the inferior vena cava. No portal vein radicles are seen, although these may be filled from a wedged hepatic venogram, even in a normal person.

This occurs because the fibrosis obstructs the retrograde injection of contrast medium into hepatic venules as well as the antegrade flow of blood and contrast medium out of the liver. The contrast medium, therefore, follows the route of least resistance to still unobstructed hepatic venules and hepatic sinusoids. Second, the increased resistance to drainage forces contrast medium into portal vein radicles (Fig. 8–9). When fibrosis becomes severe and the portal vein becomes an outflow tract from the liver, the pattern of sinusoidal filling becomes markedly unhomogeneous and the contrast medium entering portal vein radicles drains from the liver in a retrograde direction through the portal vein to portal–systemic collateral veins (Fig. 8–10).

In the preoperative evaluation for portacaval shunt operations, patients with Stage I disease are not examined since they do not have varices. Stage III patients, with severe cirrhosis and reversed portal vein blood flow, constitute 15 per cent of patients being evaluated for elective shunts and 25 per cent of patients being evaluated for emergency shunts. Therefore, most examinations occur in Stage II. In this group, additional qualitative information about the severity of obstruction to hepatic venous outflow can be gained by observing the contrast medium that is forced into portal vein radicles. In patients with lesser degrees of obstruction, the portal veins empty in an antegrade direction within 2 to 3 seconds after the end of the injection. Also, the hepatogram produced by this contrast medium is moderately dense and homogeneous. As the obstruction increases, the speed of washout of contrast medium from the portal venules decreases proportionally; in severe cirrhosis, portal vein radicles are still filled with contrast medium 10 seconds following the end of the injection. This is the stage just prior to reversal of flow in the portal vein. Also, the density of the hepatogram caused by washout of contrast medium in portal vein radicles decreases progressively as the cirrhosis becomes more advanced.

Thus, wedged hepatic venous pressure measurements and venography establish the presence and degree of portal hypertension. By grading the unhomogeneous appearance of the sinusoidal filling, some idea can be obtained about the degree of hepatic fibrosis. Finally, by observing the washout of the contrast medium that has been forced into the portal veins, an indication of the rate and direction of portal blood flow can be obtained. If flow in the portal vein is reversed, hepatofugal collateral veins, such as esophageal varices, are demonstrated.

FREE HEPATIC VENOGRAPHY. Smith et al. (1971) staged the histologic changes in

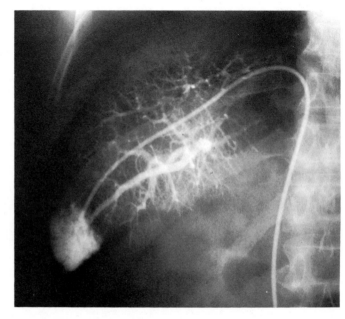

Figure 8–9. Wedged hepatic venogram in a patient with Stage II cirrhosis. The pattern of sinusoidal filling is mildly irregular. Because of increased hepatic vein resistance, contrast medium is forced into portal vein radicles, and no hepatic veins are seen. Washout of the portal vein radicles occurs in an antegrade direction, but much more slowly than normal.

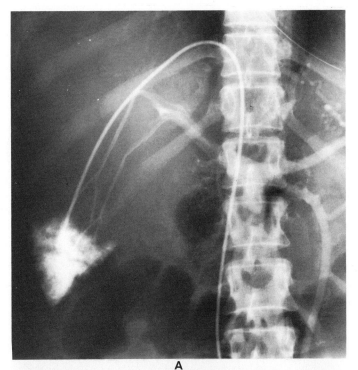

A

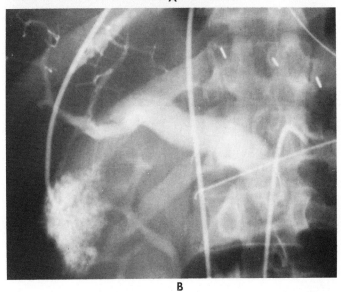

B

Figure 8–10. Wedged hepatic venograms in two patients with Stage III cirrhosis.

A. In the first patient the sinusoidal pattern is mottled. The contrast medium forced into portal vein radicles flows into the portal vein and then to the splenic, gastric and inferior mesenteric veins, indicating a reversal of flow in the portal vein.

B. In the second patient the sinusoidal filling pattern is moderately irregular. The contrast medium that has been forced through the sinusoids enters portal vein radicles and then drains both toward other peripheral portal veins radicles and centrally toward portal–systemic collateral veins.

the liver by evaluating the distortion of hepatic veins at free hepatic venography. With the catheter free in a large hepatic vein, 25 cc of contrast medium is injected rapidly. A normal free hepatic venogram is shown in Figure 8–11 (also see Fig. 2–46). The walls of the vein are smoothly tapered with fourth and fifth order branchings readily apparent. A fine reticular pattern of sinusoidal filling is seen around the terminal hepatic venules. In mild cir-

rhosis there is some loss of the branching with demonstration of only third and fourth order branches. Irregularities appear along the margins of the branches, and the sinusoidal filling is irregularly distributed through the liver. In moderate cirrhosis there is further loss of branching and lack of sinusoidal filling (Fig. 8–12). In the end stages of the disease, there is nearly complete obliteration of hepatic veins.

These angiographic findings agree with

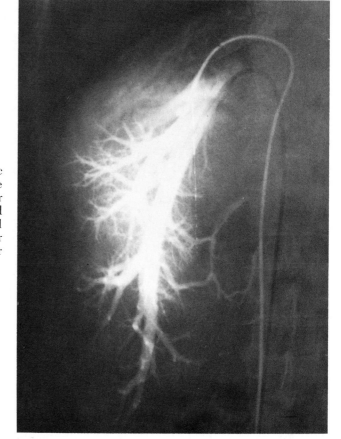

Figure 8–11. Normal free hepatic venogram. The normal hepatic veins have a generous caliber. Fourth and fifth order branchings, as well as a background speckling of sinusoidal filling, are well seen. Contrast medium refluxes to other hepatic veins, which drain to the inferior vena cava.

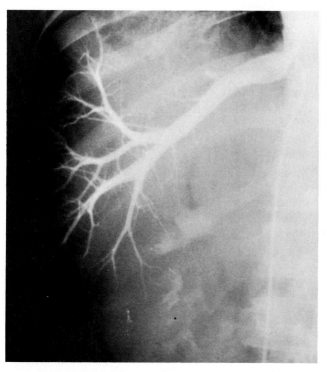

Figure 8–12. Free hepatic venogram in a patient with Stage II cirrhosis. The main hepatic vein has a normal caliber but its tributaries are narrowed, appearing squeezed and stretched. Only third and fourth order branchings are seen, and no reflux occurs into the hepatic sinusoids.

the abnormalities that Hales et al. (1959) demonstrated with injection-corrosion studies of cirrhotic livers. They found severe venous reduction in patients with cirrhosis, most marked in the hepatic veins but also affecting the portal veins. The primary cause for this reduction was fibrosis. Pseudolobules or regenerating lobules also contributed to the venous distortion. Both changes account for the abnormalities seen at free hepatic venography.

INFERIOR VENA CAVOGRAPHY. The distortion of hepatic parenchyma and regeneration of the liver that accompany advanced cirrhosis can constrict the inferior vena cava as it passes through the liver. Therefore, a measurement of inferior vena caval pressures should be a part of each hepatic venogram. These pressures should be obtained in the right atrium and in the inferior vena cava below the liver. If there is a marked discrepancy between these pressures, an inferior vena cavogram should be performed to demonstrate the cause of the gradient. Generally, the inferior vena cava is compressed as it passes through the liver. Portacaval shunts do not function well in such patients because the high inferior vena caval pressure causes a poor pressure gradient across the shunt.

Arterial Studies

Celiac angiography has four functions in the evaluation of patients with cirrhosis and portal hypertension. The first is to exclude causes of massive upper gastrointestinal bleeding other than varices. The second is to evaluate hepatic artery dynamics and to determine the extent to which hepatic arterial flow has compensated for decreased portal flow. The third is to exclude hepatoma, and the final purpose is to identify portal–systemic collateral veins, particularly esophageal varices.

EXCLUSION OF OTHER SOURCES OF MASSIVE UPPER GASTROINTESTINAL BLEEDING. Approximately 20 to 30 per cent of patients with cirrhosis and upper gastrointestinal bleeding are actually bleeding from sources other than varices. If the patient has known esophageal varices, this figure drops to about 10 per cent. The most common causes of bleeding are duodenal ulcers, gastric ulcers, hemorrhagic gastritis

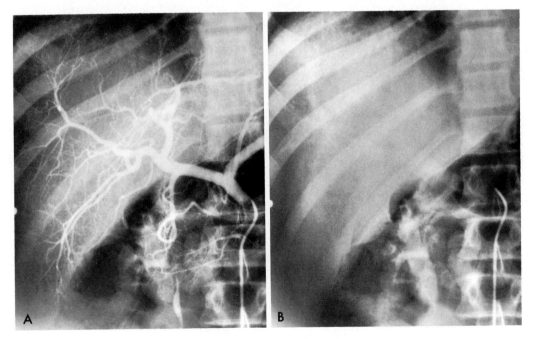

A   **B**

Figure 8–13. Celiac angiogram in a patient with Stage I cirrhosis.

A. Arterial phase. The hepatic arteries branch normally and taper progressively and smoothly toward the periphery of the liver. The appearance of these arteries is normal.

B. Venous phase. The portal vein fills from the splenic vein. The remainder of the liver has a homogeneous density.

and Mallory-Weiss tears of the esophagus. These can be detected when angiography is performed as an emergency examination during massive hematemesis. When the angiographic evaluation is done prior to elective portacaval surgery and the patient is not bleeding, such causes will not be demonstrated. The angiographic appearance of gastrointestinal bleeding is described in Chapter 6.

EVALUATION OF HEPATIC ARTERIAL HEMODYNAMICS. In Stage I cirrhosis, portal blood flow is maintained, and the hepatic arteries generally appear normal (Fig. 8–13). If the patient has fatty infiltration su-

perimposed upon early cirrhosis, the liver may be enlarged, and the hepatic arteries may appear stretched. Occasionally, hepatic blood flow is slowed in early cirrhosis (Fig. 8–14). The cause of this phenomenon is not known, but it is seen as a delayed filling of the hepatic artery branches. They may not be completely emptied by the time the portal vein is well filled. This appearance has led some authors to state that hepatic artery blood flow is decreased in cirrhosis. However, this occurs only in early cirrhosis.

As portal—systemic collateral veins divert portal flow in Stage II cirrhosis, the

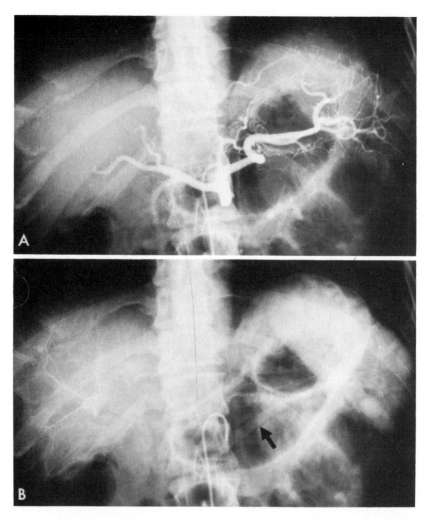

Figure 8–14. Slowed hepatic arterial blood flow in early cirrhosis. Celiac angiogram in a 30 year old man with Stage I cirrhosis.

A. Arterial phase. Contrast medium has reached the peripheral splenic and gastric arteries, but only the major hepatic artery branches are filled.

B. Venous phase. The splenic vein (➡) is well demonstrated, although the contrast medium is just filling the distal hepatic artery branches.

compensatory increase in hepatic artery blood flow to the liver can be seen on celiac or hepatic angiograms (Fig. 8–15). Thus, in most patients with moderate to severe cirrhosis, the hepatic artery and its branches are dilated, elongated and tortuous. Occasionally, the peripheral branches appear to be duplicated (Fig. 8–16). The angiographic appearance is that of two small arteries traversing side by side to the periphery of the liver, looking somewhat like railroad tracks. Viamonte and Viamonte (personal communication) have explained this appearance by showing with corrosion casts of the liver that more than one hepatic artery branch accompanies a portal vein radicle. The elongation and

tortuosity of hepatic arteries are caused by increased blood flow and occur in any artery in which this happens. Even in patients with large livers, increased hepatic artery blood flow causes some tortuosity. When the liver begins to shrink, the combination of tortuosity and retraction of the hepatic artery branches gives the characteristic angiographic appearance of advanced cirrhosis, frequently called "corkscrewing" (Fig. 8–17; also see Fig. 8–37). Unfortunately, the variation in the amount of hypervascularity that accompanies cirrhosis is wide, and correlation of any angiographic appearance of hepatic arteries with any stage of cirrhosis is difficult.

In Stage III cirrhosis, the hepatic venous

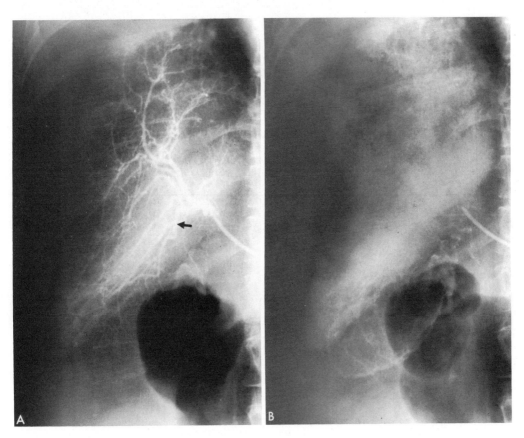

Figure 8–15. Hepatic angiogram in a 45 year old woman with Stage II cirrhosis.
A. Arterial phase. The hepatic artery branches are dilated.
The cystic artery (➡) is also dilated, as are its branches in the gallbladder.
B. Venous phase. The liver edge is separated from the abdominal wall by ascites. The hepatogram is unhomogeneously increased. Contrast medium in the gallbladder veins is dense, indicating the outline of the gallbladder. Although this is also the angiographic appearance of subacute cholecystitis, the gallbladder was carefully palpated during surgery and thought to be normal. This hypervascularization of the gallbladder and visualization of cystic veins is another manifestation of systemic arteriovenous shunting in patients with cirrhosis.

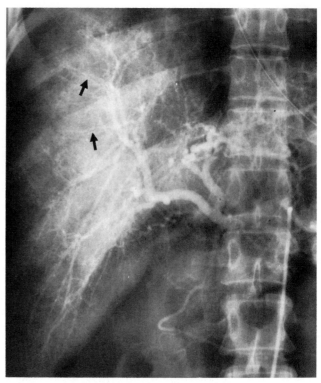

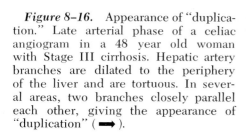

Figure 8–16. Appearance of "duplication." Late arterial phase of a celiac angiogram in a 48 year old woman with Stage III cirrhosis. Hepatic artery branches are dilated to the periphery of the liver and are tortuous. In several areas, two branches closely parallel each other, giving the appearance of "duplication" (➡).

resistance to outflow of portal vein and hepatic artery blood becomes so great that the portal vein becomes an outflow tract, and hepatic artery blood drains from the liver through the portal vein to portal–systemic collateral veins. When this situation occurs, the portal vein may be demonstrated at a selective hepatic artery injection (Fig. 8–18). The hepatic arteriogram is not as sensitive for demonstrating reversal of flow in the portal vein as a wedged hepatic venogram, which demonstrates the reversed flow at an earlier stage in the patient's disease.

Some authors have referred to the drainage of hepatic artery blood flow through the portal vein as hepatic artery–portal vein shunting. Although a controversy about the contribution of arteriovenous shunts to portal hypertension has existed over the past several years, the current general feeling is that the reversal of portal vein blood flow occurs because of the marked resistance to outflow of blood through the hepatic veins and not because of an arteriovenous shunt per se. There are, however, small arteriovenous shunts that occur throughout the body in patients with cirrhosis and

cause an increase in cardiac output. The most obvious of these are the spider nevi on the skin. They also occur in the stomach and gallbladder and are frequently seen at angiography in patients with advanced cirrhosis (Fig. 8–15). Hales et al. (1959) have demonstrated presinusoidal communications between the hepatic artery and the portal vein. Some arterial pressure may be transmitted through these to communications to the portal vein.

As portal blood flow to the liver decreases and hepatic artery blood flow increases, a reversal occurs in the normal appearance of the hepatogram phase. In the normal patient, the approximately 80 per cent of hepatic blood flow supplied by the portal vein is reflected in a dense hepatogram at splenoportography. Decreased portal blood flow results in decreased accumulation of contrast medium in the sinusoids in the capillary and venous phases. However, as the arterial flow increases, density of the hepatogram during celiac angiography increases. In patients with reversal of blood flow in the portal vein, the artery supplies all the blood to the liver, and, in these patients, the hepatogram

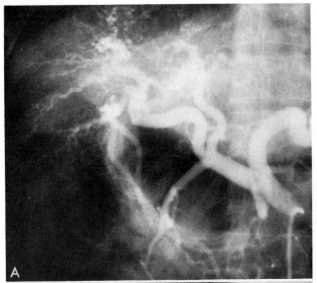

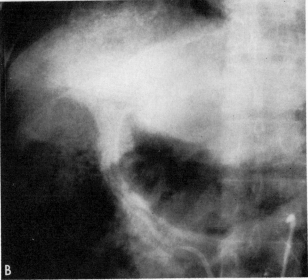

Figure 8–17. "Corkscrewing" of hepatic artery branches. Celiac angiogram in a 50 year old man with Stage III cirrhosis and a small liver.

A. Arterial phase. The hepatic artery and its branches are markedly dilated and extremely tortuous. This is the appearance of "corkscrewing."

B. Venous phase. The density of the hepatogram phase is increased. The liver is small.

phase of the arteriogram can be quite dense. Because of the varying severity of fibrosis throughout the liver, it is also frequently unhomogeneous. The density of the hepatogram phase has been used as a measure of the adequacy of the increased hepatic artery blood flow in predicting survival following portacaval shunt operations. However, the authors' experience has indicated that too much variation exists in the density of the hepatogram because of technical factors, such as KVP, for it to be a reliable criterion.

A variable that affects the appearance of the hepatic arteries in cirrhotic patients examined after a severe bout of drinking is the degree of inflammatory change or "alcoholic hepatitis" which is present in the liver (Rourke et al., 1968). As with other forms of diffuse inflammatory disease of the liver, such as viral hepatitis, this increases hepatic arterial flow and can result in a suffusion of small arteries in the liver, even when it is normal-sized or enlarged (Figs. 8–19 and 8–20). This additional insult superimposed on the patient's disease can also temporarily accentuate the course of hemodynamic changes. For example, a Stage II patient may have reversal of the blood flow in his portal vein during a bout of alcoholic hepatitis, temporarily becoming a Stage III patient. After a few weeks of

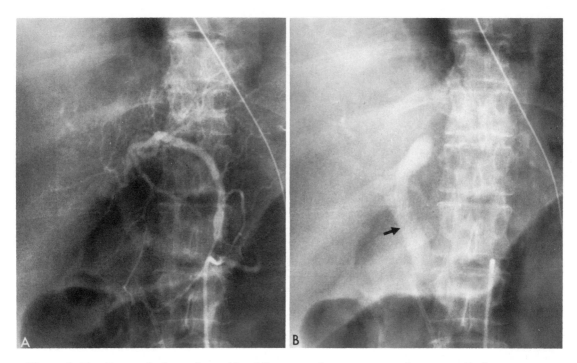

Figure 8–18. Reversal of portal vein blood flow seen during an arterial injection. Left gastric angiogram in a patient with Stage III cirrhosis.

A. Arterial phase. The left hepatic artery arises from the left gastric artery. The branches throughout the left lobe of the liver are dilated.

B. Venous phase. Contrast medium has passed through the sinusoids and is drained from the liver via the portal vein (➡).

hospital care, he may revert to Stage II. This temporary accentuation of arterial hepatic hemodynamics probably explains the approximately 10 per cent higher incidence of reversed portal vein blood flow in patients being evaluated for emergency portacaval shunts over those being evaluated for elective shunts.

Another variable in patients with portal hypertension is splenomegaly. Prediction of whether or not the spleen will be enlarged in a cirrhotic patient is impossible. Patients with mild degrees of portal hypertension may have enlarged spleens, and those with severe portal hypertension may have normal-sized spleens. Perhaps this is related to the effectiveness of the portal–systemic collateral veins in decompressing the portal system. The size of the splenic artery and splenic vein correlates directly with the size of the spleen and is independent of the degree of portal hypertension. An enlarged spleen has an increased blood flow, and the splenic artery and vein dilate to accommodate this increased flow.

It seems reasonable to postulate that the increased blood flow through an enlarged spleen must contribute to portal hypertension.

The major rationale for the angiographic evaluation of hepatic hemodynamics prior to portacaval shunt surgery has been the hope that a correlation exists between preoperative hemodynamics and postoperative survival. However, little correlation between the two has been found. The preoperative parameters that seem to correlate best with postoperative survival are those of Child's nutritional-hepatic reserve classification. The more advanced the cirrhosis preoperatively, the worse the chances for survival following a shunt operation. Moreover, the results of various series have also indicated that patients with reversed portal vein blood flow have a poor survival rate following shunt surgery. Thus, hepatic panangiography prior to shunt surgery does not give the surgeon useful predictive information. However, a preoperative knowledge of the degree of

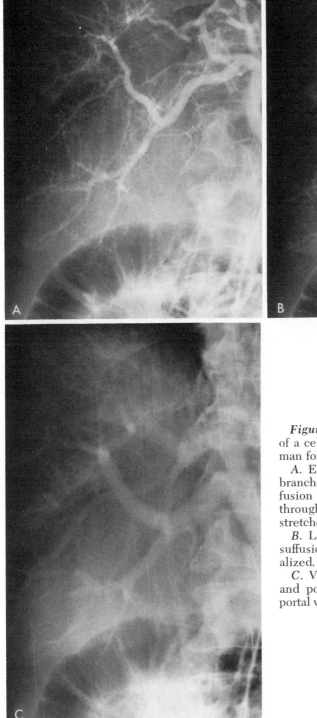

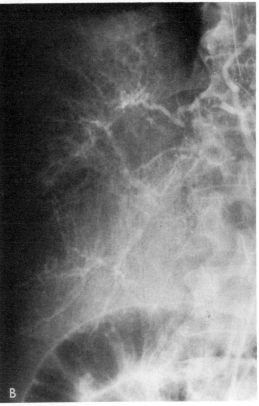

Figure 8–19. Alcoholic hepatitis. Injection of a celiacomesenteric trunk in a 40 year old man following a 2 week drinking binge.

A. Early arterial phase. The hepatic artery branches are moderately dilated, and a suffusion of small arterial branches is seen throughout the liver. These appear diffusely stretched and mildly tortuous.

B. Late arterial phase. The dilatation and suffusion of small branches can be better visualized.

C. Venous phase. The portal vein radicles and portal vein are densely opacified. The portal vein blood flow is reversed.

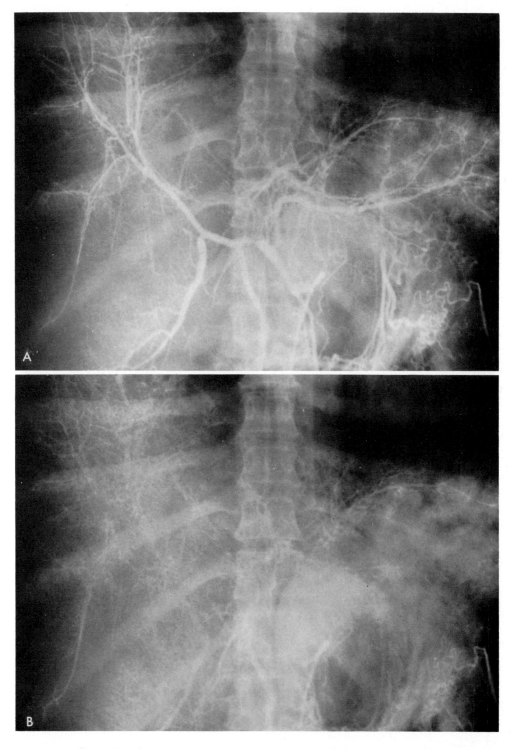

Figure 8–20. Alcoholic hepatitis. Celiac angiogram in a 37 year old woman who had been drinking steadily for 3 weeks.

  A. Arterial phase. The liver is large, and the hepatic artery branches are stretched, suggesting fatty infiltration. The terminal hepatic arteries are somewhat dilated and increased in number and have a "fuzzy" appearance, typical of alcoholic hepatitis. The major hepatic arteries are not dilated.

  B. Late arterial phase. The fuzzy, duplicated distal hepatic artery branches can be better seen.

the patient's portal hypertension, of what component of portal hypertension is due to the patient's hepatic disease (corrected sinusoidal pressure) and whether or not the portal vein blood flow has reversed are useful to the surgeon. This information can be obtained either from transhepatic portography and manometry or from wedged hepatic venography and manometry. Inferior vena caval pressure must be obtained with both methods to correct the portal pressure.

EXCLUSION OF HEPATOMA. The incidence of hepatoma in cirrhotic patients is greater than in the noncirrhotic population. The angiographic appearance of hepatoma is described in Chapter 4. When a hepatoma develops in a patient with cirrhosis, it is often more difficult to identify than in a patient with an otherwise normal liver. The diffuse form of hepatoma, particularly, may be extremely difficult to differentiate from the already diffusely abnormal cirrhotic liver on which it is superimposed (see Fig. 4–44). In general, however, a hepatoma stands out as a hypervascular mass with tumor vessels, arterial occlusions and, occasionally, arteriovenous shunting to the portal vein. Occasionally, large regenerating nodules are present in patients with cirrhosis (see Fig. 4–41) and must be differentiated from hepatomas. However, most regenerating nodules, except in postnecrotic cirrhosis, are small and have a vascularity similar to a normal liver.

DEMONSTRATION OF PORTAL–SYSTEMIC COLLATERAL VEINS, PARTICULARLY ESOPHAGEAL VARICES. Demonstration of esophageal varices is an essential part of the preoperative evaluation of the cirrhotic patient. Varices can generally be demonstrated with barium examinations and direct esophagoscopy. However, the results of these examinations are sometimes equiv-

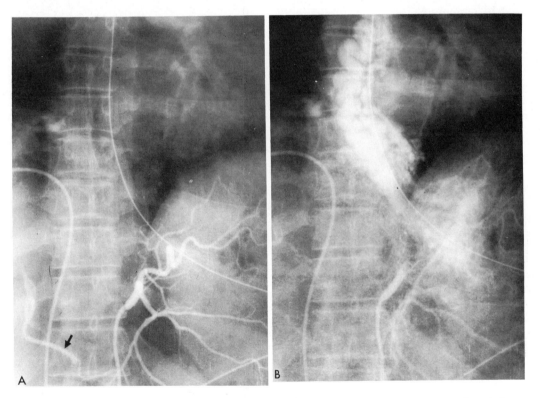

Figure 8-21. Demonstration of esophageal varices by arterial portography. A high dose left gastric angiogram in a 33 year old man with Stage II cirrhosis.

A. Arterial phase. Contrast medium floods the left gastric artery branches and refluxes through the left gastric–right gastric arterial arcade (➡) to the left hepatic artery.

B. Venous phase. Contrast medium has been forced into the veins and flows cephalad into dilated, tortuous esophageal varices.

ocal, and additional confirmatory information can be obtained by angiography. This can be done by arterial portography, transhepatic portography or splenoportography. Other portal–systemic collateral veins can also be identified during these examinations.

Arterial portography requires the injection of a high dose of contrast medium into the splenic or superior mesenteric artery. Doses up to 70 cc of 75 or 76 per cent contrast medium are injected at a rate of approximately 10 cc per second into either of these arteries. In the superior mesenteric artery the injection should be made 45 seconds after the intraarterial administration of 50 mg. of tolazoline (Priscoline) (see Chapter 10). Filming should be prolonged to at least 25 seconds since portal blood flow in patients with portal hypertension is frequently slowed. This technique generally results in good demonstration of the superior mesenteric and splenic veins. Superior mesenteric artery injections have usually been better than splenic artery injections for demonstrating esophageal varices. High dose splenic artery injections lose their advantage when the spleen is enlarged because of the marked dilution of the contrast medium. In patients with splenomegaly, long, slow injections (3 cc of 76 per cent contrast medium per second for 20 seconds) frequently give adequate opacification of the splenic vein. High dose left gastric artery injections (32 cc of 76 per cent contrast medium injected over a 4 second period) result in excellent demonstration of esophageal varices (Fig. 8–21). Empirically, the delivery of contrast medium into the vascular bed draining directly to the varices makes more sense than injecting the splenic or superior mesenteric vascular bed.

In patients with Stage II cirrhosis, the portal blood flow to the liver continues, although diminished, and the contrast medium in the venous phase of a celiac, splenic or superior mesenteric angiogram demonstrates the portal vein and some of its intrahepatic radicles. Generally, the definition of the individual portal radicles is not nearly as good as with transhepatic portography or splenoportography. In both Stage II and III cirrhosis, other portal–systemic collateral veins are demonstrated when they occur (Fig. 8–22). Occasionally,

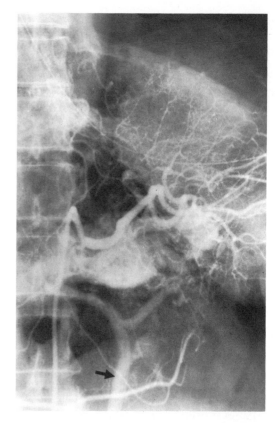

Figure 8–22. Demonstration of hepatofugal collateral veins by arterial portography. Late arterial phase of a high dose splenic angiogram in a patient with Stage III cirrhosis. The splenic artery is normal in size because the patient does not have splenomegaly. Contrast medium fills the arterial branches through the spleen and the tail of the pancreas. Contrast medium has entered the splenic vein and refluxed down the inferior mesenteric vein (➡) toward the hemorrhoidal veins.

a spontaneous splenorenal shunt can be identified.

Splenoportography

For years splenoportography was the primary angiographic method for evaluating patients with cirrhosis and portal hypertension. Even with all the other methods now available, much of the information necessary to evaluate a patient with cirrhosis or portal hypertension can be obtained with splenoportography. The measurement of splenic pulp pressure gives an accurate indication of portal pressure in patients with both postsinusoidal and presinusoidal blocks. Injection of contrast medium into the splenic pulp demonstrates the portal–systemic collateral veins which develop in patients with increased intrahepatic resistance to portal blood flow. In patients with splenic vein or portal vein thrombosis, it demonstrates the site of obstruction and the portal–portal collateral veins which regularly develop. The splenoportogram gives a good demonstration of the intrahepatic portal radicles and an assessment of the rapidity of washout of these vessels in a hepatopetal direction. When portal vein blood flow is reversed, however, the splenic and portal veins are not demonstrated.

Since the development of arterial portography, fewer splenoportograms are performed. However, the concentration of contrast medium in the portal system that can be obtained by arterial portography in patients with portal hypertension is not nearly as good as that obtained in patients with normal portal venous flow, particularly in patients with splenomegaly. Splenoportography, therefore, may still be used to evaluate the patterns of portal–systemic collateral vein development in patients with portal hypertension. In patients with splenic vein thrombosis, it may be the definitive examination. Also, because of the excellent anatomic demonstration of portal vein radicles afforded by splenoportography, it should be used routinely in the preoperative evaluation of patients who are to undergo resection of hepatic tumors (see Chapter 4).

TECHNIQUE. The same premedication is used as for angiography, and the left side of the patient's thorax and abdomen is washed with an antiseptic prior to puncture. Under fluoroscopic control, the spleen is localized and a skin wheal made with local anesthetic at a point on the skin near the lower pole in midrespiration. The entrance site on the skin, usually in the ninth or tenth intercostal space in the mid- to posterior axillary line, should allow the needle to enter the spleen near the lower pole and to be directed toward the splenic hilum (Fig. 8–23). The soft tissues are anesthetized to the peritoneum, a small stab wound is made at the site of needle puncture and a 12 gauge needle is used to make a track into the soft tissues between the ribs. The splenoportogram needle is a 6

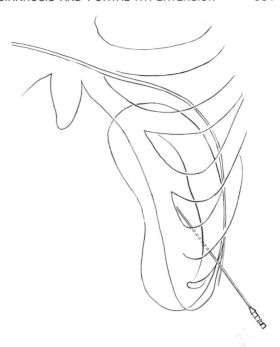

Figure 8–23. Puncture for splenoportography. The puncture site should be chosen under fluoroscopic control. It should be below the pleural reflection and low enough that the needle enters near the lower pole of the spleen and is angled toward the splenic hilum.

inch 20 gauge needle with a tight-fitting polyethylene sheath.

While the patient holds his breath in a midrespiratory phase, the splenoportogram needle and sheath are advanced rapidly into the spleen and the needle removed, leaving the sheath in place. The patient is then cautioned to take shallow respirations through the remainder of the examination. If the spleen has been entered, blood returns slowly through the sheath. The pressure is measured with a spinal manometer filled with saline, the sheath is taped in place and a small test injection of approximately 5 cc of contrast medium is made. If a proper puncture has been performed, the contrast medium spreads through the splenic parenchyma, giving a rather uneven splenogram, and drains into a splenic vein. Poor positioning of the sheath in the spleen results in a subcapsular deposition of this test injection, seen as a homogeneous collection of contrast medium which spreads slightly as the injection is made. If a subcapsular dissection is noted at the test injection, the sheath should be removed and the puncture repeated. Simply drawing the sheath back into a good position in the splenic pulp is not adequate. In this situation, an injection of contrast medium passes primarily along the track made by the needle and results in a large subcapsular deposition of contrast medium. When a new position of the sheath has been made, a second test injection is performed to ensure that the deposition of contrast medium remains in the splenic pulp.

If the sheath has a good position in the splenic pulp, the patient is moved over the angiographic changer, and an injection of 40 cc of 75 to 76 per cent contrast medium is made at a rate of 10 cc per second. Filming is done at a rate of one film per second for 15 seconds. Following injection, the catheter is removed.

The injection of contrast medium is generally painless, but the patient may have some discomfort in the left upper quadrant. Subcapsular dissections of contrast medium may result in left upper quadrant pain, occasionally radiating to the left shoulder. Following the procedure, the patient should remain in bed flat on his back for at least 6 hours.

Because contrast medium layers in the more slowly flowing veins, prone splenoportography has been recommended for more consistent demonstration of esophageal varices (Moscowitz et al., 1968). This is a reasonable approach when the patient is young and able to cooperate; however, many elderly patients have difficulty lying prone. Moreover, if the splenoportogram is performed in conjunction with other angiographic examinations, turning the patient with catheters in his femoral arteries or veins is difficult.

APPEARANCE OF THE NORMAL SPLENO-PORTOGRAM. Contrast medium flows from the collection of contrast medium in the splenic pulp through splenic vein tributaries into the splenic vein. It continues into the portal vein near the right margin of the spine and from there to the intrahepatic portal radicles (Fig. 8–24). Frequent flow defects along the course of the splenic vein are caused by an influx of nonopacified blood from the inferior and superior mesenteric veins and left gastric vein. In the normal patient, all venous flow is toward the main splenic and portal veins, and only these vessels are filled at splenoportog-

raphy. In the normal liver, the portal vein branchings are acute and are homogeneous throughout the liver. Portal vein radicles fill to the periphery of the liver. With the patient in the supine position, however, the left portal radicles often are poorly demonstrated. In the normal patient, the portal vein carries approximately 75 to 80 per cent of the hepatic blood flow, and the hepatogram that results from the splenoportogram is dense and homogeneous.

SPLENOPORTOGRAPHY IN PATIENTS WITH PORTAL HYPERTENSION DUE TO CIRRHOSIS. In Stage I cirrhosis, before portal-systemic collateral veins have developed, portal blood flow to the liver is maintained and the splenoportogram has a relatively normal appearance. As the resistance to hepatic venous outflow from the liver increases, the rate of emptying of the portal vein radicles becomes prolonged. In Stage II cirrhosis, the portal-systemic collateral veins fill with contrast medium. Most of the portal flow continues toward the liver, although the rate of empying may be significantly slowed. In addition, the fibrosis in the portal spaces accompanying advanced cirrhosis leads to distortion of the peripheral portal vein radicles in the liver, and they tend to arise more at right angles than in the normal patient. The major collateral veins which are demonstrated are the left gastric and short gastric veins to the esophageal veins, which connect with the azygos system (Fig. 8–25), the inferior mesenteric veins to the hemorrhoidal and internal iliac veins (Fig. 8–26), and communications between the splenic vein and the retroperitoneal veins along the abdominal wall and the reopened umbilical vein (Fig. 8–27). Spontaneous splenorenal shunts may also be seen. One or more of these collateral venous channels may be demonstrated.

In Stage III cirrhosis, blood flow in the portal vein, and usually in the splenic vein, is reversed, and a splenoportogram demonstrates only numerous collateral veins in the hilum of the spleen and the immediate retroperitoneum, occasionally with a spontaneous splenorenal shunt (Fig. 8–28). No demonstration of the splenic vein or of the inferior mesenteric or gastric portal–systemic collateral veins is obtained (Fig. 8–29). This appearance must not be confused with splenic vein occlusion. In splenic vein

Text continued on page 336

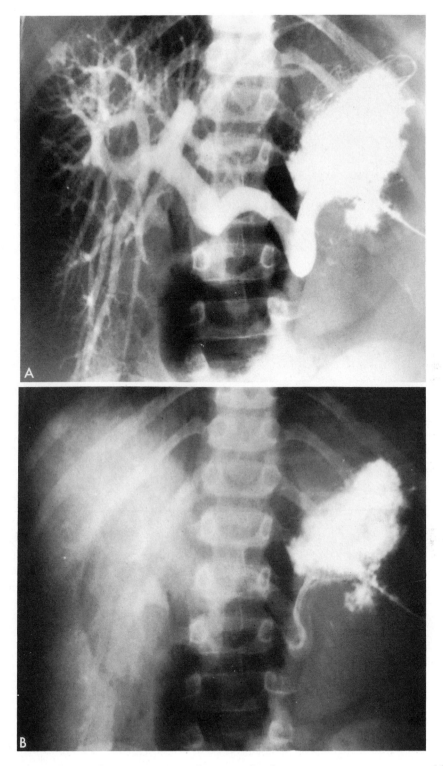

Figure 8–24. Angiographic appearance of a normal splenoportogram in a 12 year old boy with splenomegaly.

A. During injection. A large collection of contrast medium deposited in the splenic pulp flows through the splenic vein to the portal vein. No tributaries of these veins are filled. The intrahepatic portal radicles are homogeneously distributed through the liver and taper progressively toward the periphery.

B. Following injection. As the portal vein radicles wash out, a dense, homogeneous hepatogram results.

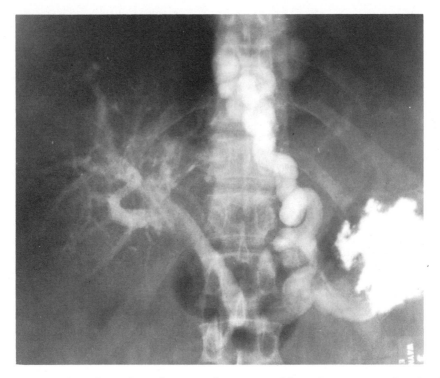

Figure 8–25. Gastric and esophageal varices demonstrated by splenoportography. A splenoportogram in a patient with Stage II cirrhosis. The contrast medium which drains to the splenic vein fills gastric and esophageal varices. Contrast medium in the portal vein continues to flow toward the liver, indicating a Stage II cirrhosis. The portal vein radicles are distorted and have fewer branches than occur in the normal person.

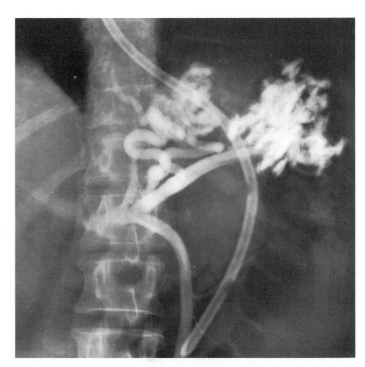

Figure 8–26. Hepatofugal blood flow in the inferior mesenteric vein demonstrated at splenoportography. Splenoportogram in a patient with advanced Stage II cirrhosis. Part of the contrast medium entering the splenic vein refluxes down the inferior mesenteric vein toward the hemorrhoidal veins. Another part enters gastric varices. A small amount continues toward the liver via the portal vein.

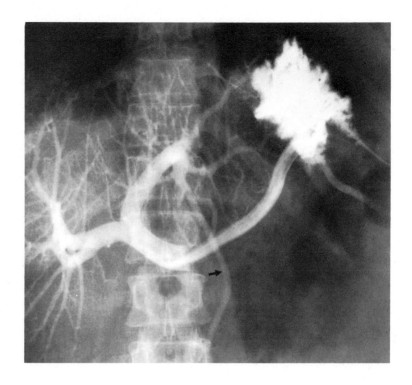

Figure 8-27. Demonstration of hepatofugal collateral development over the umbilical vein by splenoportography. Splenoportogram in a patient with Stage II cirrhosis. The portal vein branches through the liver are only moderately attenuated. Hepatopetal flow through the portal vein remains good. A dilated umbilical vein (➡) connecting with the left hepatic portal radicle takes part of the portal blood flow in a hepatofugal direction to the umbilicus and veins on the abdominal wall. Another portal–systemic collateral vein drains from the splenic hilum toward the patient's left to the abdominal wall.

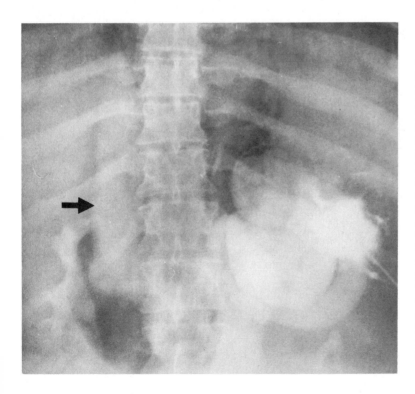

Figure 8-28. Spontaneous splenorenal shunt. Splenoportogram in a 19 year old woman with idiopathic periportal fibrosis portal hypertension and marked splenomegaly. The contrast medium drains from the splenic pulp through dilated tortuous retroperitoneal collateral veins, which communicate with the left renal vein. The contrast medium flows through the renal vein to the inferior vena cava (➡). No splenic vein is demonstrated because blood flow in this vessel is reversed. (From Redman, H. C., and Reuter, S. R.: Angiographic demonstration of portocaval and other decompressive liver shunts. Radiology 92:790, 1969.)

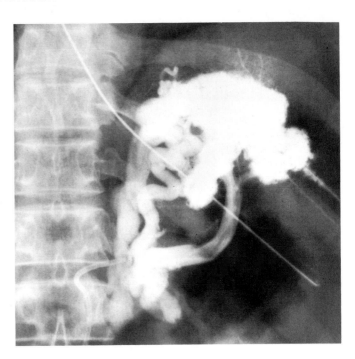

Figure 8–29. Appearance of reversal of flow in the portal vein at splenoportography. Splenoportogram in a patient with Stage III cirrhosis. The contrast medium leaving the spleen drains into large retroperitoneal veins which appear to drain toward a spontaneous splenorenal shunt. No filling is demonstrated of either the splenic or portal veins.

occlusion, portal–portal collateral veins over the gastroepiploic or gastric veins reconstitute blood flow to the portal vein. Blood flows from high to low pressure areas. With splenic vein thrombosis, portal vein pressure remains low, and collateral veins develop around the occlusion to the low pressure area. These collateral veins do not develop when flow in the portal vein is reversed because the portal vein has the highest pressure in the portal system, and all blood flows away from the portal vein.

COMPLICATIONS OF SPLENOPORTOGRAPHY. The major complication of splenoportography is bleeding from the puncture site following the examination. For this reason, splenoportograms should not be performed in patients with a prolonged clotting time. Also, because one of the mechanisms that prevents bleeding from the puncture site is tamponade of the puncture hole against the abdominal wall, splenoportograms should not be done in patients with ascites. Persistent bleeding following a splenoportogram generally requires splenectomy. In one large series, significant bleeding (500 to 2000 cc) occurred in 2 per cent of patients (Panke et al., 1959). The potential occurrence of this complication has been the major cause for the current shift to arterial portography. An emergency splenectomy in a cirrhotic pa-

tient precludes a back-up splenorenal shunt if the primary portacaval shunt thromboses, and it significantly complicates a direct portacaval shunt operation. Boijsen and Efsing (1969) have demonstrated an increased incidence of aneurysms on splenic artery branches among patients who have had a previous splenoportogram. In some of the patients, more than one aneurysm was aligned along the needle track.

Umbilical Vein Catheterization

Another method of studying the portal system is operative cannulation of the umbilical vein. Under local anesthesia, a short midline incision is made in the skin one third to one half of the way between the umbilicus and the xyphoid process. The ligamentum teres and the umbilical vein remnant within it are identified in the properitoneal fat, slightly to the right of the midline. The umbilical vein is dilated, and a catheter is passed into the left portal vein radicle to which the umbilical vein connects. Pressure determinations and injections of contrast medium can be made at this point. The injections of contrast medium should be made at moderately high rates to flood the portal system. This results in excellent demonstration of the portal–

systemic collateral veins which have developed. The method requires a minor operative intervention, and catheterization of the vein is successful in only 60 to 80 per cent of the patients in whom it is attempted. These two factors have prevented general acceptance of the method, although it does give an excellent demonstration of the portal system in patients with postsinusoidal cirrhosis without the potential hazards of splenoportography.

Transhepatic Portography

A new approach to the portal system with both diagnostic and therapeutic promise was recently reported by Lunderquist and Vang (1974). The technique is a modification of that commonly used for percutaneous transhepatic cholangiography. A needle with a Teflon sheath is introduced toward the hilum of the liver from the mid-axillary line while the patient holds his breath in a midrespiratory phase. The needle is then withdrawn from the sheath, and the patient allowed to resume quiet respirations. A syringe is attached to the sheath, which is slowly pulled back with slight negative pressure applied to the syringe. When a vein is entered, the withdrawal is stopped, and contrast medium is injected to determine whether a portal or hepatic vein has been entered. This can be determined easily by the direction of flow of the injected contrast medium. If the vein is a portal vein, a guide wire with a curved tip is introduced through the sheath into the portal venous radicle. It is best not to use straight guide wires since they tend to follow the original needle track instead of passing down the portal vein radicle. When the guide wire has been advanced into the main portal vein, the Teflon sheath is then advanced into the portal vein over the wire. Alternatively, the sheath can be withdrawn, and a catheter with a preformed shape can be introduced over the wire. When the catheter or sheath is in the main portal vein, contrast medium can be injected for portography (Fig. 8–30), and pressures can be obtained.

The advantage of transhepatic portal vein catheterization over other methods of portography is that branches of the splenic, superior mesenteric and portal veins can be catheterized selectively. Such selective

catheterizations have two important applications. The first is the ability to obtain selective samplings of blood from various pancreatic veins as part of the preoperative localization of islet cell adenomas. Using this method, Lunderquist (personal communication) has accurately localized islet cell adenomas when the pancreatic angiogram failed to reveal the site. The other potentially important application of the method is the embolization of esophageal varices in patients with cirrhosis and portal hypertension (Fig. 8–31). This approach to the control of bleeding esophageal varices is only in the early stages of development, but several investigators have used it to occlude the coronary and short gastric veins with embolic materials, tissue adhesives and sclerosing solutions. Although the results are preliminary, they indicate that the method may be superior to vasopressin infusions or Sengstaken balloon occlusion in patients with massive variceal bleeding. New portal–systemic collateral veins develop following transhepatic occlusion of the coronary and short gastric veins. Although some of these collaterals reconstitute esophageal varices, others develop internally between the portal system and retroperitoneal veins. Repeat examinations can be done to occlude newly developed esophageal collateral veins, giving internal shunts a further chance to develop. Although the preliminary results of transhepatic coronary and short gastric vein occlusion have been promising, a prolonged survival rate in patients with cirrhosis has not yet been demonstrated.

The Patient without a History of Chronic Alcoholism or Hepatitis Who Bleeds from Esophageal Varices

Occasionally a patient who has neither a history of chronic alcoholism nor the systemic sequelae of hepatic cirrhosis has massive upper gastrointestinal bleeding from esophageal varices. These may be detected during barium examinations performed at the time of the massive hemorrhage but are more often found at endoscopy or angiography. The cause of the portal hypertension and formation of

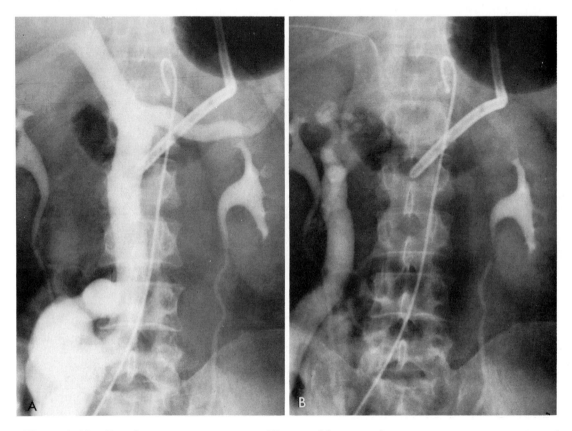

Figure 8–30. Transhepatic portogram in a 52 year old man with massive upper gastrointestinal hemorrhage.

A. Early phase. The catheter tip is in the main portal vein in the left upper corner. Although contrast medium refluxes into the splenic vein, no short gastric or coronary collateral veins extend toward the esophagus. Most of the contrast medium refluxes down a dilated superior mesenteric vein to a tangle of veins in the region of the ileocolic vein and pelvic veins.

B. Contrast medium from the pelvic veins drains via the right gonadal vein to the inferior vena cava. At autopsy, performed shortly after this study, the patient was found to have an eroded varix at the gastroesophageal junction. Thus, although he had an apparently well functioning internal shunt, it did not function adequately enough to prevent bleeding from esophageal varices.

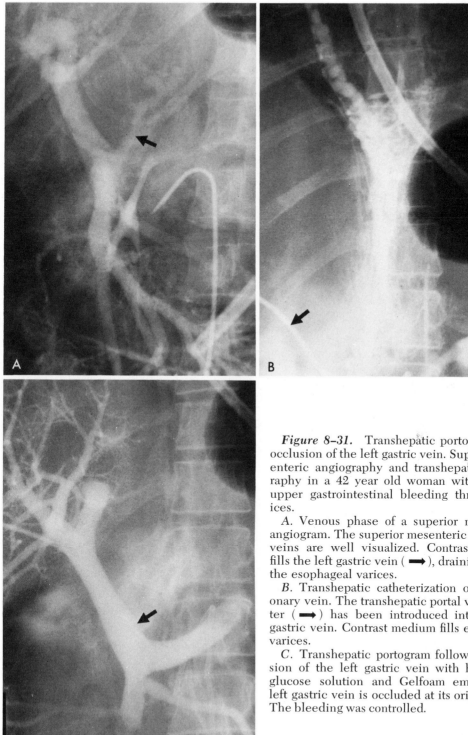

Figure 8–31. Transhepatic portography for occlusion of the left gastric vein. Superior mesenteric angiography and transhepatic portography in a 42 year old woman with massive upper gastrointestinal bleeding through varices.

A. Venous phase of a superior mesenteric angiogram. The superior mesenteric and portal veins are well visualized. Contrast medium fills the left gastric vein (➡), draining toward the esophageal varices.

B. Transhepatic catheterization of the coronary vein. The transhepatic portal vein catheter (➡) has been introduced into the left gastric vein. Contrast medium fills esophageal varices.

C. Transhepatic portogram following occlusion of the left gastric vein with hypertonic glucose solution and Gelfoam emboli. The left gastric vein is occluded at its origin (➡). The bleeding was controlled.

varices in these patients is generally a prehepatic portal block, such as occlusion of the portal or splenic vein by tumor, thrombosis or schistosomiasis. Another unusual cause is hepatic vein occlusion or the Budd-Chiari syndrome.

Presinusoidal Portal Hypertension

By far the major cause of prehepatic portal hypertension in the United States is portal vein thrombosis. This can occur in the newborn as a complication of omphalitis, or it can occur later in life as a complication of pancreatitis or tumor invasion of the portal vein. An etiology cannot be established in most patients with portal vein thrombosis. They generally come to the hospital because of variceal bleeding but do not have the general clinical appearance or history of the chronic alcoholic. Liver function studies and liver biopsies are usually normal. Angiography plays an important part in establishing the diagnosis and in providing a "road map" of the veins available for a portal–systemic decompression operation. It is essential that the surgeon have this information before undertaking a surgical procedure.

In some parts of the world, the major cause of presinusoidal portal hypertension is an infestation of the liver by *Schistosoma mansoni*. In this disease, the ova of the parasite are deposited in the intestinal wall and transported from there to the portal spaces by the portal blood flow. The ova cause fibrosis of the terminal portal vein radicles in the liver. The process of fibrosis is slow but progressive and leads to portal hypertension and to the development of portal–systemic collateral veins. Patients generally die of bleeding esophageal varices. The hemodynamics in patients with portal vein thrombosis and schistosomiasis are essentially the same. Angiography may be performed at the time of the hemorrhage, or it may be done as an elective procedure after recovery from the hemorrhage. The latter is the usual situation in these patients, since varices frequently remain unsuspected until identified during barium examinations.

PATHOLOGIC HEMODYNAMICS IN PATIENTS WITH PRESINUSOIDAL BLOCK. Patients with presinusoidal obstruction to portal vein blood flow have no intrahepatic histologic abnormality, and resistance to hepatic venous outflow is not increased. Therefore, an increase in hepatic artery blood flow compensates for the decreased portal blood flow (Fig. 8–2E). Some portal–portal collateral blood flow generally develops around the occlusion to preserve a varying degree of portal blood flow, depending on the effectiveness of the collaterals. However, most of the blood supply to the liver comes from the hepatic artery. Since resistance to the venous drainage of this arterial inflow is not increased, hepatic artery blood flow to the liver may be markedly increased. Also, the liver is generally small in patients with portal vein thrombosis. The degree of shrinkage is probably inversely related to the effectiveness of portal–portal collaterals in preserving portal blood flow. Portal hypertension develops on the splanchnic side of the block, leading to the development of portal–systemic collateral veins. Which veins develop to decompress the portal system depends upon the location and the extent of thrombosis. In some patients the thrombosis extends into the superior mesenteric, the left gastric and the splenic veins. Generally, though, the thrombosis is limited to the portal vein, and both the gastric and inferior mesenteric veins become dilated. Schistosomiasis follows the latter pattern.

ANGIOGRAPHIC APPEARANCE OF PRESINUSOIDAL BLOCK. All the angiographic methods that are applied to the evaluation of patients with cirrhosis and portal hypertension can be used to evaluate patients with portal vein thrombosis; however, the most useful are splenoportography and arterial portography.

Splenoportography. The spleen may or may not enlarge in patients with portal vein thrombosis. Splenomegaly is usually a part of advanced schistosomiasis. In portal vein thrombosis, a splenoportogram generally demonstrates the obstructed portal vein and, in addition, shows the portal–portal collateral veins which have developed through the head of the pancreas, the gallbladder and common bile duct to the intrahepatic radicles of the portal vein. These small, normally nonvisualized venous channels dilate to a marked degree and form a tangle of dilated veins which parallel the portal vein to the hilum of the liver. This appearance, shown in Figure 8–32, has been referred to as cavernomatous transformation of the portal vein (also see Fig. 8–6). Although there is some recanalization of the thrombosis, most of the channels do not represent a recanalized portal vein but result from dilatation of small veins around the portal vein. The appearance is pathognomonic for portal vein thrombosis, regardless of its cause. The portal–systemic collateral veins which develop to decompress the portal system are also demonstrated at splenoportography. These veins have the same appearance as the veins in patients with cirrhosis.

Arteriography. The arterial phase of celiac angiography in patients with presinusoidal block demonstrates the typical appearance of dilatation of the hepatic artery and its intrahepatic branches through a small liver (Fig. 8–33). The size of the splenic artery depends upon the size of the spleen, and the artery may be dilated and tortuous if the spleen is enlarged. On the venous side of the angiogram, portal–systemic collateral blood flow may be demonstrated over the gastric or inferior mesenteric veins. Left gastric angiography is the best method for demonstrating the esophageal varices. Superior mesenteric angiography following intraarterial tolazoline (see Chapter 10) is the best method for demonstrating other portal–portal collateral veins and the typical appearance of the cavernomatous transformation of the portal vein.

Celiac, high dose superior mesenteric and perhaps high dose splenic angiography should be performed in these patients to demonstrate the venous anatomy fully. It is imperative that the surgeon have an accurate knowledge of the size and the location of the splenic and superior mesenteric veins in order to perform a decompressive shunt in these patients, since the usual portacaval shunt cannot be performed (Fig. 8–34). This information is usually best obtained from the arterial studies, since only high dose superior mesenteric artery injections allow excellent demonstration of the superior mesenteric vein.

Wedged Hepatic Venography. Wedged

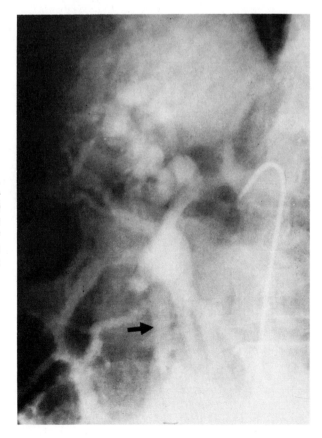

Figure 8–32. Portal vein thrombosis. Venous phase of a superior mesenteric angiogram. The superior mesenteric vein (➡) flows into a tangle of dilated collateral veins around the thrombosed portal vein to supply blood to the distal portal vein radicles. This appearance is diagnostic of portal vein thrombosis (see Fig. 8–6).

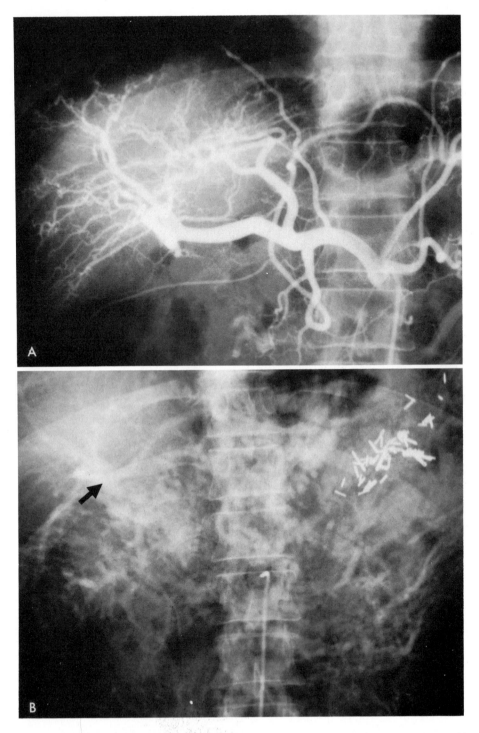

Figure 8–33. Portal vein thrombosis. Celiac and superior mesenteric angiograms in a 42 year old man who had had a splenorenal shunt because of portal vein thrombosis 20 years earlier and now has recurrent bleeding from esophageal varices.

A. Arterial phase of a celiac angiogram. The hepatic vein is dilated and supplies a number of dilated hepatic artery branches through a small liver.

B. Venous phase of a high dose superior mesenteric angiogram following injection of 50 mg of tolazoline. The splenic, superior mesenteric and portal veins are occluded. Hundreds of collateral veins throughout the abdomen bypass the occluded veins to the distal portal vein (➡).

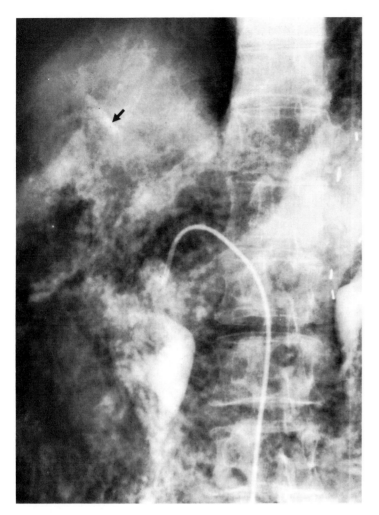

Figure 8-34. Occluded spleno-renal shunt with portal and mesenteric vein thrombosis. Venous phase of a high dose superior mesenteric angiogram in a 45 year old man who had a spleno-renal shunt because of childhood portal vein thrombosis. Hundreds of dilated collateral veins are seen throughout the mesentery. Most of these drain to small retroperitoneal veins connecting with the inferior vena cava. No superior mesenteric or portal veins are seen, so a new decompressive shunt cannot be established. Some contrast medium reaches a portal vein radicle (➡) via collateral veins around the cystic and hepatic ducts.

hepatic venography is not of much value in patients with presinusoidal block except in a negative sense. Wedged hepatic venous pressure is normal since sinusoidal pressure is not elevated. Wedged hepatic venograms demonstrate a free efflux of the contrast medium from the liver via other hepatic veins.

Hepatic Vein Occlusion

Hepatic vein occlusion, or the Budd-Chiari syndrome, is an uncommon cause of portal hypertension. The diagnosis is difficult to establish clinically, and many of the cases reported have been discovered at autopsy. Hypercoagulation states, such as occur in polycythemia vera, sickle cell anemia and secondary to the use of oral contraceptives, have resulted in hepatic vein thrombosis. Occlusion of the hepatic segment of the inferior vena cava by tumor,

such as hepatoma or hypernephroma, is another cause. However, most hepatic vein thromboses are idiopathic. The signs that bring the patient to angiography are hepatosplenomegaly and ascites, frequently accompanied by abdominal pain. The patients are usually not alcoholics, and unless the correct diagnosis is suspected, the first examinations are generally done from the arterial side. Celiac and hepatic angiography reveals an enlarged liver and spleen; the hepatic arteries are markedly stretched and bowed by the swollen liver parenchyma (Fig. 8-35). In patients with long-standing disease, the hepatic arteries may dilate and arterial–portal shunting may develop. The splenic vein is generally seen, and although the contrast medium in both the splenic and portal veins is usually of poor density, it is adequate to demonstrate the patency of these vessels. The ar-

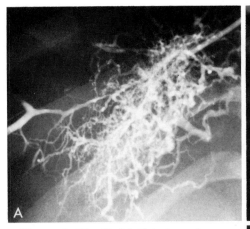
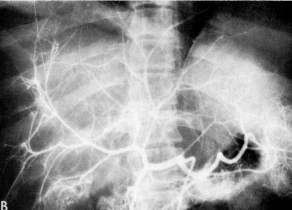

Figure 8–35. Budd-Chiari syndrome. Wedged hepatic venogram and celiac angiogram in a 17 year old woman with hepatic vein thrombosis.

A. Wedged hepatic venogram. The contrast medium forced through the sinusoids from the wedged hepatic venous catheter enters a myriad of tortuous collateral hepatic veins draining toward the inferior vena cava and toward hepatic capsular veins, demonstrating the typical "spider-web" appearance of hepatic vein thrombosis.

B. Arterial phase of a celiac angiogram. The hepatic artery branches are markedly stretched through an enlarged liver.

C. Hepatogram phase. There is dense, irregular contrast accumulation throughout the liver.

terial pattern is similar to that of alcoholic hepatitis.

The characteristic findings occur on the venous side. The first study in patients with suspected hepatic vein thrombosis should be an inferior vena cavogram, although the diagnosis is generally not considered until after the arterial examinations. The inferior vena cavogram may demonstrate occlusion of the inferior vena cava at the renal or hepatic level, with tumor extending into the cava. This appearance is generally adequate to establish a diagnosis. If the low inferior vena cava is occluded, the hepatic veins may be catheterized from above through the right atrium.

If the inferior vena cava is not occluded, the hepatic veins should be catheterized selectively and a wedged hepatic venogram performed. This gives the typical "spiderweb" appearance of the many collateral channels that develop between hepatic venules and systemic veins (Figs. 8–35 and 8–36). If all routes of access to the hepatic veins are blocked, a needle can be introduced into the liver percutaneously. Contrast medium injected into the parenchyma breaks through into the proximal hepatic venules and then fills the collateral channels, resulting in the "spider-web" pattern.

Celiac angiography demonstrates hepatosplenomegaly, and the hepatic arteries appear stretched (Fig. 8–35). The hepatogram phase of the arterial injection is dense and prolonged, and drainage of the arterial inflow of the liver via the portal vein may be demonstrated in the venous phase. In the presence of pressure induced hepatic necrosis, the hepatogram is unhomogeneous. If the disease has been present long enough, portal–systemic collateral veins develop, and high dose splenic and left gastric angiograms may demonstrate esophageal varices.

The findings at splenoportography de-

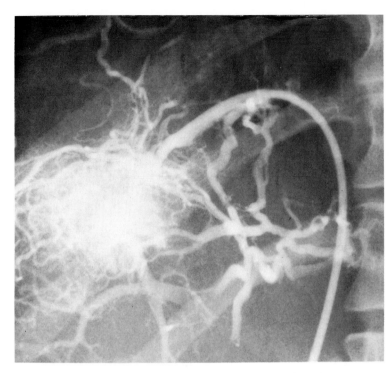

Figure 8–36. Budd-Chiari syndrome. Wedged hepatic venogram in a 14 year old girl with hepatic vein thrombosis. Contrast medium injected in the wedged position enters hundreds of small collateral veins, producing the "spider-web" appearance.

pend upon the duration of the disease. In the earlier stages, before blood flow reverses in the portal vein, the portal vein radicles appear stretched, and emptying is slowed. After blood flow in the portal vein reverses, the splenic and portal veins do not fill. Both arteriography and splenoportography may demonstrate a cause for the hepatic vein occlusion.

The Patient Who Has Had a Portal–Systemic Shunt and Has Complications Suggesting Thrombosis of the Shunt

Occasionally following a decompresive portal–systemic shunt operation, a question arises about the continued patency of the shunt, generally because the patient bleeds again or develops ascites.

Usual Hemodynamic and Angiographic Changes Following Portacaval Shunt

The postshunt angiogram varies from the preshunt study in several respects. The exact changes that occur in hemodynamics vary with the type of shunt. In a patient with a well functioning side-to-side portacaval or splenorenal shunt, the pressure in the portal system drops to about that of the inferior vena cava. In these patients, the portal vein uniformly becomes an outflow tract from the liver regardless of the direction of the portal vein blood flow preoperatively. Thus, the hepatic artery provides the entire blood supply to the liver, and the liver usually shrinks. Angiography in such patients demonstrates an increase in the arterial blood supply to the liver, generally greater than that seen prior to the shunt operation. The degree of increase appears to be greater in moderate than in advanced cirrhotic patients, presumably because the advanced cirrhotic patient has already increased his hepatic artery blood flow in response to decreased portal blood flow. Because of the small liver, the increased hepatic arterial blood flow and the patient's underlying hepatic fibrosis, the terminal hepatic artery branches appear markedly corkscrewed (Fig. 8–37). The wedged hepatic venous pressure is within the normal range, and a wedged hepatic venogram demonstrates the reversed blood flow in the portal vein to the inferior vena cava (Fig. 8–38). The hepatic veins seem to atrophy following a side-to-side portacaval shunt, and the hepat-

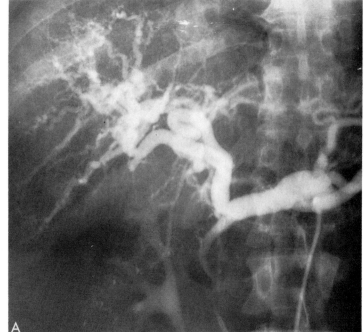

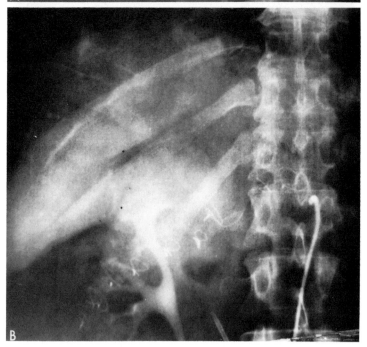

Figure 8–37. Appearance of hepatic arteries after a side-to-side portacaval shunt. Celiac angiogram in a 45 year old man.

A. Arterial phase. The hepatic artery and its branches are markedly dilated and tortuous. The liver is small.

B. Venous phase. The density of the hepatogram is homogeneously increased.

ic vein catheter wedges much closer to the inferior vena cava than preoperatively. Therefore, a larger segment of liver is filled on venograms postoperatively. With side-to-side shunts, a splenoportogram or the venous phase of a splenic angiogram demonstrates that the splenic vein communicates directly with the inferior vena cava through the shunt. The portal vein is not seen. A high dose superior mesenteric artery injection demonstrates the immediate flow of contrast medium from the superior mesenteric vein to the inferior vena cava (Fig. 8–39).

Following an end-to-side shunt, the hepatic artery also dilates, the liver shrinks

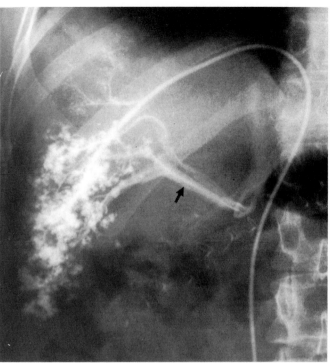

Figure 8–38. Reversed portal vein blood flow following a side-to-side portacaval shunt. Wedged hepatic venogram in a 60 year old man. Contrast medium leaving the sinusoids enters the portal vein (➡) and flows directly to the inferior vena cava. The sinusoidal filling pattern is markedly irregular. The large area of sinusoidal filling reflects the hepatic venous atrophy that occurs after portacaval shunt surgery. The catheter now wedges more proximally in the vein.

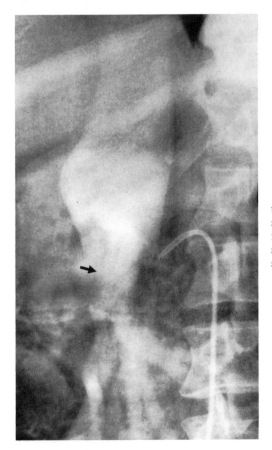

Figure 8–39. Arterial portography following a side-to-side portacaval shunt. Venous phase of a high dose superior mesenteric angiogram. The contrast medium in the mesenteric veins is well visualized, and the superior mesenteric vein (➡) empties through the shunt directly into the inferior vena cava.

and the terminal hepatic arteries have a "corkscrew" appearance. However, since the portal vein has been ligated, the portal blood flow does not reverse, and the hepatic artery inflow continues to drain from the liver via the hepatic veins. Since the hepatic veins continue to be utilized as an outflow tract, they do not atrophy, and a catheter introduced into the hepatic vein wedges in approximately the same position as preoperatively. The wedged hepatic venogram also appears similar to the preoperative examination. Surprisingly, the portal vein does not thrombose distal to the portal vein ligation, and contrast medium from the wedged hepatic venous injection frequently fills portal vein radicles. Following an end-to-side portacaval shunt, the pressure in the portal vein remains elevated. Because of this increased pressure, collateral veins develop around the ligation between the high pressure portal vein and the low pressure superior mesenteric vein. Such collaterals generally develop over the cystic and pancreaticoduodenal veins and are demonstrated at a wedged hepatic venogram (Fig. 8–40). If these collateral veins are effective in decompressing the portal vein, the wedged hepatic venous pressure drops correspondingly.

Following a Warren distal splenorenal shunt, the liver continues to be perfused by superior mesenteric blood flow. Celiac and hepatic angiograms and wedged hepatic venograms appear similar to the preoperative studies, and wedged hepatic venous pressure superior mesenteric–portal vein celiac artery injection demonstrates venous drainage of the spleen and stomach to the splenorenal shunt, while a high dose superior mesenteric artery injection demonstrates the continued perfusion of the portal vein by mesenteric blood flow. Frequently, collateral veins develop between the high pressure superior mesenteric–portal vein side of the shunt and the gastric veins, and these are demonstrated at angiography. If the surgeon has failed to ligate the middle colic vein, a markedly dilated middle colic-marginal vein anastomosis may develop to the internal iliac veins (Fig. 8–41).

Angiographic Evaluation of Patients with Occluded Portacaval Shunts

Patients in whom occlusion of a portacaval shunt is suspected can be evaluated from either the venous or arterial side. In side-to-side portacaval shunts, the thrombosis is generally soft, and the catheter can be advanced from the inferior vena cava through the occluded shunt into the portal, splenic or superior mesenteric veins (Fig. 8–42). With end-to-side shunts, only the splenic or superior mesenteric vein can be catheterized. Once the catheter is on the splanchnic side of the shunt, pressures can be obtained and the gradient across the shunt measured. An injection of contrast medium on the splanchnic side of the shunt demonstrates reconstitution of the

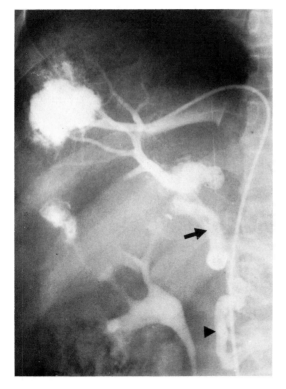

Figure 8–40. Development of collateral veins following an end-to-side shunt. Wedged hepatic venogram in a 53 year old man. The pattern of sinusoidal filling is relatively homogeneous. The contrast medium refluxes into both the hepatic and portal veins. The contrast medium entering the portal veins drains through dilated cystic (➡) and pancreaticoduodenal (▶) veins to the superior mesenteric vein. (From Reuter, S. R., and Orloff, M. J.: Wedged hepatic venography in patients with end-to-side portacaval shunts. Radiology *111*:563, 1974.)

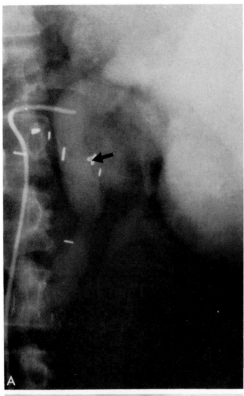

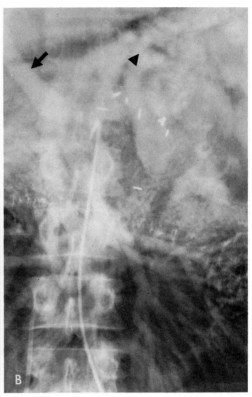

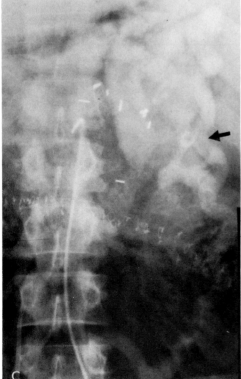

Figure 8-41. Blood flow pattern following a Warren shunt. Splenic and superior mesenteric angiograms in a 36 year old man who had had a Warren shunt for bleeding varices 4 months previously.

A. Venous phase of a splenic angiogram. The splenic vein (➡) communicates with the renal vein.

B. Early venous phase of a superior mesenteric angiogram. The contrast medium in the mesenteric veins drains predominantly toward the portal vein (➡). However, some contrast medium also enters gastric varices via reconstituted collateral veins (▶).

C. Late venous phase. A dilated middle colic vein drains from the superior mesenteric vein to the marginal vein of Drummond (➡) and then to the superior hemorrhoidal veins.

Figure 8–42. Postoperative evaluation of a side-to-side portacaval shunt from the inferior vena cava in a 48 year old man. The catheter has been introduced through the anastomosis into the hepatic limb of the shunt. In patients with side-to-side shunts, the catheter can equally well be directed into the splanchnic limb. When contrast medium is injected, many of the portal vein radicles are filled, and the contrast medium drains rapidly to the inferior vena cava. No collateral veins are seen, indicating a well functioning shunt.

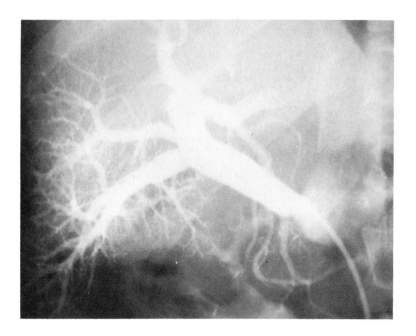

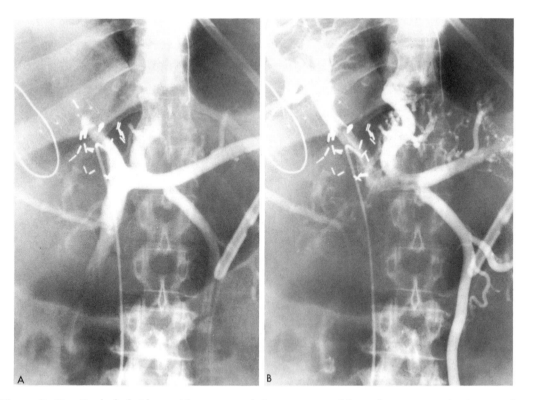

Figure 8–43. Occluded side-to-side portacaval shunt examined from the venous side. A trans-shunt catheterization of the portal system in a 43 year old man.

A. During injection, the contrast medium fills the portal, splenic, gastric and both mesenteric veins. None enters the inferior vena cava.

B. Following injection, the contrast medium has emptied from the superior mesenteric vein in an antegrade direction, and hepatopetal flow is reestablished in the portal vein. The gastric, splenic and inferior mesenteric veins have again become portal–systemic collateral veins.

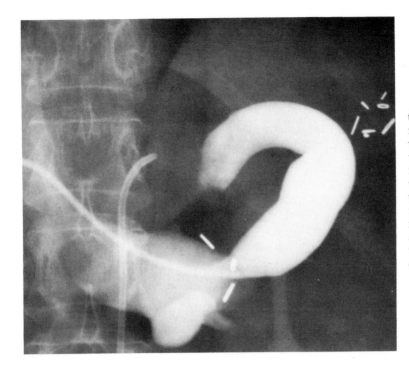

Figure 8-44. Postoperative evaluation of a splenorenal shunt from the inferior vena cava in a 38 year old woman. The catheter has been introduced through the renal vein and the anastomosis into the splenic vein. Contrast medium fills the splenic vein for a short distance retrograde and then washes out through the shunt to the inferior vena cava.

Figure 8-45. Arterial portography following an end-to-side splenorenal shunt. Venous phase of a high dose superior mesenteric angiogram in a 56 year old man. The contrast medium leaving the superior mesenteric vein drains into the splenic vein. Blood flow in the splenic vein (⟹) is reversed; contrast medium enters the left renal vein (➡) and then enters the inferior vena cava.

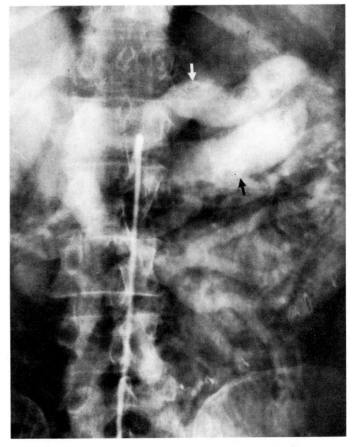

portal–systemic collateral veins via gastric or inferior mesenteric veins. In patients with side-to-side shunts, the reestablishment of antegrade flow in the portal vein may also be demonstrated (Fig. 8–43). Splenorenal shunts are difficult to evaluate from the venous side because of the angle between the splenic and renal veins (Fig. 8–44).

Arterial portography, particularly high dose superior mesenteric angiography, is useful for evaluating the blood flow dynamics in patients with suspected occlusions of decompressive portal–systemic shunts. If the shunt is open, the contrast medium in the venous phase flows freely through the shunt to the inferior vena cava (Figs. 8–39 and 8–45). If it is occluded, many collateral veins are present (Fig. 8–34); occasionally, major portal–systemic collateral veins fill. No contrast medium is seen in the inferior vena cava. High dose superior mesenteric angiography is the best method for demonstrating a mesocaval shunt. Left gastric angiography is the best method for demonstrating recurrent esophageal varices.

If the patient's spleen is still present, a splenoportogram demonstrates the portal–systemic collateral veins and may also show reestablishment of antegrade flow in the portal vein.

BIBLIOGRAPHY

Aronsen, K. F., and Nylander, G.: Use of direct portography in diagnosis of liver diseases. Radiology 88:40, 1967.

Baron, M. G., and Wolf, B. S.: Splenoportography. J.A.M.A. 206:629, 1968.

Berdon, W. E., Baker, D. H., and Casarella, W.: Liver disease in children: portal hypertension, hepatic masses. Semin. Roentgenol. 10:207, 1975.

Boijsen, E.: Selective angiography of the celiac axis and superior mesenteric artery in cirrhosis of the liver. Rev. Int. Hepat. 15:323, 1965.

Boijsen, E., and Efsing, H. O.: Aneurysm of the splenic artery. Acta Radiol. (Diagn.) (Stockh.) 8:29, 1969.

Boijsen, E., and Ekman, C. A.: Angiography in portal hypertension. J. Cardiovasc. Surg. (Torino), VII Congress International Cardiovascular Society, p. 45, 1965.

Bookstein, J. J., Appleman, H. D., Walter, J. F., et al.: Histological-venographic correlates in portal hypertension. Radiology 116:565, 1975.

Bookstein, J. J., Boijsen, E., Olin, T., et al.: Angiography after end-to-side portacaval shunt. Clinical, laboratory, and pharmacoangiographic observations. Invest. Radiol. 6:101, 1971.

Bookstein, J. J., and Whitehouse, W. M.: Splenoportography. Radiol. Clin. N. Amer. 2:447, 1964.

Braastad, F. W., Wukasch, D. C., and Jordan, P. H.: The practicality of umbilical vein cannulation in patients with and without portal hypertension. Arch. Surg., 101:32, 1970.

Conn, H. O., and Ramsby, G. R.: Angiographic technics in assessing the patency of portacaval anastomoses. Amer. J. Dig. Dis. 18:651, 1973.

Coutinho, S. G., Saad, E. A., and da Silva, J. R.: Segmental hepatic angiography. A preliminary report. Amer. J. Dig. Dis. 12:685, 1967.

Cronqvist, S., and Ranniger, P.: Spontaneous splenorenal shunts. Acta Radiol. (Diagn.) (Stockh.) 3:433, 1965.

Deutch, V., Rosenthal, T., Adar, R. et al.: Budd-Chiari syndrome: Study of angiographic findings and remarks on etiology. Amer. J. Roentgenol. 116:430, 1972.

Doehner, G. A.: The hepatic venous system. Its normal roentgen anatomy. Radiology 90:1119, 1968.

Doehner, G. A., Ruzicka, F. F., Hoffman, G., et al.: The portal venous system: Its roentgen anatomy. Radiology 64:675, 1955.

Douglass, B. E., Baggenstoss, A. H., and Hollinshead, W. H.: The anatomy of the portal vein and its tributaries. Surg. Gynec. Obstet. 91:562, 1950.

Ekengren, K., Reuterskiöld, A., and Söderlund, S.: Pre- and postoperative appearances of splanchnic veins in children with portal hypertension. Acta Radiol. (Diagn.) (Stockh.) 3:97, 1965.

Foster, J. H., Conkle, D. M., Crane, J. M., et al.: Splenoportography: An assessment of its value and risk. Amer. Surg. 179:773, 1974.

Galmarini, D., Zanoli, P. G., Riquier, G., et al.: Hepatic vein pressure determination and phlebography in the evaluation of portal hypertension. S. Afr. Med. J. 43:1011, 1969.

Göthlin, J., Lunderquist, A., and Tylén, U.: Selective phlebography of the pancreas. Acta Radiol. (Diagn.) (Stockh.) 15:474, 1974.

Hales, M. R., Allan, J. S., and Hall, E. M.: Injection-corrosion studies of normal and cirrhotic livers. Amer. J. Pathol. 35:909, 1959.

Hipoma, F. A., and Gabriele, O.: Portal venous system as a major collateral in iliac and inferior vena caval obstruction. Radiology 89:1077, 1967.

Hirooka, M., and Kimura, C.: Membranous obstruction of the hepatic portion of the inferior vena cava. Arch. Surg. 100:656, 1970.

Ingemansson, S., Lunderquist, A., and Holst, J.: Selective catheterization of the pancreatic vein for radioimmunoassay in glucagon-secreting carcinoma of the pancreas. Radiology 119:555, 1976.

Ingemansson, S., Lunderquist, A., Lundquist, I., et al.: Portal and pancreatic vein catheterization with radioimmunologic determination of insulin. Surg. Gynecol. Obstet. 141:705, 1975.

Johnson, G., Jr., Dart, C. H., Jr., Peters, R. M. et al.: Hemodynamic changes with cirrhosis of the liver: Control of arteriovenous shunts during operation for esophageal varices. Ann. Surg., 163:692, 1966.

Joly, J. G., Marleau, D., Legare, A., et al.: Bleeding from esophageal varices in cirrhosis of the liver: Hemodynamics and radiological criteria for the selection of potential bleeders through hepatic and umbilicoportal catheterization studies. Canad. Med. Ass. J. 104:576, 1971.

Kahn, P. C., O'Halloran, J. F., Jr., and Paul, R. E., Jr.: Improved portography by delayed postepinephrine celiac and mesenteric arteriography. Radiology 92:86, 1969.

Kessler, R. E., Tice, D. A., and Zimmon, D. S.: Value, complications and limitations of umbilical vein catheterization. Surg. Gynec. Obstet. 136:529, 1973.

Kessler, R. E., Tice, D. A., and Zimmon, D. S.: Retrograde flow of portal vein blood in patients with cirrhosis. Radiology 92:1038, 1969.

Kessler, R. E., and Zimmon, D. S.: Umbilical vein angiography. Radiology 87:841, 1966.

Kittredge, R. D., and Finby, N.: One aspect of splenoportography: Reversal of flow with resulting nonvisualization of the portal vein. Radiology 81:267, 1963.

Kreel, L.: Vascular radiology in liver disease. Postgrad. Med. J. 46:618, 1970.

Kreel, L., Freston, J. W., and Clain, D.: Vascular radiology in the Budd-Chiari syndrome. Brit. J. Radiol. 40:755, 1967.

Kreel, L., Gitlin, N., and Sherlock, S.: Hepatic artery angiography in portal hypertension. Amer. J. Med. 48:618, 1970.

L'Hernime, C., Paris, J. C., Quandalle, P., et al.: Spontaneous porto-caval mesenteric-gonadal anastomosis occurring in cirrhosis: A report of three cases. Ann. Radiol. (Paris) 15:823, 1972.

Lunderquist, A., and Vang, J.: Transhepatic catheterization and obliteration of the coronary vein in patients with portal hypertension and esophageal varices. New Eng. J. Med. 291:646, 1974.

Lunderquist, A., Simert, G., Tylen, U., et al.: Follow-up of patients with portal hypertension and esophageal varices treated with percutaneous obliteration of gastric coronary vein. Radiology 122:59, 1977.

Maguire, R., and Doppman, J.: Angiographic abnormalities in partial Budd-Chiari syndrome. Radiology 122:629, 1977.

Miller, F. J., Jr., Maddrey, W. C., Sheff, R. N., et al.: Hepatic venography and hemodynamics in patients with alcoholic hepatitis. Radiology 115:313, 1975.

Moreno, A. H., Ruzicka, F. F., Rousselot, L. M., et al.: Functional hepatography. Radiology 81:65, 1963.

Moskowitz, H., Chait, A., Margulies, M., et al.: Prone splenoportography. Radiology 90:1132, 1968.

Nebesar, R. A., and Pollard, J. J.: Portal venography by selective arterial catheterization. Amer. J. Roentgenol. 97:477, 1966.

Novak, D., Butsow, G. H., and Becker, K.: Hepatic occlusion venography with a balloon catheter in patients with end-to-side portacaval shunts. Am. J. Roentgenol. 127:949, 1976.

Novak, D., Butsow, G. H., and Becker, K.: Hepatic occlusion venography with a balloon catheter in portal hypertension. Radiology 122:623, 1977.

Panke, W. F., Bradley, E. G., Moreno, A. H., et al.: Technique, hazards, and usefulness of percutaneous splenic portography. J.A.M.A. 169:1032, 1959.

Peck, D. R., and Lowman, R. M.: Roentgen aspects of umbilical vascular catheterization in the newborn. The problems of catheter placement. Radiology 89:868, 1967.

Pochaczevsky, R., Calem, W. S., and Richter, R. M.: Umbilical vein portography. Its value in the diagnosis of extrahepatic portal vein obstruction and in other applications. Radiology 89:868, 1967.

Pollard, J. J., and Nebesar, R. A.: Altered hemodynamics in the Budd-Chiari syndrome demonstrated by selective hepatic and selective splenic angiography. Radiology 89:236, 1967.

Pollard, J. J., Nebesar, R. A., and Mattoso, L. F.: Angiographic diagnosis of benign diseases of the liver. Radiology 86:276, 1966.

Popper, H., Elias, H., and Petty, D. E.: Vascular pattern of the cirrhotic liver. Amer. J. Clin. Path. 22:717, 1952.

Price, J. B., Jr., Voorhees, A. B., Jr., and Britton, R. C.: Operative hemodynamic studies in portal hypertension. Significance and limitations. Arch. Surg. 95:843, 1967.

Rachlin, L., Hansen, R. H., and Carolan, J. J.: Umbilical vein catheterization and cirrhosis. Surg. Gynec. Obstet. 130:272, 1970.

Raffensperger, J. G., Shkolnik, A. A., Boggs, J. D., et al.: Portal hypertension in children. Arch. Surg. 105:249, 1972.

Ramsay, G. C., and Britton, R. C.: Intraparenchymal angiography in the diagnosis of hepatic veno-occlusive diseases. Radiology, 90:716, 1968.

Redman, H. C.: The Budd-Chiari syndrome: Angiography and its complications. J. Can. Assoc. Radiol. 26:271, 1975.

Redman, H. C., and Reuter, S. R.: Angiographic demonstration of portocaval and other decompressive liver shunts. Radiology 92:788, 1969.

Redman, H. C., Reuter, S. R., and Miller, W. J.: Improvement of superior mesenteric and portal vein visualization with tolazoline. Invest. Radiol. 4:24, 1969.

Reuter, S. R., and Chuang, V. C.: The location of increased resistance to portal blood flow in obstructive jaundice. Invest. Radiol. 11:54, 1976.

Reuter, S. R., Berk, R. N., and Orloff, M. J.: An angiographic study of the pre- and postoperative hemodynamics in patients with side-to-side portacaval shunts. Radiology 116:33, 1975.

Reuter, S. R., and Orloff, M. J.: Wedged hepatic venography in patients with end-to-side portacaval shunts. Radiology 111:563, 1974.

Reynolds, T. B., Ito, S., and Iwatsuki, S.: Measurement of portal pressure and its clinical application. Amer. J. Med. 49:649, 1970.

Rösch, J., and Dotter, C. T.: Extrahepatic portal obstruction in childhood and its angiographic diagnosis. Amer. J. Roentgenol. 112:143, 1971.

Rosenberg, R. F., and Sprayregen, S.: The hepatic artery in cirrhosis: An angiographic pathophysiologic correlation. Angiology 25:499, 1974.

Rourke, J. A., Bosniak, M. A., and Ferris, E. J.: Hepatic angiography in "alcoholic hepatitis." Radiology 91:290, 1968.

Rousselot, L. M., Ruzicka, F. F., and Doehner, G. A.: Portal venography via the portal and percutaneous splenic routes. Anatomic and clinical studies. Surgery 34:557, 1953.

Ruzicka, F. F., and Rossi, P.: Arterial portography: Patterns of venous flow. Radiology 92:777, 1969.

Smith, G. W., Westgaard, T., and Björn-Hansen, R.: Hepatic venous angiography in the evaluation of cirrhosis of the liver. Ann. Surg. 173:469, 1971.

Tavill, A. S., Wood, E. J., Kreel, L., et al.: Budd-Chiari syndrome: Correlation between hepatic scintigraphy and clinical, radiologic, and pathologic findings in 19 cases of hepatic venous outflow obstruction. Gastroenterology 68:509, 1975.

Tylen, U., Simert, G., and Vang, J.: Hemodynamic changes after distal splenorenal shunt studied by sequential angiography. Radiology 121:585, 1976.

Viamonte, M., Jr., Danner, P., Warren, W. D., et al.: A new technique for the assessment of hyperkinetic portal hypertension. Radiology 96:539, 1970.

Viamonte, M., Jr., LePage, J. R., Russell, E., et al.: The hemodynamics of diffuse liver disease. Sem. Roentgenol. 10:187, 1975.

Viamonte, M., Jr., Martinez, L., Parks, R. E., et al.: Liver shunts. Amer. J. Roentgenol. 102:773, 1968.

Viamonte, M., Jr., and Viamonte, M.: Liver circulation. Crit. Rev. Clin. Radiol. 27:214, 1974.

Viamonte, M., Jr., Warren, W. D., and Fomon, J. J.: Liver panangiography in the assessment of portal hypertension in liver cirrhosis. Radiol. Clin. N. Amer. 8:147, 1970.

Viamonte, M., Jr., Warren, W. D., Fomon, J. J., et al.: Angiographic investigations in portal hypertension. Surg. Gynec. Obstet. 130:37, 1970.

Warren, W. D., Fomon, J. J., Viamonte, M., et al.: Spontaneous reversal of portal venous blood flow in cirrhosis. Surg. Gynec. Obstet. 126:315, 1968.

Warren, W. D., Fomon, J. J., Viamonte, M., et al.: Preoperative assessment of portal hypertension. Ann. Surg. 165:999, 1967.

Warren, W. D., and Muller, W. H., Jr.: A clarification of some hemodynamic changes in cirrhosis and their surgical significance. Ann. Surg. 150:413, 1959.

Warren, W. D., Restrepo, J. E., Respess, J. C., et al.: The importance of hemodynamic studies in management of portal hypertension. Ann. Surg. 158:387, 1963.

Widrich, W. C., Robbins, A. H., Nabseth, D. C., et al.: Portal hypertension changes following selective splenorenal shunt surgery. Evaluation by percutaneous transhepatic portal catheterization, venography, and cinefluorography. Radiology 121:295, 1976.

Chapter 9

MAJOR EQUIPMENT USED IN VISCERAL ANGIOGRAPHY AND RADIOGRAPHIC TECHNIQUE

Placing the tip of a catheter in the proper visceral artery orifice is only one part of producing a successful angiogram. All too frequently, the mechanics of catheterization are overstressed by beginning angiographers, while the other aspects of the examination, such as the sequential filming of the arterial, capillary and venous phases, are slighted. Although the principles of good radiographic technique can be violated without serious consequence when many parts of the body are examined, strict adherence to good radiography must be maintained during angiography.

MAJOR EQUIPMENT USED IN ANGIOGRAPHY

A detailed discussion of the engineering of angiographic equipment, radiographic generators or rapid film changers is not within the scope of this book. However, we are frequently asked by practicing radiologists what the minimum requirements for radiographic equipment are in visceral angiography. Most departments planning an angiographic special procedures room want a multipurpose room, in which neurologic, cardiac, visceral and peripheral angiographic examinations can be performed. The equipment requirements for these various types of angiography are, of course, different. Biplane capability is recommended for neuroradiology, and in cardiac angiography cinefluorographic recording is necessary. Angiography of the abdominal vessels requires neither. The equipment that is chosen, therefore, depends on the special procedures for which the room will be used.

Radiographic Generators

The optimum contrast differentiation between the contrast medium in the blood vessels and the surrounding tissues is obtained in almost all patients using a KVP of as close to 70 as possible. With this KVP, standard film–screen combinations require about 50 to 100 MAS for proper film exposure. In order to avoid motion unsharpness, 100 milliseconds is the longest exposure time that should be used for visceral work. Therefore, a generator with a minimum output of 800 to 1000 MA is required. It should be either a three-phase, twelve-pulse rectified or a secondary contacting generator. Single phase generators are no longer recommended since they would require high-speed film–screen combinations and KVP ranges of 90 to 100 for obese patients.

Radiographic Tubes

Recent, significant advances in tube design allow greater heat storage and dissipation in the tube anode, increasing the allowable milliamperage at which the tubes can be operated during serial angiography. The two most important advances are high-speed rotation of the anode and decreased angulation of the target. High-speed rotation markedly improves the capacity of the anode for instantaneous heat loading. At the same time, the angulation of the target has been changed from the traditional 17 degrees to 10 to 12 degrees, spreading the cathode beam over a greater anode surface while maintaining the same effective focal spot. With these innovations, 1 mm focal

spots can be used under most angiographic conditions up to 100 MAS generator output, significantly decreasing the geometric distortion of the radiographic system. Changing from a 2 mm conventional tube to a 1 mm tube with high-speed rotation and decreased target angle is the single most important, inexpensive change that can be made to improve the quality of the angiographic image. There is no longer any reason to have a 2 mm focal spot tube in a visceral angiographic installation. In some cardiac angiography suites, 2 mm focal spots are still used since they can be loaded with 1500 MA. The resulting exposure times are very short, in the range of several milliseconds. Other changes in tube design to allow further loading capabilities of tubes are being researched at present. These include increasing the diameter of the anode and altering the anode alloy. Hopefully, the day is not far off when a 0.6 mm focal spot can be used for most visceral angiographic procedures. A careful check of the effective focal spot size at the actual technique used during angiography is important. The actual focal spot size may be larger than specified because manufacturers do not measure the focal spot size at clinical MA ranges.

Angiographic Film Changers

Rapid serial film changers must be used for visceral angiography. Manually operated cassette tunnels holding three to four films or hand-pulled changers are not adequate. The three basic types of rapid film changers in general use for abdominal angiography are cassette changers, cut film changers and roll film changers. Each has certain advantages and disadvantages which must be weighed in choosing one for a specific angiographic installation. Whichever type is chosen, the field size must be 14 × 14 inches in order to include the entire superior mesenteric vascular bed.

Cassette Changers

Two types of cassette changers are available. One uses modified metal radiographic cassettes; the other, vacuum packed cardboard cassettes. Both have excellent screen contact. The advantages of the former are a relatively low price and a relatively simple design, decreasing mechanical problems. However, the cassettes are 11 × 14 inches, too small for general use in visceral angiography. There are only 12 cassettes, and the programming is not versatile. The vacuum cassette changer has the advantages of the metal cassette changer and, in addition, has a 14 × 14 inch field size, is versatile in programming and can be used for a full angiographic series. Its major disadvantage is the increased amount of time required to load and unload the vacuum cassettes.

Cut Film Changers

The major advantage of the cut film changer for angiographic work is the ease with which the films can be handled following exposure of the angiographic series. This is particularly important during more sophisticated catheterizations when the findings of one series will determine the next step. In this instance, selected films from the arterial, capillary and venous phases can be developed first and then a decision made about how to proceed. With roll film, the entire angiographic series must be developed before a decision can be made. Screen contact may be a problem with both cut and roll film changers, but can be excellent if these are kept in good adjustment. Screen contact should be checked at least once a month, and if found faulty, should be adjusted.

Roll Film Changers

The major advantage of roll film changers is the speed with which the changers can be run. Films can be exposed at a rate of 6 per second, while cut film changers are generally limited to 2 to 4 per second. This is important in angiocardiography but has little use in visceral angiography. A rate of film change greater than 2 per second is rarely necessary in gastrointestinal angiography. The main problems with roll film changers involve the handling, viewing and storage of the rolls. Because of these problems, most angiographers have the frames of the film cut apart with a paper cutter prior to viewing. To date, only one roll film changer has been developed with a 14 × 14 inch film size. This particular changer features a device that cuts the roll after the exposures. Although the changer is loaded with a roll of film, it delivers cut films.

See-Through Film Changers

Both cut and roll film changers are now being developed with built-in image intensifiers. This arrangement of film changer and intensifier has advantages over the more traditional installations. First, one tube is eliminated from the system, since a single tube is used for both fluoroscopy and filming of the angiographic series. Second, the patient does not move between fluoroscopy and filming. Finally, the exposures of the angiographic series can be monitored on television and videotape at the same time they are recorded on film. Catheter recoil or subintimal injection occurring during the examination can therefore be seen immediately, the injection discontinued and corrections made to allow for a successful angiogram.

The major disadvantage of the current see-through changer is the large amount of scatter from the patient, caused by using the overhead tube for fluoroscopy. This results in several times the radiation dosage to the examiner as compared with conventional under-the-table fluoroscopy. Most of the scatter can be removed with curtain shields and aprons, but these are bulky and interfere with the smooth performance of the examination. Another disadvantage is that generally only a single port, small field image intensifier can be used. Also, in order to keep the patients' radiation exposure to reasonable levels, it is important to remove the radiographic screens from the roentgen beam during fluoroscopy. All in all, the advantages of well-designed see-through changer systems may outweigh their disadvantages.

Angiographic Tables

Several types of angiographic tables are manufactured for use in angiographic installations. Some of these have specialized options which adapt them to cardiac, neurologic or magnification angiography. These include rotating cradle tops, adjustable headboards and a motor-driven eleva-tion of the table top. In visceral angio-graphy, most of these options are not required. A simple floating table top with good longitudinal and lateral motion is ade-quate, though the elevating table top is im-portant if direct serial magnification angio-graphy is to be done.

Image Intensification and TV Monitors

All modern angiographic installations should have both image intensification and television display of the intensified image. Catheterizations can be performed using image intensification with a mirror display, but manipulating a catheter at the patient's groin while trying to look into a mirror cen-tered over the patient's upper abdomen is awkward. In cardiac and neurologic angio-graphy, the television display is even more important; with cardiac angiography, cine recording of the intensified image is neces-sary. Because of recent improvements in image intensifier resolving power, more and more medical centers are using 100/105 mm cameras for some of the film-ing usually done with rapid film changers. The advantages of 100/105 mm cameras are: there is a lower radiation dose to the patient, patients do not need to be moved during fluoroscopy and filming and there is a considerable saving in film cost.

Film–Screen Combinations

Some controversy exists about the use of high-speed film with slower speed screens versus slower film with high-speed screens in angiography. Until recently, this contro-versy was theoretical, but the introduction of high-resolution, high-speed screens with rare earth phosphors, excellent resolv-ing power and improved high-speed film has made both options possible. Either method will probably result in excellent angiograms. It is apparent, however, that limits exist to the speed to which a film–screen combination can be pushed. For ex-ample, if extremely fast film is used with ultra high-speed screens, so few photons

are required to produce the desired film density that serious quantum mottle occurs on the radiographs. A film–screen combina-tion must be chosen that has enough speed to allow latitude in the exposure technique but yet avoids too much speed and the resulting quantum mottle.

At the other end of the spectrum, slower screens and slower film should not be com-bined. Although this may result in "more beautiful" angiograms, the amount of radia-tion that patients receive during such an angiographic procedure is considerable. The film–screen combination chosen should balance the highest film quality with the lowest patient exposure.

Injectors

Modern motor-powered injectors regu-late the flow rates. The injection rate (of course limited by the capacity of the cath-eter) and the duration of injection can be dialed directly on the injector. Flow regu-lation is done by an electronic feedback mechanism between the flow and the pres-sure, modifying the pressure throughout the injection to maintain the flow at a con-stant rate. This type of injector is particu-larly useful in gastrointestinal angiography, since visceral angiographers generally make their own catheters in a variety of lengths rather than using the preformed catheters used in cardiac angiography. Moreover, it is constricting to be limited to a few catheters of given length, diameter and number of side holes. Maximum flexi-bility of approach is desirable. These injec-tors are quite accurate in the injection ranges generally employed in gastrointes-tinal angiography. They have enabled angiographers to achieve angiograms in which the injection rate approximates the flow of the artery being injected. Gas-propelled and motor-driven injectors with which flow rate cannot be regulated should no longer be used.

Grids

High-quality grids must be used in angiography. These should have ratios of

10:1 and should be at least 100 line with aluminum spacing.

Rotating grids are currently being used in visceral angiography in some medical centers. These have some advantages over stationary grids, since small linear structures, such as blood vessels, which run in the same plane as stationary grid lines, are poorly visualized. As we look at smaller and smaller vessels, the elimination of grid lines becomes important. This is particularly so in direct serial magnification angiography.

RADIOGRAPHIC TECHNIQUE

Excellent radiographic technique is essential in angiography. Vascular motion must be stopped, and good contrast must be maintained. A violation of any of the following principles of good radiographic technique will result in loss of detail.

Collimation

The field of irradiation should be limited as closely as possible to the organ being examined. This is one of the most important principles in angiographic technique. All possible scattered radiation must be eliminated to assure good contrast and to improve the sharpness of the blood vessels. The more selective the injection of contrast medium, the closer the field must be collimated. With close collimation, the examiner should mark the center of the field being examined on the patient's skin, identifying this point at fluoroscopy. This must be done in the phase of respiration in which the angiographic series is exposed.

A high-quality collimator is also extremely important in obtaining excellent angiograms and should have a lead iris diaphragm extending into the x-ray tube to help reduce off-target irradiation.

Exposure Factors

Angiographic examinations in the abdomen should be exposed as close to 70 KVP as possible. This provides the ideal contrast between the contrast medium in the arteries and the adjacent soft tissues. When the KVP drops below 70, the films become too black-white; above 80 they begin to become gray.

The milliamperage of the generator should generally be the maximum that the tube will tolerate. Most modern x-ray tubes will allow a 1 mm focal spot to be loaded with 800 to 1000 MA.

The exposures in angiographic procedures should be at the shortest possible time to give the desired density to the film at 70 KV. The pulsation of blood vessels leads to indistinctness of the vascular margin, and although the excursion of the visceral vessels during systole and diastole is not nearly as great as of vessels near the heart, definite cephalocaudad motion of the celiac artery and its branches occurs during the heart cycle. With a 1000 MA three-phase generator, exposures can generally be kept below 50 milliseconds in an average patient.

Fixed KV radiography should be used in visceral angiography. In fact, both the KV and MA are fixed for most patients. The KV should be 70 KVP and the MA the maximum allowed by the tube rating chart. The variable is the time, and the density of the film can be altered by increasing and decreasing the exposure time. In obese patients the time should not be increased above 100 milliseconds. When this exposure time is reached, the KV should be increased to achieve further film density.

Object–Film Distance

Since the patient must lie supine on the angiographic table, the organ that is being examined is anywhere from 10 to 40 cm from the film. Prone angiography is generally impractical, even when an anterior structure is being examined, so the geometric distortion due to patient anatomy must be accepted. The distance between the film changer and the angiographic table top, however, can be minimized. Some film changers can be elevated with a motor-driven mechanism, and care should be taken to oppose the changer and the table top before filming. Generally the changer must be elevated and depressed each time the patient is moved from the fluoroscopic to the filming position, since the bar supporting the front end of the angiographic table will not clear the elevated changer. If no elevation mechanism is present on the changer, it should be placed in the fixed position that allows the least amount of clearance by the moving angiographic table. Taking care to minimize the object–film distance is one of the small but important things an angiographer can do to improve angiographic images.

Filming Sequence

The sequence of filming depends on the blood flow in the vascular bed being investigated and on the information that is desired. Thus, in a lateral aortogram, two films per second for 2 or 3 seconds will adequately delineate the orifices of the celiac, superior and inferior mesenteric arteries. However, studies of the celiac and superior mesenteric vascular beds require observance of the contrast medium as it passes through arteries, capillaries and veins. In this instance, several films need to be taken during the arterial phase, fewer during the capillary phase and even fewer during the venous phase. We generally expose two films per second for 3 to 4 seconds, one film per second for 3 to 4 seconds and one film every third second for 15 seconds. Such a series would contain all the available information. The final choice of a filming sequence is up to the individual angiographer. However, extension of the filming into the venous phase is essential, and this requires 23 to 25 seconds.

The "Tailored" Angiogram

A standard angiogram does not exist. Each angiographic examination must be individualized to the patient and his suspected disease. In some instances, all the necessary information may be obtained with a single anteroposterior celiac injection. In others, both the celiac and superior mesenteric arteries must be injected, followed perhaps by superselective injections. Individualizing the examinations requires observation of each film series before proceeding to the next. As mentioned under the section about angiographic film changers, this is best accomplished by using cut films, since a film from each phase of the angiogram can be developed prior to the remainder of the examination, decreasing the waiting time between the angiographic series. Tailoring the examination also allows for modifications of a patient's position or corrections of radiographic technique which might not have been optimum on a previous injection. Most important, however, it allows for a complete, definitive examination at a single sitting.

Preliminary Film

A preliminary exposure should be taken of the area to be examined prior to beginning the catheterization procedure. This allows the angiographer to modify the radiographic technique before the first angiographic series and to adjust the position of the patient relative to the film changer in order to include the required information. The preliminary film should be exposed in the same phase of respiration in which the angiogram is to be performed. The preliminary film also reveals the presence of residual barium from a previous gastrointestinal examination prior to catheter insertion so that the angiogram can be delayed until the barium is removed.

It is also useful to expose the first film of each angiographic series prior to the injection of contrast medium. This allows use of the subtraction technique in selected instances. Although subtraction is not frequently used in visceral angiography, we have found it very useful in the evaluation of the venous phase. This can generally be accomplished with the more sophisticated injectors by delaying the start of injection 0.2 to 0.4 second after the initiation of the filming series.

Total Systems Performance

Careful attention must be given to every aspect of the equipment, from focal spot size, radiographic technique and film–

screen combination to proper function of the automatic film processor in order to be sure there is no weak link in the system which would reduce the final image quality.

Direct Serial Magnification Angiography

Many neuroradiologists routinely do lateral cerebral angiograms with direct magnification, and a few angiographers routinely use direct serial magnification for renal angiography. However, in the gastrointestinal tract, magnification angiography will probably never become a routine procedure. The organs being examined are too large to magnify two times on a 14 × 14 film. Therefore, a preliminary examination of the celiac, superior mesenteric or inferior mesenteric circulation must always precede a magnification study.

Direct serial magnification has value in selected situations in visceral angiography, particularly when it is combined with superselective injection of contrast medium into the organ being evaluated. In the pancreas questionable abnormalities of the pancreaticoduodenal arcades and smaller branches can generally be classified as either normal or abnormal. Similarly, in the liver direct serial magnification is of value in defining more clearly subtle arterial abnormalities in patients with suspected tumors, particularly cholangiocarcinomas. Although the major usefulness of magnification angiography is enlargement of the arteries and veins, a side benefit comes from modification of the geometry that results from placing the patient nearer the tube. Thus, in any of the visceral organs in which several layers of arteries are superimposed, the increased divergence of the roentgen beam causes the vessels to be spread farther apart, and superimposition becomes less of a problem in interpretation of the angiograms. This is particularly helpful in evaluating bowel angiodysplasias and in the pancreas generally.

One of the major factors limiting the use of magnification angiography in the gastrointestinal tract has been tube design. The conventional tubes allowed neither adequate focusing of the electron beam nor heat storage capacity by the anode. By developing new anode alloys and by decreasing the target angle, manufacturers have increased the loading capacities of microfocus tubes. At present there is a great deal of research being done in tube design, and hopefully the new cathodes and anodes being evaluated will result in a microfocus tube that can be loaded adequately for visceral magnification. A by-product of this research should be development of a tube that will allow the routine use of a 0.6 mm focal spot for conventional angiography. Another problem has been the NEMA specifications that were developed to describe focal spot size. These have allowed manufacturers to pass off as 0.3 mm focal spots, tubes that in reality have a focal spot of 0.45 mm in one diameter. Moreover, the focal spots are measured by manufacturers at unrealistically low MA levels. As the MA is increased into the clinical range, there is considerable "blooming" of the focal spot size. Whenever an angiographer receives a new magnification tube, it is essential that he measure the focal spot immediately so that the tube can be returned if it is not satisfactory.

Prior to purchasing tubes and equipment for direct serial magnification angiography, it would probably be useful for any radiologist to discuss the equipment with an angiographer who has had some experience using the technique. The literature in the field is highly technical and not particularly helpful to persons planning an angiographic suite. The tube purchased should depend on the type of magnification intended. For example, if no more than two times magnification is desired, little improvement in resolution is achieved by going below a focal spot 0.3 mm in diameter, whereas three to four times magnification requires a focal spot in the range of 0.1 mm. Generally speaking, little additional information is obtained in clinical gastrointestinal angiography by magnifying more than two times, although three to four times magnification has proven very useful in renal angiography.

Two primary methods have been developed for doing magnification angiography. The original, and most generally used, is the air gap technique. An alternative method is the short distance–rotating grid technique. Each has advantages and disadvantages.

The air gap technique uses the conventional 100 cm focal spot–film distance; the organ to be examined is placed approximately halfway between the focal spot and film. Generally, this gives about 25 to 30 cm air gap between the patient and the film, and this is adequate to clean up most of the scattered radiation. However, it does not clear up all scattered radiation, and magnification films made with an air gap technique frequently appear somewhat gray. A rotating grid can be used with the air gap technique to clean up the scatter, but this increases the radiation necessary to produce the same density. Most angiographers who perform direct serial magnification angiography with the air gap technique become accustomed to the slightly decreased contrast on the film and feel that it does not interfere with the diagnostic information. The major advantage of the air gap technique is that it can be done simply, particularly if an elevating angiography table is available. Several manufacturers now supply such a table. The patient can be elevated, the grid removed from the film changer and the examination performed.

The short distance–rotating grid technique also has advantages and disadvantages. The major advantages are that the short distance, generally 65 cm from focal spot to film, decreases the amount of MAS necessary to produce an equivalent amount of darkening on the film, and the MA can be kept to near 50 MA. With the currently available tubes, this prevents "blooming" of the focal spot, and the effective focal spot size remains small. At the same time, the rotating grid cleans up scattered radiation, and the resulting radiographic images have excellent contrast and clarity. The disadvantage of the method is the relatively high skin dose, although it is confined to a small segment of skin. In order to produce approximately 1.6 to 1.8 times magnification, the collimator of the tube is on the patient's skin. Since the Bureau of Radiation Health regulations forbid placing the anode closer than 12 inches to the patient's skin, further magnification can only be obtained by increasing the object–film distance. Since the rotating grids must be specially focused for the short focal spot–film distance, any significant variance in the object–film distance increases the focal spot–film distance as well, and grid cut-off

may become a problem. Also, increasing the focal spot–film distance increases the necessary MA and defeats, in part, the advantages to be obtained from the short distance technique. Finally, the rotating grids which are currently available are driven by compressed air which must be available in the angiographic suite. The amount of noise that the rotating grids made in the early days of development has been considerably decreased with improved design.

In summary, direct serial magnification is an important adjunct to gastrointestinal angiography. It should not be used as a routine method but should be used to resolve questions that are raised on conventional angiograms. It is most useful when combined with superselective injections of contrast medium into the vascular bed being evaluated. Which technique for magnification the angiographer chooses depends on individual preference; both produce satisfactory examinations with existing technology. A great deal of investigation is currently being done in tube design, and, hopefully, tubes will be developed soon that are more suitable than those currently available.

BIBLIOGRAPHY

Amplatz, K.: New rapid roll-film changer. Radiology 90:130, 1968.
Amplatz, K.: Simple Bucky diaphragm for high speed angiography. Invest. Radiol. 2:387, 1967.
Billing, L., Bogren, H., and Seldinger, S. I.: Selective renal angiography utilizing 70 mm image intensifier fluorography. Medicamundi 14:55, 1968.
Boijsen, E., Holm, T., and Kaude, J.: Comparative angiographic studies using 70 mm intensifier fluorography and serial film changer. Medicamundi 14:120, 1968.
Bookstein, J. J., and Powell, T. J.: Short-target-film rotating-grid magnification. Comparison with air gap magnification. Radiology 104:399, 1972.
Bookstein, J. J., and Voegeli, E.: Critical analysis of magnification radiography. Radiology 98:23, 1971.
Bull, K. W., Curry, T. S., III, Dowdey, J. E., et al.: The cut-off characteristics of rotating grids. Radiology 114:453, 1975
Doi, K., and Imhof, H.: Noise reduction by radiographic magnification. Radiology 122:479, 1977.
Felson, B., and Schmidt, O. E. W.: The significance of grid ratio in clinical radiography. Radiology 75:925, 1960.
Fischer, H., Roller, G., and Hubbard, P.: An analysis of several factors influencing injection rates in angiography. Radiology 83:396, 1964.
Hoffman, J. R., Staiger, J. W., Wollan, R. O., et al.: The Minnesota special procedure room. Radiology 98:551, 1971.
Komar, N., Courtney, N., and Fischer, H. W.: Studies

with an angiographic injector of automatic flow-rate control design. Radiology 90:981, 1968.

Moore, R., Krause, D., and Amplatz, K.: Flexible grid-air gap magnification technique. Radiology *104*: 403, 1972.

Moseley, R., Jr., Holm, T., and Williams, H.: Composite Modulation Transfer Functions of Image Intensi-fier-Television Systems. *In* Diagnostic Radiologic Instrumentation. Springfield, Illinois, Charles C Thomas, Publisher, 1965.

Ovitt, T. W., Moore, R., and Amplatz, K.: The evalua-tion of high-speed screen-film combinations in angiography. Radiology *114*:449, 1975.

Rao, U. V. G., and Clark, R.: Radiographic magnifica-tion versus optical magnification. Radiology *94*:196, 1970.

Stanton, L., Matsumoto, K., Pyenson, J., et al.: A new test object for evaluating resolution in serial angi-ography. Radiology 93:1190, 1969.

Stein, H. L.: Direct serial magnification renal arteri-ography: a clinical study. J. Urol. *109*:964, 1973.

Stucky, J. P., Schad, N., and Pircher, L.: Die Entwick-lung moderner Kontrastmittelinjecktoren. Acta Radiol. (Suppl.) (Stockh.) *270*:155, 1967.

Viamonte, M., Jr., and Hobbs, J.: Automatic electric injector. Development to prevent electromechan-ical hazards of selective angiocardiography. Invest. Radiol. 2:262, 1967.

Wold, G. J., Scheele, R. V., and Agarwal, S. K.: Evalua-tion of physician exposure during cardiac catheter-ization. Radiology 99:188, 1971.

Chapter 10

PHARMACO-ANGIOGRAPHY

VASOCONSTRICTOR DRUGS
  Pharmacology
    Epinephrine
    Norepinephrine
    Vasopressin
    Angiotensin
  Angiographic Uses
    Enhancement of Tumor Demonstration
    Redistribution of Blood Flow
    Slowing Venous Blood Flow to Improve
      Retrograde Phlebography
VASODILATOR DRUGS
  Pharmacology
    Tolazoline

    Papaverine
    Epinephrine
    Histamine
    Acetylcholine Chloride
    Glucagon
    Contrast Medium
    Bradykinin
    Prostaglandins
  Angiographic Uses
    Improve Venous Visualization
    Dilate Spastic Vessels
THERAPEUTIC PHARMACOANGIOGRAPHY
  Tumor Infusion

Pharmacoangiography is a term used to describe angiography performed following the modification of blood flow by vasoactive drugs. This technique can be very useful in certain diagnostic situations to improve visualization of arterial or venous abnormalities. Both vasoconstrictor and vasodilator drugs are used. The vasoconstrictor drug most commonly used with angiography in the United States is epinephrine. Angiotensin, norepinephrine and vasopressin are also available. The more common vasodilator drugs are tolazoline and contrast medium. Papaverine, bradykinin, acetylcholine chloride, histamine, glucagon, and several of the prostaglandins have also received some evaluation. Some drugs, such as epinephrine, have a biphasic effect, and the angiogram can be performed during either the vasoconstrictor or vasodilator phase. Others, such as vasopressin, cause constriction in one vascular bed and dilatation in another.

The vasoactive drugs are injected through the catheter used for the angiogram. The doses used are much lower than those needed to achieve the same effect by intravenous administration. Therefore, selective intraarterial administration of these vasoactive drugs into the celiac or superior mesenteric arterial bed usually causes little systemic response. Some of the drugs are metabolized in the liver; all are markedly diluted before reaching the systemic circulation. The lack of systemic effect from selective intraarterial injections has been the most important factor in the development of pharmacoangiography.

A maximum angiographic effect is obtained by injecting the contrast medium at the height of arterial drug response. This time is known for the drugs in common use but has not been evaluated for all the drugs that are available. Similarly, the minimum drug dose necessary to cause the desired arterial response should be used. Some doses are known because of an accumulation of clinical information, but others have not been accurately determined. In some instances, drug dosages and optimum injection time for contrast medium have been extrapolated from animal experiments.

The mechanism of action of the vasoactive drugs currently used in pharmacoangiography is widely varied. Some, such as histamine, have an unknown form of action. Others, such as vasopressin and bradykinin, act directly on vascular smooth muscle. Epinephrine and norepinephrine stimulate the alpha and beta adrenergic receptors. The alpha receptors are innervated by autonomic fibers; the beta receptors are not. The alpha receptors cause vasoconstriction; beta receptors cause vasodilatation. The response to these drugs depends on the ratio of alpha and beta receptors in the vascular bed, the dose level and the time of observation. The beta response appears to be longer lasting than the alpha response. Both alpha and beta receptors can be selectively blocked by appropriate drugs. For example, Dibenzyline will block the alpha response, propranolol, the beta.

VASOCONSTRICTOR DRUGS

Pharmacology

Epinephrine

Epinephrine is both an alpha and a beta adrenergic stimulator, but the alpha (constrictor) component tends to override the beta (dilator) component unless the injected vascular bed has few alpha receptors. The visceral arteries all show some degree of constriction following an intraarterial injection of epinephrine. The degree of response varies greatly from artery to artery and from patient to patient. In the celiac bed, the hepatic, splenic, left gastric and gastroduodenal arteries constrict more than the inferior phrenic and intrapancreatic arteries. Differential constriction is apparent when the dose of epinephrine is from 5 mcg to 15 mcg, but is often obscured by larger doses. The superior and inferior mesenteric arterial branches to the bowel constrict rather uniformly, while the pancreatic branches of the superior mesenteric artery are less responsive. The constriction in the mesenteric arteries is less than that in the celiac artery. An injection of 2 to 3 mg of propranolol, a beta adrenergic blocker, into the superior mesenteric artery prior to the epinephrine injection produces consistent vasoconstriction (Steckel et al., 1968). Prolonged or repeated use of epinephrine can lead to escape from alpha receptor control and subsequent vasodilatation. While this is a factor in therapeutic usage, it is not important in the diagnostic setting.

Norepinephrine

Norepinephrine, a catecholamine closely related to epinephrine, also stimulates the alpha adrenergic receptors strongly and the beta receptors weakly. While it consistently causes vasoconstriction, this is less marked than the vasoconstriction seen following a comparable dose of epinephrine. Vasodilatation is also less prominent. Its effect is blocked by adrenergic blockaders. Vasoconstriction is transient following a single arterial injection. Systemic side effects have not been significant at the dosage levels used for clinical pharmacoangiography. Norepinephrine has been especially useful as an adjunct to pancreatic angiography (Boijsen, 1971).

Vasopressin

Vasopressin is an octapeptide which has both antidiuretic and vasoconstrictor properties and is produced in the neurohypophysis. Most commercially available preparations are assayed in pressor units. The antidiuretic function causes reabsorption of water in the distal renal tubules independent of electrolytes. Vasoconstriction is caused by a direct action on the vascular contractile elements in the arterioles and, especially, in the precapillaries. This response is longer lasting than that seen with epinephrine. Vasopressin does not affect the alpha receptors, and its action is not affected by adrenergic blocking agents. Blood pressure is not altered in normal, nonanesthetized patients with an intraarterial vasopressin administration at the dosage levels used in pharmacoangiography. Bowel cramps may occur, caused by increased bowel motility. The drug is apparently deactivated rapidly by the liver and the kidneys. It is probably this rapid deactivation that keeps the antidiuretic effect from being a serious problem during selective superior mesenteric arterial administration in diagnostic angiography. Fluid balance, bradycardia and coronary vasoconstriction are significant factors in therapeutic infusions, and patients must be monitored carefully for these complications (see Chapter 6). It should always be remembered that the effect of vasopressin does not lyse immediately with the cessation of drug infusion.

Angiotensin

Angiotensin is a naturally occurring decapeptide which causes marked vasoconstriction, probably by direct action on vascular smooth muscle in the smaller arterioles. It is a more potent vasoconstrictor than either epinephrine or norepinephrine. Kaplan and Bookstein (1972) used angiotensin in a series of human celiac and superior mesenteric angiograms. They found it to be a potent vasoconstrictor in the smaller arteries of the hepatic and superior mesenteric distribution. In particular, constriction of the superior mesenteric artery was profound. The intrapancreatic arteries were less affected than the other arteries evalulated. In their series, no significant increase in blood pressure occurred, and bradycardia was not observed. The drug effect was gone in 1 to 2 minutes. Tumor vessels did not constrict with angiotensin. No adverse side effects occurred, though tachyphylaxis was demonstrated after repeated intraarterial injections. The systemic effects of angiotensin include an increase in arterial pressure, a decrease in cardiac output and bradycardia. These side effects should be watched for when the drug is used in pharmacoangiography.

Angiographic Uses

Enhancement of Tumor Demonstration

Initially, pharmacoangiography was used to enhance the demonstration of renal cell carcinomas. Intraarterial injections of epinephrine, 3 to 5 mcg, cause constriction of the non-neoplastic arteries and allow more selective filling of the tumor with contrast medium. With experience it has become apparent that renal cell carcinoma can almost always be definitively diagnosed without epinephrine. Epinephrine-enhanced renal angiography is now generally reserved for patients with hematuria and no indication of tumor on conventional renal angiograms

To date, the use of vasoconstrictor drugs for tumor enhancement has not been widespread in the visceral vascular bed. There are several series that report improved visualization of pancreatic or hepatic carcinomas and hepatic metastases following either epinephrine or angiotensin. Ekelund and Lunderquist (1974) found improved diagnostic information in 70 per cent of patients in a series done with angiotensin. Greater filling of smaller arteries was the reason for increased information. Epinephrine has been specifically useful in determining the extent of carcinoid tumors (Goldstein, 1976). Epinephrine can constrict the feeding arteries to a tumor (Fig. 10–1), and therefore the smallest effective dose should be used. Vasoconstrictor drugs often have some value in tumor demonstration, but they should not be used without a control angiogram since vasoconstriction may introduce arterial irregularities, making interpretation difficult (Fig. 10–2).

The epinephrine dose in visceral angiography depends upon the size of the vascular bed injected but varies between 5 and 20 mcg. Doses over 20 mcg tend to cause a generalized arterial constriction which obscures tumor vascularization. A norepinephrine dose is from 5 to 10 mcg. Angiotensin doses range between 0.5 and 5 mcg. Since vasopressin is generally infused, little data is available about its effect on visceral arteries following a single injection. An infusion of 0.2 pressor unit per minute (Nusbaum et al., 1968) generally causes a marked decrease in the superior mesenteric blood flow. Complete cessation of blood flow can sometimes be achieved with 0.4 pressor unit per minute. Data for the celiac and inferior mesenteric arteries are incomplete; however, an infusion of 0.1 to 0.2 pressor unit in the celiac artery causes good vasoconstriction.

Doppman (1969) demonstrated that the neovascularity of granulation tissue is not responsive to vasoconstrictor drugs in animals. While there are several case reports of nonresponsive inflammatory tissue in man, especially renal abscesses, the arteries in some inflammatory tissue are known to constrict. Active vasoconstriction of arteries in inflammatory tissue surrounding colonic carcinomas has been observed following epinephrine (Fig. 10–3). This is demonstrated by cessation of arteriovenous shunting and marked constriction of the vasa recta in the inflamed bowel. In chronic pancreatitis, the pancreatic arteries seem to be more than normally affected by epinephrine (Boijsen and Redman, 1967)

A
B

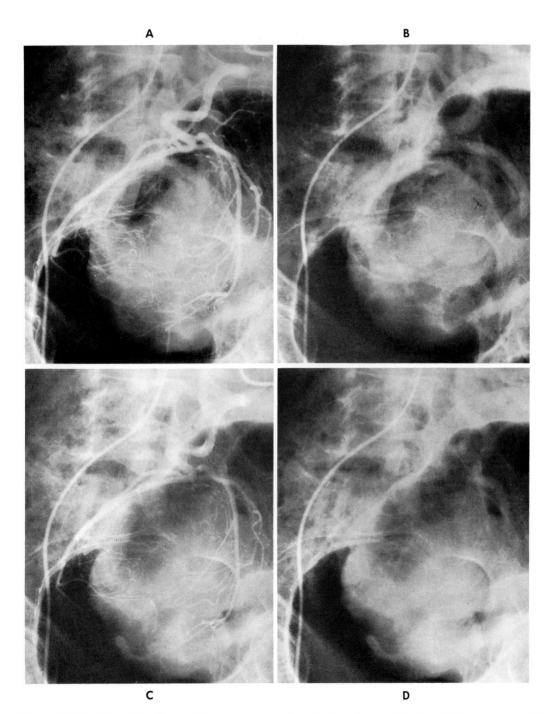

C
D

Figure 10–1. Sigmoid villous adenoma pre- and postepinephrine injection. Inferior mesenteric angiogram in a 69 year old man with a massive sigmoid villous adenoma.

A. Preepinephrine. Arterial phase. The large sigmoid mass receives many arterial branches from the dilated inferior mesenteric artery.

B. Venous phase. There is dense venous drainage.

C. Postepinephrine. Arterial phase following epinephrine, 10 mcg. Arterial supply to the tumor is diminished, and fine detail is lost.

D. Venous phase. Venous return is diminished.

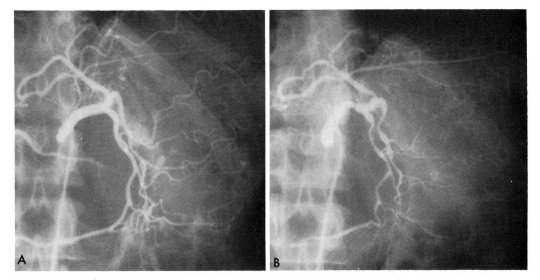

Figure 10-2. Gastric bleeding pre- and postvasopressin infusion. Left gastric angiogram.

A. Preinfusion angiogram. Arterial phase. The left gastric artery and its branches are all regular. A bleeding site is seen in the gastric fundus.

B. Postinfusion study. Arterial phase following vasopressin, 0.2 pressor unit per minute. The left gastric artery and its branches are constricted and have many luminal irregularities. No bleeding is seen. The multiple irregularities could be misinterpreted if a preliminary angiogram is not obtained before drug injection or infusion.

Redistribution of Blood Flow

Arterial blood flow can be redistributed within a given vascular bed because of the varied responses of the individual arteries to vasoconstriction. For example, celiac blood flow can be redistributed toward the pancreas by performing celiac angiography 20 to 30 seconds following administration of 10 to 15 mcg of epinephrine into the celiac artery (Fig. 10–4). The peripheral splenic and hepatic arterial branches constrict, and the majority of the bolus enters the common hepatic artery, gastroduodenal artery and its pancreatic branches. Even superselective splenic or gastroduodenal angiography for pancreatic disease can often be enhanced by pharmacoangiography (Fig. 10–5). Similarly, the demonstration of adrenal tumors can be improved by epinephrine-enhanced celiac angiography because of the lesser effect on the inferior phrenic arteries. Angiotensin is effective in increasing the flow through the pancreatic arcades when appropriate superselective injections cannot be made (Kaplan and Bookstein, 1972).

Vasoconstrictors can be used to slow blood flow in high flow states, such as that seen in some arterial collaterals, hypervascular neoplasms and, most commonly, cirrhosis. When arterial blood flow exceeds 15 to 20 cc per second in the celiac or superior mesenteric artery, it is difficult to make a selective injection approximating the rapid flow. The contrast medium is diluted so that the smaller arteries cannot be evaluated, and the venous phase is often equally poor. Vasoconstrictors will slow the arterial blood flow enough to permit adequate arterial and venous demonstration.

To date, 5 to 15 mcg of epinephrine is used for redistributing blood flow. Too large a dose decreases the differential effect because of more generalized vasoconstriction, while too small a dose does not cause any significant vasoconstriction.

Slowing Venous Blood Flow to Improve Retrograde Phlebography

Intraarterial vasoconstrictors can be used to slow the arterial input to a vascular bed markedly while the veins are injected in a retrograde manner. This method is used primarily in the renal circulation (Olin and Reuter, 1965). The washout of contrast medium from veins is slowed, and the con-

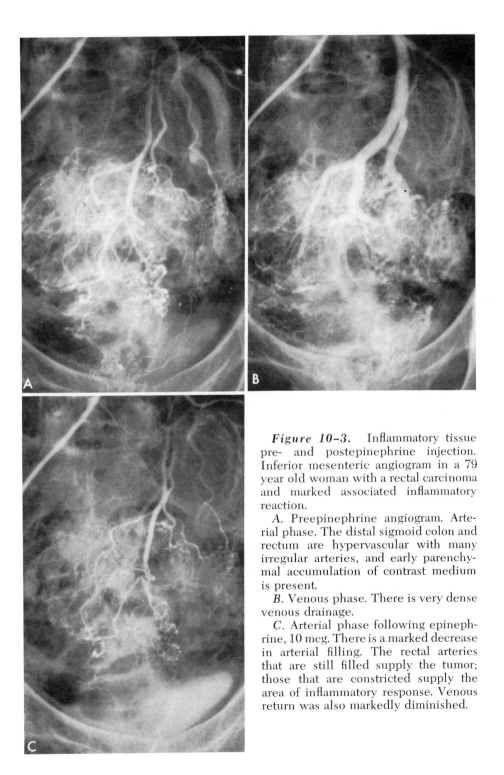

Figure 10–3. Inflammatory tissue pre- and postepinephrine injection. Inferior mesenteric angiogram in a 79 year old woman with a rectal carcinoma and marked associated inflammatory reaction.

A. Preepinephrine angiogram. Arterial phase. The distal sigmoid colon and rectum are hypervascular with many irregular arteries, and early parenchymal accumulation of contrast medium is present.

B. Venous phase. There is very dense venous drainage.

C. Arterial phase following epinephrine, 10 mcg. There is a marked decrease in arterial filling. The rectal arteries that are still filled supply the tumor; those that are constricted supply the area of inflammatory response. Venous return was also markedly diminished.

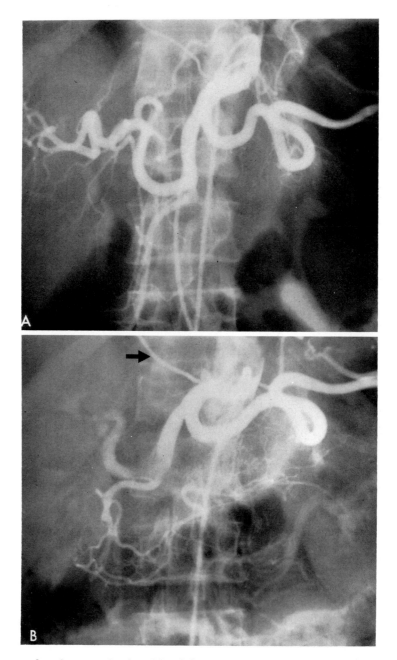

Figure 10–4. Redistribution of celiac blood flow following epinephrine injection. Celiac angiogram in a 54 year old woman.

A. Preepinephrine angiogram. Arterial phase. The peripheral hepatic arterial branches are filled. Though the gastroduodenal artery is filled, few intrapancreatic arteries are seen.

B. Arterial phase following 10 mcg of epinephrine. The pancreatic arcades are well demonstrated, while the intrahepatic arteries are not filled. The right inferior phrenic artery is dilated (➡).

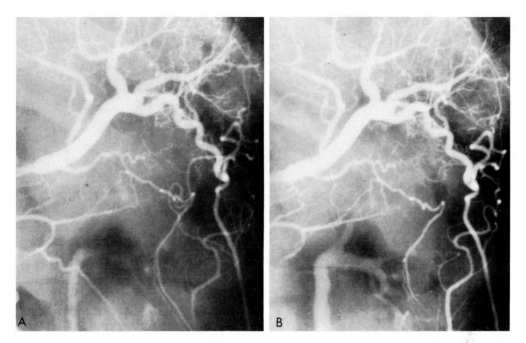

Figure 10–5. Epinephrine enhancement of superselective splenic angiography. Splenic angiogram in a 45 year old man.

A. Preepinephrine angiogram. Arterial phase. The pancreatica magna artery and a few finer branches are demonstrated.

B. Arterial phase following epinephrine, 6 mcg. Though little response is seen in the splenic arterial branches, an increased number of arteries are filled in the tail of the pancreas. The epiploic arteries are also better filled.

trast medium fills more peripheral veins. This method has little current application to the visceral circulation, but hepatic veins may be better demonstrated by combining retrograde hepatic venous injections with celiac or superior mesenteric arterial infusions of a vasoconstrictor. In the kidney, the dose used to cause maximum slowing is 0.2 mcg of epinephrine per kilogram body weight, with a maximum of 20 mcg. In the celiac and superior mesenteric circulations, doses of 20 to 30 mcg of epinephrine usually markedly slow arterial blood flow.

VASODILATOR DRUGS

Pharmacology

Tolazoline (Priscoline)

Tolazoline is a transiently effective adrenergic blocking agent which causes arterial dilatation by direct action on the arterial vascular bed. While tolazoline can cause hypotension and tachycardia, these side effects do not occur with the intraarterial doses used in pharmacoangiography. Injection of contrast medium following tolazoline may cause increased discomfort and mild bowel cramps. Dilatation is more prominent in the superior mesenteric artery than in the celiac artery, and the improvement of visualization of the superior mesenteric veins is more marked than that of the splenic vein.

Papaverine

Papaverine is a short-acting, smooth muscle relaxant, with a direct effect on the arterial wall. It appears to have no significant side effects when injected into the superior mesenteric artery. The effect is variable, but blood flow can be increased by as much as 30 per cent. Slight bowel cramps may occur.

Epinephrine

Epinephrine is a biphasic drug affecting both alpha and beta receptors. Following vasoconstriction there is usually a vasodilatation phase accompanied by hyperemia. This phase generally begins about 90 seconds after an epinephrine injection into the celiac circulation and lasts up to 15 minutes. The intensity of vasodilatation varies from patient to patient. Kahn et al. (1969) described an infusion technique utilizing the vasodilatory phase following an epinephrine injection. In contrast to most other vasodilators, epinephrine causes equally improved visualization of the veins in the celiac and the superior mesenteric circulations.

Histamine

Histamine acid phosphate causes arterial dilatation and increased blood flow. The mechanism of this action is unclear. Histamine does not cause a consistent or significant increase in blood flow and is not widely used.

Acetylcholine Chloride

Acetylcholine chloride in small doses causes superior mesenteric arterial dilatation with associated increase in blood flow. Since it acts on smooth muscle, bowel cramps often occur. Currently, no preparation for intravascular human use is available in the United States. Preliminary studies in Europe suggest that acetylcholine chloride is less effective than bradykinin for improvement of venous visualization.

Glucagon

Glucagon has recently been used experimentally to cause splanchnic vasodilatation and increased venous visualization (Danford and Davidson, 1969). Clinical application has been too limited to judge usefulness at this time.

Contrast Medium

The angiographic contrast media cause a very brief decrease in blood flow followed by vasodilatation and an increase in blood flow of 30 to 60 per cent in the superior mesenteric artery. This property is used by some angiographers to increase blood flow. We have found this technique less effective than the use of either tolazoline or bradykinin. It also increases the total volume of contrast medium used, an important factor when several angiographic series are planned.

Bradykinin

Bradykinin is a naturally occurring polypeptide which is an important blood flow regulator. It acts directly on smooth muscle and is rapidly deactivated by the liver. While it can cause hypotension, this has not been observed during pharmacoangiography. Dilatation of the celiac artery equals that of the superior mesenteric artery, but venous visualization is less markedly enhanced in the celiac vascular bed. Bradykinin is probably the most consistent drug available for improving venous visualization. It is widely used for this purpose in Europe, but has not received approval of the Food and Drug Administration in the United States.

Prostaglandins

The prostaglandins are biologically active fatty acids found in man and other mammals. Several groups of prostaglandins cause relaxation of vascular smooth muscle, and laboratory and clinical trials suggest that prostaglandins E_1 and F_2 may be superior to bradykinin for enhancing venous visualization. The duration of action is longer in the superior mesenteric vascular bed, and side effects are minimal. These drugs are not yet available for general clinical use in the United States. European clinical experience in both peripheral and superior mesenteric angiography has shown significant improvement in arterial visualization in the first instance and significant improvement in venous demonstration in the second.

Angiographic Uses

Improve Venous Visualization

A common use of vasodilators in visceral angiography is to increase the concentration of contrast medium in veins. The increased blood flow that accompanies vaso-dilatation allows a larger volume of contrast medium to be injected per unit time, resulting in a larger bolus reaching the venous vascular bed at a given time. Demonstration of visceral veins is important in the angiographic evaluation of several gastrointestinal abnormalities. In patients with portal hypertension, esophageal varices and other hepatofugal collaterals can be identified. Portal and splenic vein thrombosis and collateral veins can be demonstrated (Fig. 10–6). Postoperative patency of por-

tacaval and other decompressive liver shunts can be evaluated (Fig. 10–7). Venous visualization is important in the diagnosis and determination of operability of gastric and pancreatic tumors. In our experience, bradykinin is the most reliable drug for enhancing venous visualization. Tolazoline is the best substitute available in the United States, though some authors prefer a priming dose of contrast medium. Table 10–1 lists the adult doses of the more commonly used drugs and indicates the optimum time for injection of contrast medium.

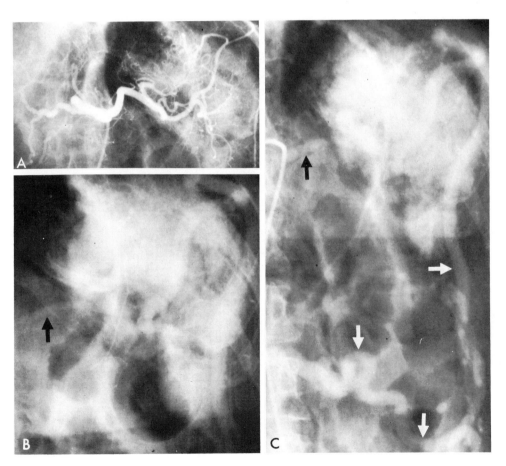

Figure 10–6. Splenic venous collaterals pre- and posttolazoline. Celiac angiogram in a 79 year old woman with a large pancreatic carcinoma.

A. Arterial phase. The gastroduodenal, common and proper hepatic and splenic arteries are all encased by neoplasm. Smaller arteries in the tail of the pancreas are also involved.

B. Venous phase pretolazoline. The splenic vein is faintly visualized (➡). It is narrowed and displaced. A collateral vein drains caudally, but its distal course could not be followed.

C. Venous phase following tolazoline, 60 mg. The splenic vein (➡) is better visualized, and the collateral venous channel can be followed peripherally (⇒).

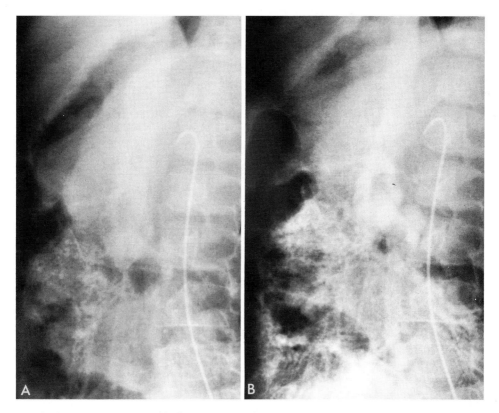

Figure 10–7. Improvement of the venous phase of superior mesenteric angiography with tolazoline.

A. Maximal venous phase following conventional mesenteric angiography. Although the inferior vena cava is well demonstrated, the superior mesenteric vein, the shunt itself and the peripheral superior mesenteric veins are poorly visualized.

B. Maximal venous phase following 25 mg tolazoline. The inferior vena cava is well demonstrated, and there is marked improvement in the demonstration of the superior mesenteric veins and the shunt. (From Redman, H. C., and Reuter, S. R.: Angiographic demonstration of portacaval and other decompressive liver shunts. Radiology 92:789, 1969.)

Dilate Spastic Vessels

Occasionally, a patient in shock will have an angiographic procedure. The redistribution of blood flow during shock results in splanchnic vasoconstriction, and the arteries appear irregular and abnormal. Vasodilators reverse this constriction temporarily and allow for better arterial visualization (Fig. 10–8).

THERAPEUTIC PHARMACOANGIOGRAPHY

The most important and widespread use of therapeutic pharmacoangiography is in the control of gastrointestinal hemorrhage. This has been covered in Chapter 6. There are two other situations in which the angiographer may be called upon to assist in therapy of a patient. These include vasodilation in patients with reversible mesenteric

TABLE 10–1. Doses of Vasodilator Drugs and Time at which Maximum Effect Occurs

	ADULT DOSE	TIME OF MAXIMUM EFFECT
Tolazoline	50 mg	40– 50 seconds
Papaverine	60 mg	90–150 seconds
Epinephrine	16–24 mcg	7– 10 minutes
Contrast medium	20–30 cc	20– 30 seconds
Bradykinin	8–10 mcg	40– 50 seconds

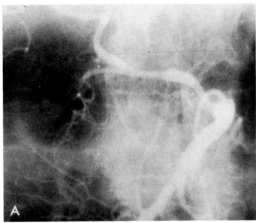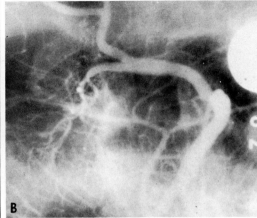

Figure 10–8. Shock simulating atherosclerosis, pre- and posttolazoline. Superior mesenteric angiogram in a 55 year old man with massive upper gastrointestinal hemorrhage.

A. Pretolazoline angiogram. Arterial phase. The replaced right hepatic artery is markedly irregular. Very few arteries to the bowel are seen. They are fine and irregular.

B. Arterial phase following tolazoline, 50 mg. The right hepatic artery appears normal. The bowel branches are now filled, as are some pancreatic branches.

arterial vasoconstriction secondary to shock or cardiac failure (see Chapter 3) and infusion of tumors with chemotherapeutic agents.

Tumor Infusion

Chemotherapeutic agents have been infused into tumors by catheter for several years. These catheters have generally been introduced into the tumor arterial supply at operation. More recently, catheters have been placed in the appropriate superselective position by the percutaneous technique using the brachial, axillary or femoral artery. Thrombosis and aneurysm formation of the infused artery are not uncommon complications of long term infusion therapy (see Fig. 3–25C). Except for making the thrombosed artery inaccessible for repeat infusion, few serious problems develop. Thrombosis or hemorrhage at the catheterization site is uncommon even when catheters, such as Kifa thin-walled red (ID:OD = 1.4:2.2), have been left in place 2 or more weeks, and the procedure has been repeated several times. Percutaneous placement obviates the need for general anesthesia. Serial angiograms in these perfusion patients often show hypervascu-larity in the perfused areas after 1 to 2 weeks of chemotherapy.

BIBLIOGRAPHY

Abrams, H. L., Boijsen, E., and Borgström, K. E.: Effect of epinephrine on the renal circulation. Radiology 79:911, 1962.

Athanasoulis, C. A., Waltman, A. C., VanUrk, H., et al.: Blood flow measurement with the spillover technique during intra-arterial drug infusion. Radiology 109:717, 1973.

Beránck, I., Belán, A., and Vosmik, J.: Artielle Pharmacoportographie bei Pfortaderdruck. Fortschr. Röntgenstr. 120:673, 1974.

Boijsen, E.: Personal communication, 1971.

Boijsen, E., and Redman, H. C.: Effect of bradykinin on celiac and superior mesenteric angiography. Invest. Radiol. 1:422, 1966.

Boijsen, E., and Redman, H. C.: Effect of epinephrine on celiac and superior mesenteric angiography. Invest. Radiol. 2:184, 1967.

Burch, G. E., and DePasquale, N. P.: Bradykinin. Amer. Heart J. 65:116, 1963.

Carlson, L. A., Ericsson, M., and Erikson, U.: Prostaglandin E_1 (PGE_1) in peripheral arteriographies. Acta Radiolog. (Diag.) (Stockh.) 14:583, 1973.

Cen, M., and Rosenbusch, G.: Zöliakographie mit Adrenalin. Fortschr. Röntgenstr. 111:82, 1969.

Cho, K. J., Chuang, V. P., and Reuter, S. R.: Prostaglandin E as a pharmacoangiographic agent for arterial portography. Radiology 116:207, 1975.

Conn, H. O., Ramsby, G. R., and Storer, E. H.: Hepatic arterial escape from vasopressin-induced vasoconstriction: An angiographic investigation. Amer. J. Roentgenol. 119:102, 1973.

Danford, R. O., and Davidson, A. J.: The use of glucagon as a vasodilator in visceral angiography. Radiology 93:173, 1969.

Davis, L. J., Anderson, J. H., Wallace, S., et al.: The use of prostaglandin E₁ to enhance the angiographic visualization of the splanchnic circulation. Radiology 114:281, 1975.

Dencker, H., Göthlin, J., Hedner, P., et al.: Superior mesenteric angiography and blood flow following intra-arterial injection of prostaglandin F₂α. Amer. J. Roentgenol. 125:111, 1975.

Doppman, J. L., Fried, L. C., and DiChiro, G.: Absent constrictive response of wound vessels to intra-arterial vasopressors: Angiographic observations. Radiology 93:57, 1969.

Dotter, C. T., and Rösch, J.: Communication to Western Angiography Society, February 1971.

Ekelund, L. and Lunderquist, A.: Pharmacoangiography with angiotensin. Radiology 110:533, 1974.

Ekelund, L., Laurun, S., and Lunderquist, A.: Comparison of a vasoconstrictor and a vasodilator in pharmacoangiography of bone and soft-tissue tumors. Radiology 122:95, 1977.

Erikson, U., Fagerberg, S., Krause, U., et al.: Angiographic studies in Crohn's disease and ulcerative colitis. Amer. J. Roentgenol. 110:385, 1970.

Finnerty, F. A.: Hemodynamics of angiotensin in man. Circulation 25:255, 1962.

Goldstein, H. M., Thaggard, A., Wallace, S., et al.: Priscoline-augmented hepatic angiography. Radiology 119:275, 1976.

Green, H. D., and Kepchar, J. H.: Control of peripheral resistance in major systemic vascular beds. Physiol. Rev. 39:617, 1959.

Hawkins, I. F., Kaude, J. V., and MacGregor, A.: Priscoline and epinephrine in selective pancreatic angiography. Radiology 116:311, 1975.

Kahn, P. C.: Contrast-vascoconstrictor mixtures in angiography. Amer. J. Roentgenol. 105:772, 1969.

Kahn, P. C.: Selective angiography of the inferior phrenic arteries. Radiology 88:1, 1967.

Kahn, P. C., and Callow, A. D.: Selective vasodilatation as an aid to angiography. Amer. J. Roentgenol. 94:213, 1965.

Kahn, P. C., Frates, W. J., and Paul, R. E.: The epinephrine effect in angiography of gastrointestinal tract tumors. Radiology 88:686, 1967.

Kahn, P. C., O'Halloran, J. F., and Paul, R. E.: Improved portography by delayed postepinephrine celiac and mesenteric arteriography. Radiology 92:86, 1969.

Kaplan, J. J., and Bookstein, J. J.: Abdominal visceral pharmacoangiography with angiotensin. Radiology 103:79, 1972.

Kaude, J., and Wirtanen, G. W.: Celiac epinephrine enhanced angiography. Amer. J. Roentgenol. 110:818, 1970.

MacGregor, A. M. and Hawkins, I. F., Jr.: Selective pharmacodynamic angiography in the diagnosis of carcinoma of the pancreas. Surg. Gynec. Obstet. 137:917, 1973.

Meng, C.-H., and Elkin, M.: Angiographic study of the effect of vasopressors on renal vascularity (metaraminol). Amer. J. Roentgenol. 95:323, 1965.

Nusbaum, M., Baum, S., Kuroda, K., et al.: Control of portal hypertension by selective mesenteric arterial drug infusion. Arch. Surg. 97:1005, 1968.

Nusbaum, M., Baum, S., Sakiyalak, P., et al.: Pharmacologic control of portal hypertension. Surgery 62:299, 1967.

Olin, T. B., and Reuter, S. R.: A pharmacoangiographic method for improving nephrophlebography. Radiology 85:1036, 1965.

Redman, H. C., Reuter, S. R., and Miller, W. J.: Improvement of superior mesenteric and portal vein visualization with tolazoline. Invest. Radiol. 4:24, 1969.

Ross, G.: Effects of epinephrine and norepinephrine on the mesenteric circulation of the cat. Amer. J. Physiol. 212:1037, 1967.

Sancetta, S. M.: General and pulmonary hemodynamic effects of pure decapeptide angiotensin in normotensive man. Circ. Res. 8:616, 1960.

Schmarsow, R., and Peters, P. E.: The pancreatographic effect during pharmacoangiography of the pancreas. Acta Radiolog. (Diag.) (Stockh.) 16:73, 1975.

Steckel, R. H., Ross, G., and Grollman, J. H.: A potent drug combination for producing constriction of the superior mesenteric artery and its branches. Radiology 91:579, 1968.

Steckel, R. J., Tobin, P. L., Stein, J. J., et al.: Intra-arterial epinephrine protection against radiation nephritis. Radiology 92:1341, 1969.

Stein, H. L.: The diagnosis of traumatic laceration of the spleen by selective arteriography, direct serial magnification angiography, and intra-arterial epinephrine. Radiology 93:367, 1969.

Texter, E. C.: Small intestinal blood flow. Amer. J. Dig. Dis. 8:587, 1963.

Texter, E. C., Chou, C.-C., Merrill, S. L., et al.: Direct effects of vasoactive agents on segmental resistance of the mesenteric and portal circulation. J. Lab. Clin. Med. 64:624, 1964.

Tibblin, S., Koch, N. G., and Schenk, W. G.: Splanchnic hemodynamic responses to glucagon. Arch. Surg. 100:84, 1970.

Wholey, M. H., Stockdale, R., and Hung, T. K.: A percutaneous balloon catheter for the immediate control of hemorrhage. Radiology 95:65, 1970.

INDEX

Note: Page numbers in *italics* refer to illustrations. Page numbers followed by (*t*) refer to tables.

377